ANATOMY, PHYSIOLOGY, PATHOLOGY AND BACTERIOLOGY

for Students of Physiotherapy
Occupational Therapy and
Gymnastics

ANATOMY, PHYSIOLOGY, PATHOLOGY AND BACTERIOLOGY

for Students of Physiotherapy Occupational Therapy and Gymnastics

C. F. V. SMOUT
M.D., M.R.C.S., L.R.C.P.

Emeritus Professor of Anatomy, University of Birmingham
formerly Examiner to the Chartered Society of Physiotherapy

R. J. S. McDOWALL
M.D., D.Sc., M.R.C.P., F.R.C.P.(E)

Emeritus Professor of Physiology, University of London
Examiner to the Royal College of Surgeons of England and of Edinburgh

B. T. DAVIS
M.B., Ch.B., M.C.Path.

Assistant Dean, University of Birmingham
Faculty of Medicine and Dentistry

FIFTH EDITION

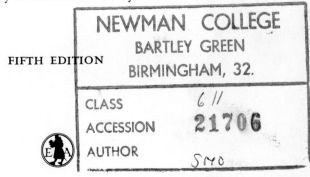
Edward Arnold (Publishers) Ltd   London

© *C. F. V. Smout, R. J. S. McDowall*
and B. T. Davis, 1968

First published	...	1944
Reprinted	...	1945
Second edition	...	1947
Reprinted	1948,	1949
Third edition	...	1956
Reprinted	...	1960
Fourth edition	...	1962
Fifth edition	...	1968

SBN: 7131 4129 8

PRINTED IN GREAT BRITAIN BY
WILLIAM CLOWES AND SONS, LIMITED, LONDON AND BECCLES

PREFACE

It is probably true to say that most students who will be reading this book for the first time were not born when it was first published. It is gratifying to record that the popularity of the book does not wane with the passing of the years, as a glance at page iv will show. Periodically the authors strive to keep the book up to date, and now that the time has come to produce a 5th edition, this opportunity has been welcomed. The Physiology section is particularly well served by Professor McDowall, who writes with his usual awareness of the needs of the student of Physiotherapy. Dr. Jacoby, the clarity of whose histological drawings are a noted feature, is now the Professor of Anatomy (Histology) at Cardiff. We have added in this edition for the first time a section on Pathology and Bacteriology, which has been framed strictly in accordance with the Syllabus of the Chartered Society. For this purpose we have introduced a new author, Dr. B. T. Davis, who is not only a specialist in his subject but a writer of repute.

Previous editions have been criticised for the fact that the section on Physiology occupies rather less than half that on Anatomy. This discrepancy is more apparent than real, for the major portion of the letterpress is in the Physiology section. The subject of Anatomy is more easily mastered if extensive use is made of visual aids, and full advantage has been taken of this, for in that section no less than 274 of the 306 illustrations are to be found.

We hope that the 5th edition will prove even more useful than its predecessors.

C. F. V. Smout

Birmingham 1968.

CONTENTS

ANATOMY

CHAPTER I

HISTOLOGY

Under the heading Histology, the *microscopic structure* of the various components of the human body will be described. We should realise that structure is intimately related to function and that if we are to understand how the body works we must commence with an appreciation of its architecture.

The human body originates from a single cell; that cell divides and becomes two cells, which in turn divide and become four cells, and so on until at one stage of our existence we have the shape of a segmented sphere.

From this simple beginning the human *body* is developed and shaped with amazing rapidity.

In spite of the manifold complexities of the body its basal anatomical unit is the *cell*, for all the tissues of the body, including muscles and nerves, and all the organs, including blood vessels and skin, are composed chiefly of cells. It becomes essential that these structures should be supported and nourished, and so a connecting tissue (connective tissue) is developed which not only forms a support but also contains the blood vessels which carry nutrition to the cells.

Each cell is composed of a variable quantity of protoplasm (*cytoplasm*) within which is a *nucleus* (except in the mature red blood cell). The nucleus is essential for the life of the cell, the cytoplasm is both a food store and workshop, for it is here that all the specialised functions of the cell take place.

Cells perform a variety of *functions*. They may secrete, e.g., the cells of many glandular organs; they may be responsible for movement, e.g., muscle cells; they may transmit impulses, e.g., nerve cells; they may carry essential material to other cells, e.g., the red blood corpuscles which carry oxygen; they may destroy harmful bacteria, e.g., the white blood corpuscles; or they may be capable of reproducing another organism, e.g., the reproductive cells. Nearly all cells, by a process of division, can multiply, and in this way worn out cells are replaced and damaged tissue is repaired.

Epithelium

The surface of the body is covered and the hollow organs (e.g., the intestinal tract and the ducts of glands) lined by a layer or layers of cells called *epithelium*. The interior of blood vessels, lymph vessels and serous membranes are lined by a layer of cells called *endothelium*.

The *functions* of these membranes may be purely protective or they may in addition secrete or excrete.

Epithelium is divided into two groups—simple, consisting of a single layer of cells, and compound, consisting of several layers.

The common types of simple epithelium are as follows:—

(i) **Squamous epithelium** consists of a layer of flat cells with flat nuclei. It lines, for instance, the alveolar spaces in the lungs and covers the glomeruli of the kidneys. *Endothelium* (fig. 22) is morphologically very similar to this type of epithelium but is of different embryonic origin.

These types of covering facilitate a speedy exchange of dissolved substances. The growth of squamous epithelium is stimulated by mechanical irritation producing, for instance, "the horny hands of toil." Squamous epithelium tends to grow in excess over a scar which may become keloid or horny. This disappears with time as the fibrous tissue in the wound shrinks and the stimulation of the skin is reduced.

(ii) **Cubical epithelium** consists of a layer of cubical cells with round nuclei. It is found, for instance, in the thyroid gland and in the tubules of the kidney.

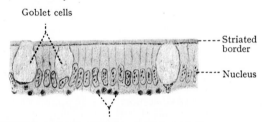

Goblet cells

Striated border

Nucleus

Lymphocytes migrating through epithelium

FIG. 1.—Columnar epithelium from the small intestine.
(From an original drawing by F. Jacoby.)

(iii) **Columnar epithelium** consists of a layer of columnar cells with oval nuclei. At certain places, individual cells become modified to

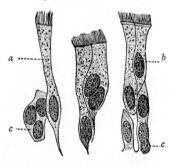

FIG. 2.—Teased ciliated epithelium from the human trachea. (Cadiat.)
(a) Large fully formed cell. *(b)* Shorter cell. *(c)* Developing cells with more than one nucleus.

form mucus secreting cells. From their shape some are known as *goblet cells*. This type of epithelium is particularly well seen in the gastro-intestinal tract where it is furnished with a so-called striated border.

Cubical and columnar epithelium are frequently adapted for secretory functions. They are always very active and, in addition to producing various secretions, they play an important part in selective absorption as in the small intestine and tubules of the kidney.

(iv) **Ciliated columnar epithelium** consists of columnar cells from which numerous hair-like processes emerge on the free surface. These processes are continually in action causing the movement of mucus and foreign particles. This type of epithelium is seen in the respiratory passages and in some of the reproductive organs.

The common types of compound epithelium are as follows:—

(i) **Stratified squamous epithelium** consists of several layers of cells. The deepest layers are columnar but the cells tend to become flattened as they reach the surface. The cells are connected by protoplasmic bridges. This type of epithelium is found in the mouth, pharynx, oesophagus, certain parts of the reproductive organs and in the eye. Stratified squamous epithelium which in its upper layers has become keratinised (horny) forms the surface of the skin and is thus highly protective.

(ii) **Transitional epithelium** consists of several layers of cells, flat on the surface and pear-shaped in the deeper layers. It is found in the urinary tract (kidney, ureter and bladder) and is also protective.

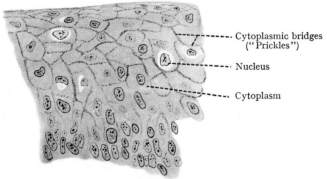

Cytoplasmic bridges ("Prickles")

Nucleus

Cytoplasm

FIG. 3.—Stratified squamous epithelium (vertical section).
(*From an original drawing by F. Jacoby.*)

The various types of epithelium frequently rest upon a *basement membrane* and are supported by *connective tissue* called the *corium* or *tunica propria*.

The Connective Tissues

Connective tissue is widespread throughout the body and it functions as a generalised framework supporting the more important structures. While in other tissues of the body cells predominate and the ground substance (matrix) is relatively small, the feature of connective tissue is that the ground substance is abundant and the cells relatively scanty.

The cells of connective tissue are classified as *macrophages* or scavengers and are part of the reticulo-endothelial system in the body. The most common are the fibroblasts and histiocytes. In addition there are granular cells called mast cells which act like glands and liberate histamine and heparin. They are especially prevalent in the lungs. Histamine is liberated in persons hypersensitive to foreign proteins (anaphylaxis) or by certain drugs (histamine releasers).   Heparin (originally isolated from the liver) is especially concerned with the maintenance of the fluidity of the blood. There are also non-granular cells called plasma cells.   All these connective tissue cells are concerned with dealing with bacteria which may have gained access to the connective tissue.

The connective tissue matrix may be homogeneous (e.g. hyaline cartilage) but it is usually fibrous in nature.

The widespread generalised form of loose connective tissue is called areolar tissue; the more specialised forms are adipose tissue, fibrous tissue, elastic tissue, cartilage and bone.

Areolar tissue consists of a matrix in which there are bundles of white fibres and a loose network of yellow elastic fibres, cells, blood vessels, etc.   It has

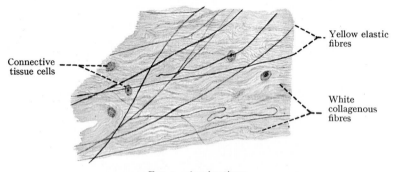

FIG. 4.—Areolar tissue.
(*From an original drawing by F. Jacoby.*)

a wide distribution throughout the body and is found beneath the skin in the subcutaneous tissues, between the muscles and around and within the viscera.   One of its features is that areolar tissue stores water between the fibres and even in the fibroblastic cells themselves.

Adipose tissue consists of masses of specialised connective tissue cells in

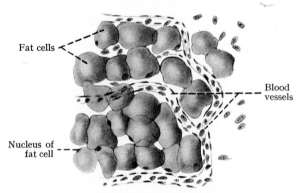

FIG. 5.—Adipose tissue.
(*From an original drawing by F. Jacoby.*)

which each individual cell is filled with a large fat globule. It is widely distributed but tends to concentrate in certain regions of the body, e.g. the buttocks, abdominal wall, mesentery, great omentum, around the kidneys and in the bone marrow.

Fibrous tissue consists of densely packed white fibres with connective tissue cells between them. These bundles of fibres are composed of collagen, which is a fibrous protein rich in glycine, proline and hydroxyproline. Its fibres are 1–200 μ in diameter. They may run parallel or they may interlace. The feature of fibrous tissue is its toughness, hence it is found ensheathing other structures, e.g. joints, forming the capsule and ligaments; glands, forming the gland capsule; bone, forming the periosteum; nerves, forming the perineurium, and muscles, forming the epimysium. It also forms tendons, deep fascia and aponeuroses. To the naked eye it has a characteristic silver-grey appearance. It does not stretch with sudden tension, but if tension is sustained it will elongate.

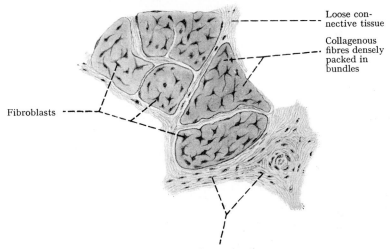

Loose connective tissue

Collagenous fibres densely packed in bundles

Fibroblasts

Connective tissue

FIG. 6.—Cross section of tendon showing dense white fibrous tissue.
(*From an original drawing by F. Jacoby.*)

Fibrous tissue is laid down in any tissues after mechanical or bacterial injury. Blood clots and effusions are said to become "organised" when they are invaded, first by blood vessels and then by fibroblasts which form the fibres. For this an adequate supply of vitamin C is necessary, otherwise wounds do not heal strongly. New fibrous tissue on which there is no tension tends to shrink, and this is responsible for unsightly scars in the skin. At first the scar is red because of its vascularity but eventually it becomes white as the fibrous tissue grows. Fibrous tissue also causes adhesions between parts of the body which are normally mobile. This occurs in the abdomen after peritonitis and also in various inflammatory states such as arthritis. As a result, the joints become fixed, and it is an important province of physiotherapists to "break down" such adhesions by frequent stretchings, but sometimes the services of the surgeon are necessary, especially in old standing cases.   These facts emphasise the importance of early movement, active and passive, after injury.

Elastic tissue consists predominantly of elastic fibres, yellow in colour, which give it elasticity.   It is found in the ligamentum nuchae and ligamenta flava of the vertebral column and also in the vocal cords, lungs, trachea and bronchi and in the walls of blood vessels.   Its fibres are more elastic than collagen and have only about 1/10th its breaking strength.   On x-ray diffraction it is quite different from collagen, and the electron microscope shows no periodicity in its fibres.   The matrix appears to consist of fibrous proteins. It must be understood that muscles are also very elastic.

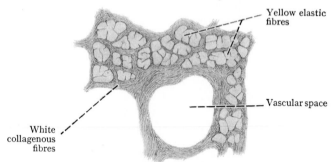

Yellow elastic fibres

Vascular space

White collagenous fibres

Fig. 7.—Transverse section of the ligamentum nuchae showing yellow elastic tissue.
(*From an original drawing by F. Jacoby.*)

Cartilage (gristle) is an avascular connective tissue in which the ground substance has hardened.   Three types are described, viz., hyaline cartilage, white fibro-cartilage and yellow elastic fibro-cartilage.

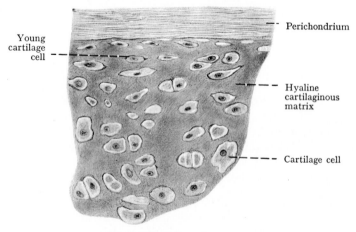

Perichondrium

Young cartilage cell

Hyaline cartilaginous matrix

Cartilage cell

Fig. 8.—Hyaline cartilage.
(*From an original drawing by F. Jacoby.*)

Hyaline cartilage is the most freely distributed type. It is covered except in the joints by a tough membrane called the *perichondrium* which is responsible for its formation and nutrition. Hyaline cartilage contains oval or flattened cells often in groups of two or more in a homogeneous matrix in which no fibres are to be seen. It covers the articular surfaces of bones, forms the costal cartilages, part of the nasal septum and the cartilages of the respiratory passages. A deposition of lime salts tends to occur in the hyaline cartilage of certain parts of the body as age advances.

White fibro-cartilage consists of a cartilaginous matrix with cartilage cells superimposed by dense layers of white fibrous tissue. It is found as discs within joint cavities and between the vertebrae.

Yellow elastic fibro-cartilage consists of cartilage cells in a hyaline matrix and yellow elastic fibres forming a meshwork around the cells. It is found in the external ear and parts of the larynx.

Bone

Bone is connective tissue in which a specific collagenous ground substance is formed and impregnated with calcium salts. In the long bones there is an outer layer of compact bone, cancellous bone at either end and a large

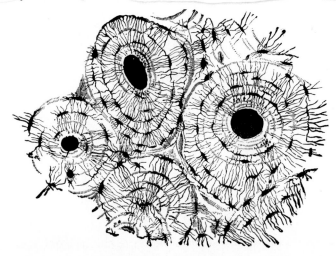

Fig. 9.—Transverse section of compact bony tissue (of humerus). Three of the Haversian canals are seen, with their concentric rings; also the lacunae, with the canaliculi extending from them across the direction of the lamellae. The Haversian apertures, lacunae and canaliculi, were filled with air and debris in grinding down the section, and therefore appear black in the figure, which represents the object as viewed with transmitted light. The Haversian systems are so closely packed in this section that scarcely any interstitial lamellae are visible. × 150. (Sharpey.)

central medullary cavity in the shaft. The articular surfaces are covered by hyaline cartilage, elsewhere the bone is enveloped in a tough membrane called the *periosteum*.

Compact bone consists of a series of *Haversian systems* made up of concentric layers of bone called *lamellae* surrounding a central canal, called an *Haversian canal* in which are blood vessels, nerves and lymphatics. The lamellae contain small spaces called *lacunae* in which bone cells are situated. The lacunae are connected with the central Haversian canal and with one another by small channels called *canaliculi*. Between the Haversian systems there are additional bony lamellae called *interstitial lamellae*.

Cancellous bone consists of a network of bony lamellae with large spaces between them which contain bone marrow.

Most bones are preceded by hyaline cartilage, but a few are preceded by membrane (e.g., certain skull bones). This transformation from cartilage to bone or from membrane to bone is due to the activity of bone-forming cells called *osteoblasts*, some of which are actually converted into bone cells in the process. Other cells called *osteoclasts* destroy bone tissue and are responsible not only for shaping the bone, but also for tunnelling the medullary cavity.

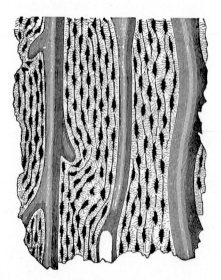

Fig. 10.—Longitudinal section from the human ulna, showing Haversian canals, lacunae and canaliculi. (Rollett.)

Muscle Tissue

Muscle consists of 20 per cent. protein and of 80 per cent. salt solution. The colour is due to the pigment *myoglobin* which contains iron and is capable of holding oxygen. The muscle proteins form a weak gel. About 40 per cent. of the total protein consists of *myosin* and about 20 per cent. of *myogen*.

Muscle exists in three forms: (i) skeletal, voluntary or striped; (ii) involuntary, smooth or unstriped; (iii) cardiac which is also involuntary.

Skeletal Muscle. A muscle is made up of numerous muscle fibres arranged in bundles. Each bundle is surrounded by a sheath of connective tissue called the **perimysium,** which is prolonged inwards between the fibres forming the *endomysium.* The bundles are bound together by further connective tissue called the *epimysium* (part of the deep fascia).

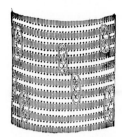

FIG. 11. — Longitudinal section of skeletal muscle showing alternate light and dark bands. (Schafer.)

Each muscle fibre, which should be regarded as an enormously elongated multi-nucleated cell, is made up of numerous longitudinally arranged contractile units called *myofibrils* in which are seen the characteristic bands of light and dark substances. When muscles contract the light bands flow into the dark bands while the dark bands become narrower. The electron microscope has, however, shown that the subject is more complex than appears at first sight. The muscle fibre, whose many nuclei are lying at the periphery, is surrounded by a sheath called the *sarcolemma.* The fibres of striped muscle are somewhat cylindrical and do not branch. It is these light and dark bands which give skeletal muscle its striated appearance, hence it is known as *striped muscle* (figs. 11 and 12).

In most animals some muscles are redder than others depending on the amount of myoglobin they contain. In man most muscles are mixed, the redder fibres generally lying in the deeper parts of the muscles. They are concerned with the maintenance of sustained activity and therefore predominate in the postural muscles.

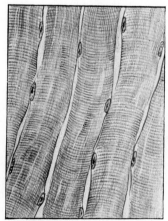

FIG. 12.—Longitudinal view of skeletal muscle fibres.

Note cross striation and peripherally situated nuclei.

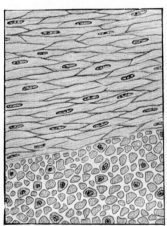

FIG. 13.—Unstriped muscle cut longitudinally (above) and transversely (below).

Note in the upper part, spindle-shaped individual muscle fibres, some showing a nucleus.

Capillaries and nerves are numerous. The motor nerves terminate in so-called *end-plates* (fig. 19) by which impulses are conveyed from the central nervous system to cause the muscle to contract. Besides these nerves there are also sensory nerves in the muscle fibres which convey afferent impulses to the brain, giving information as to the degree of tone in the muscle (fig. 20).

Unstriped muscle is made up of spindle-shaped cells, each with a central oval nucleus. There are no transverse striations, but each cell shows faint longitudinal striation due to contractile elements (myofibrils). There is no sarcolemma.

Unstriped muscle is innervated by non-medullated nerve fibres from the autonomic nervous system.

DIFFERENCES BETWEEN THE THREE TYPES OF MUSCLES

Voluntary muscle	Involuntary muscle	Cardiac muscle
Cross-striped separate fibres	No cross striations, also called smooth muscle	Cross-striped fibres connected together
Under voluntary control	Not under voluntary control	Not under voluntary control
Not normally rhythmically contractile	Slow rhythmical contractions	Rapid rhythmical contractions
Controlled by the pyramidal system of nerves	Controlled by the autonomic system	Controlled by the autonomic system
Not much affected by drugs	Easily affected by drugs	Easily affected by drugs
Contraction of individual fibres (all or none)	Contraction of groups of fibres	Contraction of whole heart (all or none) in the lower animals, e.g. frog

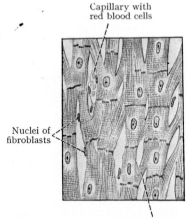

Capillary with
red blood cells

Nuclei of
fibroblasts

Interconnecting
bridge

FIG. 14.—Longitudinal section of cardiac muscle showing its syncytial arrangement.

Note cross striation and centrally placed nuclei.

Cardiac muscle consists of an interlacing of branching, somewhat rectangular, cells. Each cell has a central nucleus; there are no cell boundaries and no sarcolemma. The cells exhibit transverse striations but are involuntary. By interlacing with each other the muscle forms what is known as a *syncytium* and this is important in that impulses can pass readily between the muscle fibres, causing either the atria or ventricles to contract as a whole.

In the ventricles beneath the lining membrane of the heart there are some special muscle fibres which are associated with the conducting system (*vide* p. 361). These are known as *Purkinje fibres*. They are larger than ordinary heart muscle fibres, do not branch so frequently, and they contain contractile cross-striated myofibrils at their periphery only.

Nervous Tissue

Nervous tissue is designed to receive and transmit impulses and is so highly specialised that it has lost the power of reproducing itself. Repair of nerve cells does not, therefore, occur.

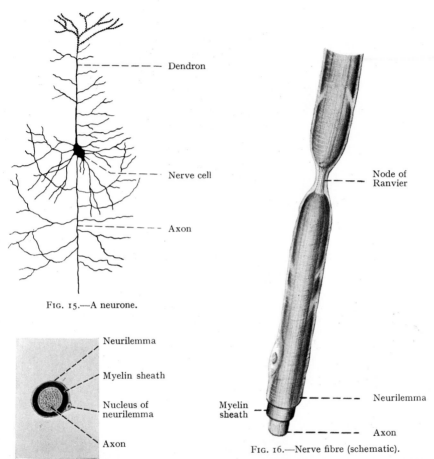

Fig. 15.—A neurone.

Fig. 17.—A nerve fibre in transverse section.

Fig. 16.—Nerve fibre (schematic).

It is made up of *nerve cells* of varying size, from which *nerve processes* or fibres emerge. A nerve cell and its processes are known as a neurone. The nerve cells and their processes in the central nervous system are surrounded by a specialised supporting tissue called *neuroglia*.

Bundles of nerve fibres, bound together by connective tissue and lying outside the central nervous system, constitute what are commonly called "nerves" or nerve trunks (fig. 18).

Each *nerve cell* consists of a cell body containing a nucleus and one process which conducts impulses from the cell, called the *axis cylinder* or *axon*, and a varying number of other processes called *dendrites* or *dendrons* which conduct impulses towards the cell.

The protoplasm within the nerve cell is responsible for the maintenance of both the cell and its processes. Each nerve cell has a spherical or oval nucleus and its protoplasm has a granular appearance due to the presence within it of a number of small bodies called *Nissl's granules*. These granules disappear when the cell is fatigued.

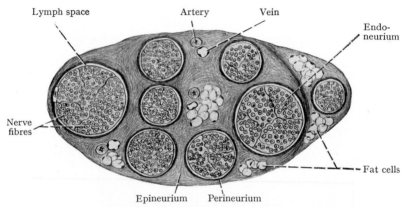

FIG. 18.—Transverse section of a nerve trunk showing the nerve fibres in bundles. These are bound together by connective tissue called the epineurium. Each bundle is surrounded by a sheath called the perineurium and the individual nerve fibres within the bundles are supported by the endoneurium.

Nerve cells congregate mainly in the grey matter of the brain and spinal cord, but they are also found in the ganglia of the peripheral nervous system.

According to the number of processes given off, a nerve cell is classified as unipolar, bipolar or multipolar.

Multipolar cells predominate in the brain and spinal cord. They vary considerably both in shape and size, some of the commonest being the *stellate* and *pyramidal* cells found in the cerebral cortex and the anterior horn cells in the spinal cord.

The function of nerve cells is to receive nervous impressions and to send impulses which are transmitted by the nerve processes to the effector organs. All conscious activity depends on the proper functioning of nerve cells.

Nerve fibres are found in the brain, spinal cord and the peripheral nerves. They may be medullated or non-medullated.

Medullated fibres have a *myelin sheath* around the axon called the *medullary sheath* (fig. 16). Myelin is a fatty substance composed of lipoids. The medullary sheath is surrounded by a delicate membrane called the *neurilemma* or *nucleated sheath of Schwann*. The myelin sheath is interrupted at intervals. These interruptions are called the *nodes of Ranvier* and are confined to the peripheral nerves. They are not present in the central nervous system. The neurilemma has no such clefts but is a continuous membrane. Nerve fibres in the central nervous system have no neurilemma.

Non-medullated fibres of peripheral nerves are enclosed in neurilemma but have no myelin sheath and appear grey in colour. They are present in the autonomic nervous system and innervate glands, involuntary muscle, blood vessels and lymphatics.

Fibres running from the sympathetic to the spinal nerves are called *grey* rami communicantes for they are non-medullated; fibres running from the spinal nerves to the sympathetic are called *white* rami communicantes for they are medullated.

Axons terminate by branching and end either as free fibres or in special end-organs, e.g., the motor end-plates in muscles and the encapsulated nerve endings in the skin (fig. 29). The sensory nerve endings in muscle (fig. 20) register the degree of tension in, or the length of, the muscle fibres.

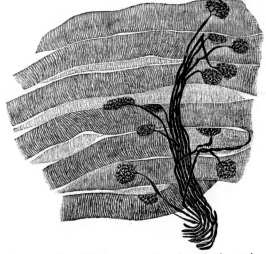

FIG. 19.—Specialised nerve-endings in striped muscle. (Motor end-plates.) × 170. (Szymonowicz.)

Dendrons, with the exception of the long sensory nerve fibres, are characteristically short and branching. They form synapses with terminations from other nerve cells.

Synapses are the points of contact between neurones. It is important to realise that they are capable of conducting an impulse in one direction only, viz., from the termination of the axon of one neurone to the dendrons or the cell body of another. It is probable that these terminals do not come into direct contact and it is believed that the gap at the synapse is bridged by the transmission of chemical substances.

The Cells of the Blood (see also p. 352)

The cells of the blood consist of two kinds, red and white blood *corpuscles*. In addition there are some small bodies called blood *platelets*. All are suspended in a fluid called the blood *plasma*.

In the human body there are about 6,500 c.c. of blood, but this varies with the body weight. In each cubic millimetre of blood in the resting body there are about 5,000,000 red cells (rather less in women), 8,000 white cells and 250,000 platelets. These cells float freely in the blood stream.

The red cells are called *erythrocytes* and each red cell is a biconcave non-nucleated disc (about $\frac{1}{3000}$ inch in diameter) which owes its colour to the fact that it contains within it the iron-containing pigment haemoglobin. A feature of the red cells is their elasticity, for they can be compressed easily and then quickly regain their shape when the pressure is released. This

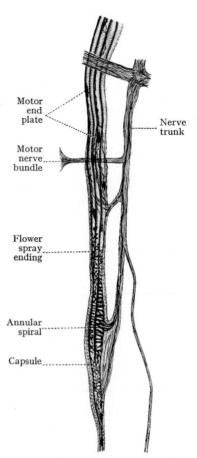

Motor
end
plate

Nerve
trunk

Motor
nerve
bundle

Flower
spray
ending

Annular
spiral

Capsule

FIG. 20.—Sensory nerve ending in muscle.   (Redrawn from Ruffini.)

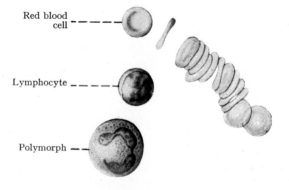

Red blood
cell

Lymphocyte

Polymorph

FIG. 21.—Blood cells.

enables them to pass through fine blood vessels with a diameter smaller than themselves. The average life of a red cell is 100/120 days and new cells are formed during adult life in the red marrow of the flat bones, particularly the ribs, the skull and the pelvis. Red cells perform the most important function of carrying oxygen from the lungs to the tissues.

The white cells are called *leucocytes* and are nucleated. There are several varieties of white cells, but by far the commonest are the *polymorphonuclear neutrophil leucocytes* which are usually known by the abbreviated term "polymorphs." Their characteristic is that the nucleus in each cell is lobulated. They perform the useful function of ingesting foreign bodies and harmful bacteria and are thus spoken of as "phagocytes." The other predominant white cell is the *lymphocyte* and its characteristic is that its nucleus almost fills the cell, thus the cytoplasm is small in amount. Lymphocytes increase in certain chronic diseases, e.g., tuberculosis.

Polymorphs are derived from the red bone marrow; lymphocytes from

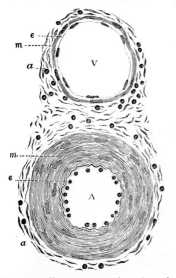

FIG. 22.—Transverse section through a small artery and vein. × 350. (Klein and Noble Smith.)

(*a*) Tunica adventitia; (*m*) tunica media; (*e*) tunica intima with endothelium.

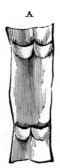

FIG. 23.—A. Vein opened showing valves.

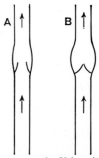

FIG. 24.—A. Vein with valves open. B. Vein with valves closed, showing ballooning of the vein above.

the lymphoid tissue scattered through the body, particularly the lymph nodes, the spleen and the tonsil.

Platelets are minute protoplasmic elements which perform a useful function in hastening or initiating the clotting of blood. They are probably derived from the red bone marrow.

The Blood Vessels (figs. 22, 23 and 24)

The chief blood vessels are the arteries, capillaries and veins.

Arteries are composed of three layers: an outer layer called the *tunica* *adventitia* consisting of connective tissue, a middle layer called the *tunica media* composed mainly of smooth muscle and yellow elastic tissue in varying proportions, and an inner layer called the *tunica intima* composed of connective tissue and endothelium.

Capillaries are small tubes (normally about the diameter of a red cell) consisting of a single layer of endothelial cells.

Veins are made up of a thick tunica adventitia with a weak tunica media, lined by a tunica intima.   Veins have valves which are usually composed of two cusps although sometimes there are three.   These valves are formed by a prolongation inwards of the tunica intima.

Lymphatic Vessels

Lymphatic vessels resemble veins structurally, but their walls are thinner. A tunica adventitia is present only in the larger vessels, the tunica media is weak and there is a lining which constitutes the tunica intima.   Valves are more numerous than in veins, giving the vessels a beaded appearance.

Lymphatic nodes are small kidney-shaped organs which lie in the path-

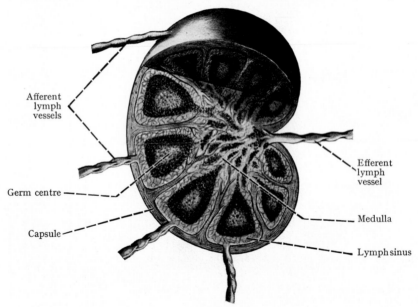

Afferent lymph vessels

Efferent lymph vessel

Germ centre

Medulla

Capsule

Lymph sinus

FIG. 25.—A lymph node on section (diagrammatic).
(*Redrawn from "The Tissues of the Body," by permission of Sir Wilfrid Le Gros Clark.*)

way of lymphatic vessels.   They are often referred to as lymphatic *glands*, but the term *node* is more acceptable because we should avoid the impression that they secrete.

Lymph nodes perform the dual function of filtering lymph and forming lymphocytes.   Each node consists of a connective tissue *capsule* from which septa extend into the interior of the node, dividing it into numerous segments.   Each segment consists of a lymph follicle in the centre of which is a *germ centre* where lymphocytes are formed and around the lymph follicle there is a *lymph sinus* which is continuous with *afferent lymph vessels*. These vessels are numerous and they enter the node on its convex surface.

The central portion of the node is called the *medulla* which contains cords of lymphocytes and lymph sinuses. A single *efferent lymph vessel* leaves the node on its concave aspect at the *hilum*.

Carcinoma (cancer) spreads by lymphatic vessels and soon infiltrates lymphatic nodes. Septic infections may also be carried by the lymphatic vessels and cause the nodes to become inflamed.

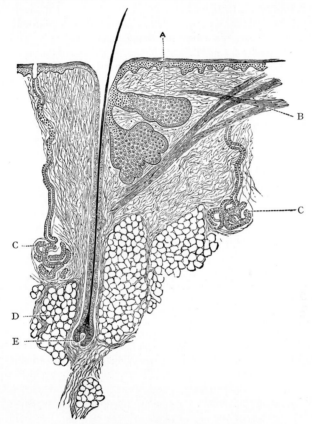

FIG. 26.—Vertical section of skin. (Klein.)

A. Sebaceous gland opening into hair follicle. B. Muscle fibres. C. Sweat gland. D. Subcutaneous fat. E. Fundus of hair follicle with hair papilla.

The Skin (figs. 26 and 27)

The skin is a protective covering for the body. It contains the terminations of many sensory nerves by which the body is informed of the varying conditions of its environment.

The structure of the skin. The skin varies in thickness in different parts of the body. The variation is between 0·1 mm. and 4 mm., being thickest in the palms of the hands and the soles of the feet.   It consists of an outer layer of stratified squamous epithelium called the *epidermis* and an inner layer of connective tissue called the *dermis* or *corium.*

The epidermis in those regions where the skin is thick and well-developed is seen to consist of four layers.

(i) *The stratum Malpighii* (or germinativum) is the deepest layer of the epidermis.   In its deeper part new cells are formed which are gradually pushed towards the surface of the skin and are eventually shed.   The predominant cell in this layer is called the prickle cell for it has spikes in the form of protoplasmic bridges between the cells.   In the deepest layers of this stratum the cells may contain granules of melanin pigment.   This dark pigment varies in intensity in different regions of the body, and while much more abundant in the coloured races it is present to some extent in the white races and may become increased in response to irritation especially by sunlight.

(ii) *Stratum granulosum* or granular layer is often absent, and even where the skin is thick it usually consists of a single layer of cells only.   The intracellular granules are made up of a substance called eleidin.

(iii) *Stratum lucidum* or transparent layer is also inconstant.   Here the eleidin granules have disappeared and the cellular content is gradually being transformed into keratin.

(iv) *Stratum corneum* or horny layer.   The nuclei and cellular structures have disappeared and are replaced by flattened horny flakes rich in keratin, which is a sulphur-containing compound.   These flakes are continually being shed or worn away and are replaced by the proliferation of cells from the deepest layer of the epidermis.   This layer becomes thickened in response to mechanical stimulation and is best seen in the palms and soles.

The epidermis is avascular but is nourished by tissue fluid which permeates the intercellular spaces of the Malpighian layer from the subpapillary plexuses in the dermis.   Free nerve endings are present in the epidermis where they are situated for the most part in the Malpighian layer, but in certain sensitive parts of the body, e.g., the tips of the fingers, they may reach as far as the stratum granulosum.

The dermis (cutis vera or corium) is a supporting and nourishing tissue for the epidermis.   It consists chiefly of collagenous fibres with an admixture of elastic tissue.   This elastic tissue allows the skin to stretch during body movements and to move freely over underlying structures.   The dermis projects into the epidermis as the dermal papillae, and these can be seen as ridges on the surface of the skin in certain regions, e.g., the palms and soles. In these papillae are nerve endings, capillary loops from the subpapillary plexuses, and also lymphatic vessels (fig. 27).

Beneath the dermis is the *superficial fascia* containing a variable quantity of fat which acts as a padding.

Nails are developed as a modification of the stratum lucidum and are produced by extreme keratinisation of the area involved.   They grow from a mass of epithelium known as the nail-bed or matrix.

Hairs are derived from the epidermis and their roots lie in pits called the *hair follicles* into the extremity of which a dermal papilla projects containing

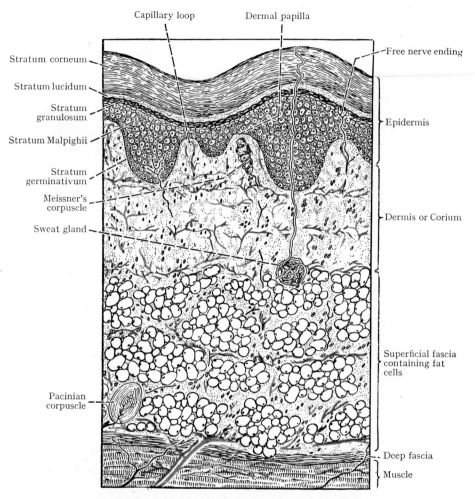

Capillary loop   Dermal papilla

Stratum corneum

Free nerve ending

Stratum lucidum

Stratum
granulosum

Epidermis

Stratum Malpighii

Stratum
germinativum

Meissner's
corpuscle

Dermis or Corium

Sweat gland

Superficial fascia
containing fat
cells

Pacinian
corpuscle

Deep fascia

Muscle

FIG. 27.—A vertical section through the skin (schematic).

[facing page 18]

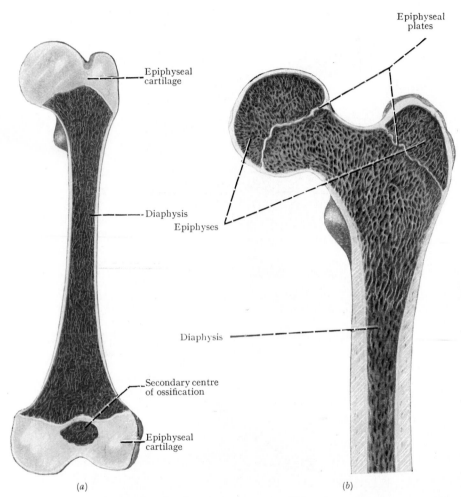

Epiphyseal
cartilage

Epiphyseal
plates

Diaphysis

Epiphyses

Diaphysis

Secondary centre
of ossification

Epiphyseal
cartilage

(a)   (b)

FIG. 32 (a)—A coronal section through the femur of a child aged seven months.

(b)—A coronal section through the upper end of the femur of a child aged twelve years.

blood vessels and nerves. To each follicle some fibres of smooth muscle are attached which are capable of causing the hairs (in certain animals) to "stand on end." The same condition is seen in man in the form of the roughened skin which occurs on exposure to cold ("goose skin"). Hairs protect the underlying area, retard heat loss and in some animals are acutely sensitive. They tend to grow in response to mechanical irritation.

Sebaceous glands are found in most parts of the skin. They are pear-shaped structures, with a stem representing the duct of a gland, opening into a hair follicle. They secrete a fatty substance called *sebum* which acts as a lubricant for the hairs and covers the surface of the body with a greasy secretion. This is mildly antiseptic and performs the important function of rendering the skin waterproof and controlling the shedding of the surface epithelium. Blockage of the ducts of sebaceous glands leads to the formation of comedones (blackheads), pustules (if infected), acne or sebaceous cysts.

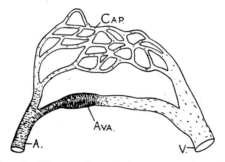

Fig. 28.—Diagram of an arterio-venous anastomosis.
(*Redrawn from the "Tissues of the Body," by permission of Sir Wilfrid Le Gros Clark.*)
Ava. Arterio-venous anastomosis; A. Artery; V. Vein; Cap. Capillary.

Sweat glands are numerous in the skin in most regions of the body. Each gland consists of a characteristically coiled tube which ascends from the deepest layers of the dermis and passes through the epidermis to the surface of the skin. These glands are of two types: (1) large glands derived from hair follicles and confined to certain regions of the face, the axillae and the sex organs; (2) small glands derived from the epidermis which have a wide distribution throughout the body. The ceruminous glands which secrete the wax in the ear passages and the mammary glands are examples of large sweat glands which have become specialised for a specific purpose.

Blood supply to the skin. A feature of the blood supply to the skin is the subpapillary plexus in the dermis (fig. 27) which gives the skin its colour. From this plexus capillaries pass forward into the dermal papillae in the form of loops. These loops can be seen in the living subject with the aid of a microscope when the superficial layers of the skin are made transparent with oil.

A further feature of the blood vessels in the skin is the presence in certain regions in warm-blooded animals, including man, of a large number of arterio-venous anastomoses (fig. 28). In this way the blood can be short-circuited without having to pass through the capillaries and thus rapid adjustments can be made in the circulation to suit the varying needs of the body.

Innervation of the skin.   Mention has already been made of the free nerve endings in the skin; these are associated with the sensation of pain and may be quite superficial, e.g., in the cornea of the eye.   Besides these there are certain specialised end-organs consisting of nerve-endings encased within a fibrous capsule of varying thickness.   Thus there are the oval corpuscles of Meissner and the disc-like endings of Merkel, both of which are associated with touch; the lamellated corpuscles of Pacini and bulbous corpuscles of Krause, both associated with pressure and Ruffini's end-organs associated with the perception of heat; the latter are not encapsulated (figs. 27 and 29).

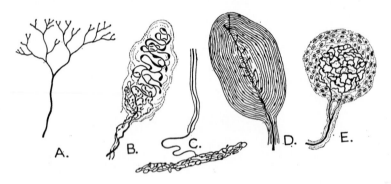

FIG. 29.—Nerve-endings in skin.

A. Free nerve ending; B. Meissner's corpuscle; C. Ruffini's end-organ; D. Pacinian corpuscle; E. Krause's end-bulb.

The functions of the skin is further referred to in the Physiology section (p.431) but a summary can be appended here.   The skin is concerned with:—
Protecting the underlying structures.

Receiving sensations from without, from which nerve impulses are set up. These are passed to the central nervous system via the free and encapsulated nerve endings situated in the deeper layers of the skin.

Storing blood.   The skin is believed to retain about a litre of blood which is stored in the subpapillary plexuses where it circulates slowly but is available for use in an emergency.

Regulating temperature.   The temperature of the body is chiefly regulated by adjusting the calibre of the peripheral vessels.   The hair retains heat. Evaporation of sweat is a means whereby the body temperature is lowered.

Secreting sweat and sebum.

Excreting water and salts contained within the body fluids.   This function may be of value when the kidneys become inefficient.   If sweating is excessive too much salt may be lost.

Breathing.   Very little respiration occurs through the skin in man, but it is quite appreciable in certain animals (frog).

CHAPTER II

OSTEOLOGY

Introduction. For purposes of description the body is consider ̷ ̷ ̷
being in the *anatomical position*. It is very important to keep this constantly in mind to ensure consistency of description. In this position the subject is regarded as standing with the palms of the hands, as well as the head and eyes, facing forward.

In describing the position of certain structures the following planes are constantly referred to:—

The median plane, which is a vertical plane equivalent to the mid-line of the body. It thus bisects the body into two symmetrical (right and left) halves.

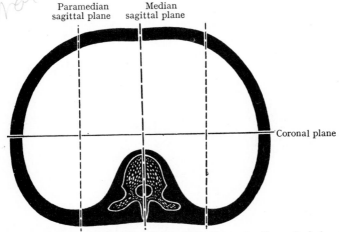

Fig. 30.—A transverse section through the trunk, illustrating the vertical planes.

The sagittal plane, which is the median plane or any vertical plane parallel to the median plane.

The coronal plane, which is any vertical plane at right angles to the median plane.

The transverse plane, which is any horizontal plane.

Structures lying nearest to the mid-line are said to be *medial*; those lying farthest from the mid-line are said to be *lateral*. The terms *superior* and *inferior* explain themselves, but in describing the limbs the terms *proximal* and *distal* are substituted respectively. The terms *anterior* and *posterior* are used instead of front and back respectively. The term *volar* may be used to indicate the anterior aspect of the forearm and hand.

In anatomy the terms *arm* and *leg* refer only to *parts* of the upper and lower limbs. The upper limb is divided by the shoulder, elbow and wrist

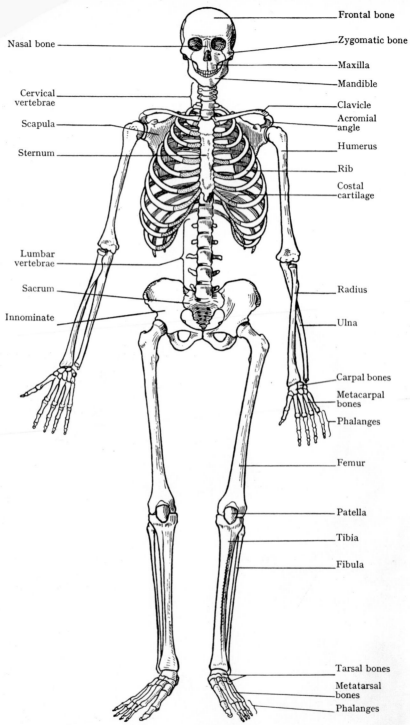

Frontal bone

Nasal bone

Zygomatic bone

Maxilla

Mandible

Cervical
vertebrae

Clavicle

Acromial
angle

Scapula

Sternum

Humerus

Rib

Costal
cartilage

Lumbar
vertebrae

Sacrum

Radius

Innominate

Ulna

Carpal bones

Metacarpal
bones

Phalanges

Femur

Patella

Tibia

Fibula

Tarsal bones

Metatarsal
bones

Phalanges

FIG. 31.—The bony skeleton.

22

joints into the *shoulder, arm, forearm* and *hand*.   The lower limb is divided by the hip, knee and ankle joints into the *hip, thigh, leg* and *foot*.

That part of anatomy which deals with the skeleton is known as *Osteology*, and osteology forms the very basis of anatomy.   In attempting to master this important branch of medical science, something more is required than the mere reading of a text-book.   The reader will find that he is just wasting time, unless, as he reads, he works out for himself *with bone in hand* the various features under consideration.

The bony skeleton is divided into an *axial skeleton* made up of the bones of the trunk, head and neck, and an *appendicular skeleton* made up of the bones of the limbs (also called appendages or extremities).

Functions of the Bony Skeleton

(i) The bony skeleton is the main supporting structure of the body and presents rigid surfaces for the attachment of muscles, ligaments and fascia.

(ii) The bones are linked together by joints, and this enables them to act as levers for the muscles.   Under ordinary circumstances the bone from which the muscle originates remains more or less fixed when the muscle contracts, and the bone into which the muscle is inserted performs the movement.

(iii) The skeleton forms a protective case for many organs of the body. Thus, the skull encloses the brain; the vertebral column, the spinal cord; the pelvis, the bladder and lower part of the alimentary tract as well as the female reproductive organs; while the bony thorax resembles a light packing-case consisting of a series of laths (the ribs) which, while not hampering the movements of respiration, protect such vital organs as the heart, lungs, liver, spleen and to some extent the kidneys and stomach.

(iv) The skeleton acts as a storehouse for calcium which is essential for the activity of organs.

Classification of the individual bones

Bones are classified as *long bones* (most bones of the limbs), *short bones* (bones of the wrist and ankle), *flat bones* (bones of the skull) and *irregular bones* (bones of the face and vertebral column).

The general structure, form and growth of bone

The long bones are described as consisting of a *shaft*, an *upper* (*proximal*) and a *lower* (*distal*) *end*.   The extremities of such bones take part in the formation of *joints* and are covered with a special *articular cartilage*; the whole of the remainder of the bone is enveloped by a thin membrane which is closely adherent to the surface called the *periosteum*.   Near the middle of the shaft there is a *nutrient foramen* which transmits an artery, companion veins, nerves and lymphatics into the interior of the bone.   There are numerous smaller foramina at the extremities which transmit blood vessels, but here the veins predominate.

If a long bone is sectioned longitudinally, it is seen to consist of an outer framework of hard *compact bone*; a central *medullary cavity* in the shaft, filled, in the recent state, by red bone marrow before puberty and by yellow bone marrow (fat) after puberty; while the extremities are seen to consist of *cancellous (spongy) bone* in the interstices of which is red bone marrow during the period of growth (up to 25 years of age) and yellow bone marrow afterwards.

If a longitudinal section is made through a growing long bone in a young adult, a well marked white line is seen at either end which clearly differentiates shaft from extremities. This white line is composed of cartilage and is known as the *epiphyseal plate* (fig. 32 (*b*), facing p. 19). The shaft of the bone between the two epiphyseal plates is known as the *diaphysis*, and the extremities bounded by the epiphyseal plates as the *epiphyses*.

Usually a long bone develops an epiphysis at each end in this way, but the ribs, clavicles, metacarpals and phalanges are notable exceptions for they have an epiphysis at one end only.

A bone grows in *length* by new bone which is laid down in the region of the epiphyseal plate. A bone grows in *circumference* by new bone which is laid down beneath the periosteum.

Bone is a form of connective tissue which has been hardened by the deposition of lime salts in a definite pattern within its interstices. These lime salts are absorbed from the food and for this vitamin D is necessary. Besides this *inorganic* matter bone is made up of *animal* or *organic* matter, and while the former is responsible for its hardness the latter is responsible for its limited elasticity and flexibility.

The development and repair of bone

All the bones of the body are developed from embryonic connective tissue called "mesenchyme." In the case of most bones this mesenchyme chondrifies, i.e., is replaced by cartilage, before it ossifies, i.e., is replaced by bone. A few bones, notably those at the vault and sides of the skull and also the clavicle, do not pass through this stage of chondrification but are developed from membrane.

A long bone consists primarily of a rod of cartilage cells surrounded by a thin membrane called the *perichondrium*. The perichondrium later becomes the *periosteum*. Bone commences to be laid down in the centre of the cartilaginous rod forming what is called the "*primary centre of ossification.*" This centre grows towards the extremities of the bone; thus the shaft or diaphysis consists at one stage of bone, and the extremities or epiphyses of cartilage (fig. 32 facing p. 19). Bone is laid down by bone-building cells called *osteoblasts*. These are active within the primary centre and also immediately beneath the periosteum. While osteoblasts are busy laying down new bone, other cells called *osteoclasts*, which are bone destroyers, are busy trimming the newly formed bone and giving it shape. Osteoclasts also tunnel the bone centrally, and in this way a *medullary cavity* is formed which rapidly fills with red bone marrow. Later, one or more secondary centres of ossification appear in the epiphyses (fig. 32 (*a*)) and these by proliferation and through the agency of the osteoblasts gradually convert the epiphyseal cartilage into bone, leaving the narrow epiphyseal plate intervening between diaphysis and epiphysis (fig. 32 (*b*)).   When eventually the epiphyseal plate disappears and diaphysis joins epiphysis, growth ceases.

Repair of the bone after injury takes place by direct bone formation from the periosteum, and this is known as *callus*.

THE SKULL

The skull is made up of a number of separate bones united at fixed joints called *sutures*.   The lower jaw is an exception for it is united to the skull by a movable joint.

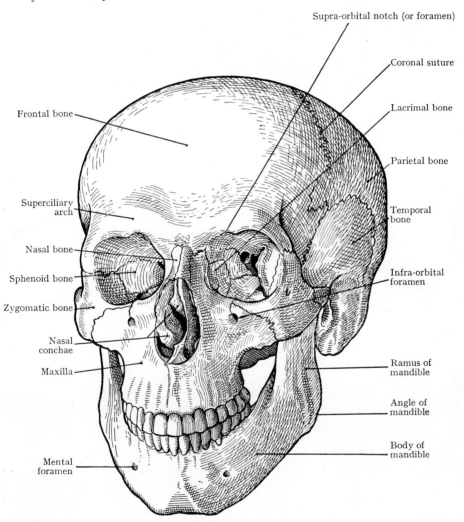

Supra-orbital notch (or foramen)

Coronal suture

Lacrimal bone

Frontal bone

Parietal bone

Temporal bone

Superciliary arch

Nasal bone

Sphenoid bone

Infra-orbital foramen

Zygomatic bone

Nasal conchae

Maxilla

Ramus of mandible

Angle of mandible

Body of mandible

Mental foramen

Fig. 33.—The skull viewed from the front.

For purposes of description the bones of the skull are divided into the bones of the cranium and the bones of the face. The upper part of the cranium is known as the *vault* and the lower part as the *base* of the skull.

When viewing the skull from the front (fig. 33) the *frontal bone* with its *superciliary arches* can be seen and also the *eye sockets* or *orbits* bounded by the frontal bone superiorly, the *zygomatic bone* and part of the sphenoid laterally, the ethmoid and lacrimal bones medially, and the maxilla inferiorly; the *nasal bones* forming the bridge of the nose; the *nasal cavity* divided into two by the bony nasal septum; the *conchae* jutting into the nasal

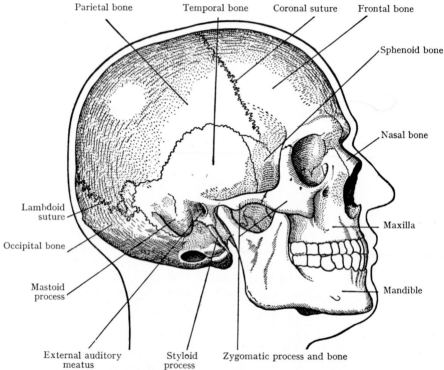

Parietal bone   Temporal bone   Coronal suture   Frontal bone

Sphenoid bone

Nasal bone

Lambdoid suture

Maxilla

Occipital bone

Mastoid process

Mandible

External auditory meatus   Styloid process   Zygomatic process and bone

FIG. 34.—The right side of the skull.

cavity from the lateral wall; the *maxilla* or upper jaw; the *zygomatic bone* forming the prominence of the cheek; the *mandible* consisting of a body which lies in the horizontal plane and two rami which lie in the vertical plane, the body being united with the ramus at the angle of the jaw.

Four foramina are present on the front of the skull and all are of importance because they transmit sensory branches of the Vth cranial nerve as they pass to supply the skin of the face. These foramina are the *supra-orbital notch* or *foramen* above the orbit, the *infra-orbital foramen* below the orbit, a *foramen in the zygomatic bone* and the *mental foramen* in the mandible.

When viewing the skull from the side (fig. 34) the frontal bone is seen separated from the parietal bone by the *coronal suture* and the parietal bone from the occipital bone by the *lambdoid suture*. Parts of the sphenoid and temporal bones complete the side-wall. The *zygomatic process, external*

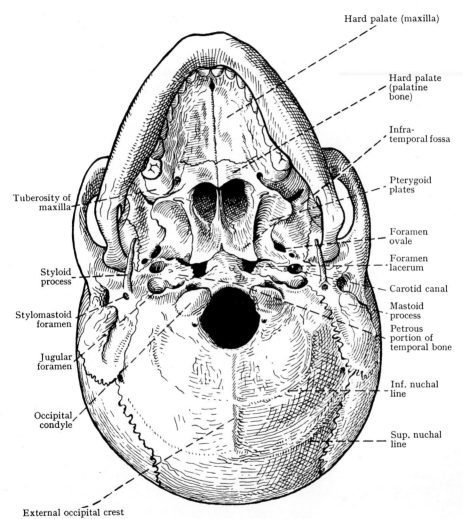

FIG. 35.—The skull viewed from below.

auditory meatus, mastoid process and *styloid process*—all parts of the temporal bone—should be located on this aspect of the skull.

When viewing the skull from below (fig. 35) the palatine processes of the maxillae and parts of the palatine bones are seen, forming the *hard palate*; behind this is the posterior aspect of the nasal cavity bounded laterally by the *medial pterygoid plates* and among the numerous foramina which present themselves between the posterior aspect of the nose and the foramen magnum, the student should locate the *foramen ovale*, the *foramen lacerum*, the *carotid canal*, the *jugular foramen* and the *stylomastoid foramen* as these are all related to the cranial nerves which will later come under consideration. The following bony landmarks should also be located: the *infratemporal fossa*, the *medial* and *lateral pterygoid plates*, the *tuberosity of the maxilla*, the

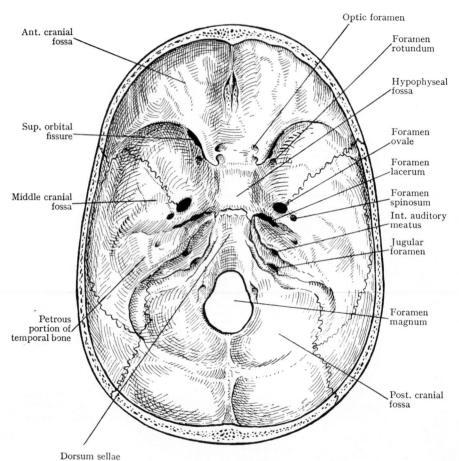

FIG. 36.—The interior of the base of the skull (floor of cranial cavity).

petrous portion of the temporal bone, the *styloid process*, the *mastoid process* and the *occipital condyles*, the *external occipital protruberance* and *crest* and the *nuchal lines* on the occipital bone.

   When viewing the floor of the cranial cavity (fig. 36) the following foramina should be located: the *superior orbital fissure*, the *foramen rotundum*, the *foramen ovale*, the *foramen lacerum* and the *jugular foramen*.

   The floor of the cranial cavity is seen to be divided into three fossae, the

anterior cranial fossa separated from the m
wing of the sphenoid bone, the *middle cranial*
petrous portion of the temporal bone, and the
behind this.

The Mandible consists of a *body* and two *rami* which
the jaw. Surmounting each ramus is the *coronoid process*
condyloid process with its articular surface posteriorly, while
two processes is the *mandibular notch* (fig. 37).

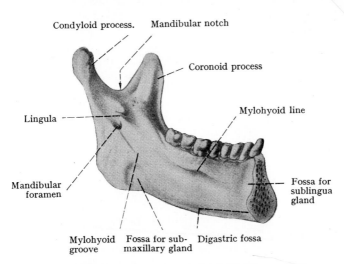

Condyloid process.   Mandibular notch

Coronoid process

Mylohyoid line

Lingula

Mandibular
foramen

Fossa for
sublingua
gland

Mylohyoid   Fossa for sub-   Digastric fossa
groove   maxillary gland

FIG. 37.—The medial aspect of the left half of the mandible.

On the inner side of the ramus is the *mandibular foramen*, while running downwards and forwards from this is the prominent *mylohyoid groove*.
Above the mylohyoid groove anteriorly is the *mylohyoid line* and below this
line anteriorly is the *digastric fossa* (fig. 37).

The four muscles of mastication are inserted into this bone—the *masseter
muscle* into the lateral aspect of the ramus; the *temporalis muscle* into the
coronoid process; the *lateral pterygoid muscle* into the condyle; and the
medial pterygoid muscle into the medial aspect of the angle (see pp. 123 and
124 for further details).

THE VERTEBRAL COLUMN (fig. 38)

There are 33 individual vertebrae in the vertebral column made up of
7 cervical, 12 thoracic or dorsal, 5 lumbar, 5 sacral and 4 coccygeal.
In the sacral and coccygeal regions the vertebrae are fused together, elsewhere they are separated by fibro-cartilaginous *intervertebral discs*.
The vertebrae from different regions present individual peculiarities but
all are constructed on the same general plan.

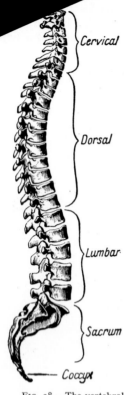

Cervical

Dorsal

Lumbar

Sacrum

Coccyx

FIG. 38.—The vertebral
column.

A typical Vertebra (from the mid-thoracic region, fig. 39) will be seen to consist of a mass of bone, the *body*, from which two bars of bone called the *pedicles* project backwards. The margins of the pedicles are notched and in the articulated vertebral column these form *the intervertebral foramina* which transmit the spinal nerves. From the pedicles two thin plates of bone called the *laminae* pass medially and backwards, and these are united in the mid-line by the prominent *spine*. At the junction of pedicle and lamina a bar of bone known as the *transverse process* projects laterally. On this process in the thoracic region there is a facet for articulation with the tubercle of a rib. Near the root of each transverse process lie the *superior* and *inferior articular processes* which articulate with similar processes on the adjacent vertebrae. Body, pedicles and laminae bound a space called the *vertebral foramen* which is occupied by the spinal cord and its coverings. Pedicles, laminae and spine constitute the *vertebral arch*.

A typical Cervical Vertebra (fig. 40) presents all the above features but can be distinguished by the following characteristics: The spine is bifid, there is a foramen for the vertebral vessels in each transverse process called the foramen transversarium, the vertebral foramen is triangular, the body is small and its upper and lower surfaces are concavo-convex with synovial joints on either side.

The first, second and seventh cervical vertebrae being atypical require special consideration.

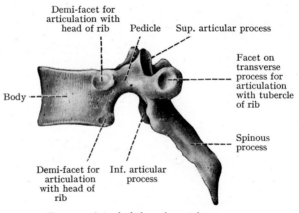

Demi-facet for
articulation with
head of rib   Pedicle   Sup. articular process

Facet on
transverse
process for
articulation
with tubercle
of rib

Body

Spinous
process

Demi-facet for   Inf. articular
articulation   process
with head of
rib

FIG. 39.—A typical thoracic vertebra.

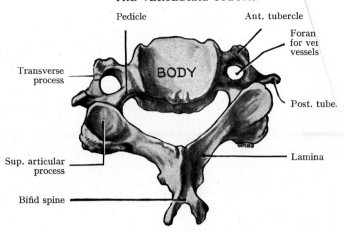

Pedicle

Ant. tubercle

Foran
for ver
vessels

Transverse
process

BODY

Post. tube.

Sup. articular
process

Lamina

Bifid spine

FIG. 40.—A typical cervical vertebra.

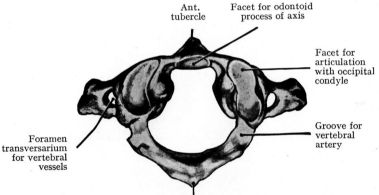

Ant.
tubercle

Facet for odontoid
process of axis

Facet for
articulation
with occipital
condyle

Foramen
transversarium
for vertebral
vessels

Groove for
vertebral
artery

Post. tubercle (rudimentary spine)

FIG. 41.—The atlas.

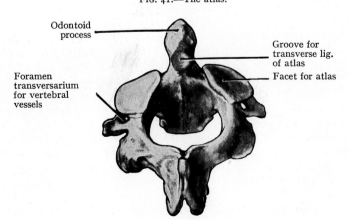

Odontoid
process

Groove for
transverse lig.
of atlas

Foramen
transversarium
for vertebral
vessels

Facet for atlas

FIG. 42.—The axis.

The first Cervical Vertebra or *atlas* (fig. 41) has no body and no spinous process. It is merely a ring of bone, on the superior surface of which are two large semilunar articular facets. Here the bone articulates with the occipital condyles, forming the atlanto-occipital joints at which nodding movements of the head take place.

The second Cervical Vertebra or *axis* (fig. 42) is readily distinguished by the peg-like odontoid process which surmounts the body. The odontoid process represents the body of the atlas which has fused with the axis. At the atlanto-axial joint, rotation of the head takes place.

The seventh Cervical Vertebra is called "the vertebra prominens" because its spine is longer than that of any other cervical vertebra. Another feature of its spine is that it is not bifid. The transverse process is relatively large but the foramen transversarium within it is very small for it transmits only a small vein.

A typical Thoracic Vertebra (fig. 39) has already been described. Its

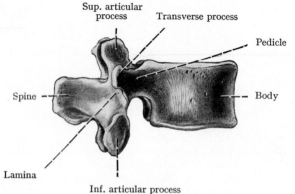

Fig. 43.—A typical lumbar vertebra.

distinguishing features are the demi-facets on the body for articulation with the heads of ribs and the whole facet on each transverse process for articulation with the tubercle of a rib. Less pronounced features are the heart-shaped bodies and the oblique spines. The first thoracic vertebra has a whole facet on the upper part of its body for the first rib and a half facet on the lower part of its body for the upper facet on the head of the second rib. The tenth, eleventh and twelfth vertebrae have one facet for the head of the corresponding rib. The eleventh and twelfth vertebrae have no facets on their transverse processes.

A typical Lumbar Vertebra (fig. 43) has a large kidney-shaped body with a triangular vertebral foramen, short pedicles, long and slender transverse processes, thick laminae and a horizontal spine. It may be distinguished by the absence of facets for ribs and the absence of foramina in the transverse processes. It presents one important positive feature, viz., the horizontally directed quadrate spine. These vertebrae are larger than those from any other region.

The **Sacrum** (figs. 44 and 45) is made up of five vertebra
The upper half of its lateral border presents an *auricula.*
articular surface which articulates with a similar surface on the
bone. This sacro-iliac joint is most important, since it is callec
support the weight of the whole of the upper part of the body v
transmitted through this joint to the pelvis and lower limbs. The sa
forms the posterior wall of the pelvis. Its anterior and posterior surfa
present the *anterior* and *posterior sacral foramina* which transmit the anterior
and posterior rami of the sacral nerves respectively and also the sacral vessels.

The bone is tunnelled by the *sacral canal* which contains nerve roots, the
filum terminale of the spinal cord and the terminal part of the sheath of the
spinal cord (dura and arachnoid mater) which ends at the level of the second
piece of the sacrum.

The upper part or base of the sacrum presents a superior articular facet
which articulates with the fifth lumbar vertebra. The anterior margin of
this facet is prominent and is called the *sacral promontory*. The bone forming
the remainder of the base is known as the *lateral mass* of the sacrum and on it
is a shallow groove occupied by the lumbosacral trunk.

Certain important muscles are attached to the bone, viz., the iliacus, piriformis and coccygeus in front and the multifidus, sacrospinalis and gluteus
maximus behind.

The ligaments attached to the bone are all concerned with the stabilisation
of the sacro-iliac joint and include, besides the capsule of the joint, the
anterior sacro-iliac ligaments in front, the long and short posterior sacro-iliac
ligaments behind, the interosseous sacro-iliac ligaments on the upper part of
the lateral border, and the sacrospinous (small sacrosciatic) ligament and the
sacrotuberous (great sacrosciatic) ligament on the lower half of the lateral
border (figs. 95 and 96).

The **Coccyx** consists of a variable number of rudimentary vertebrae
(usually four) fused together. The levator ani muscle is attached to its
lateral border and the sphincter ani externus to its tip.

THE BONES OF THE THORAX

The **Sternum or Breast Bone** (fig. 46) consists of an upper part called
the *manubrium* which is succeeded by a larger part called the *body*, and the
body finally ends below in the *xiphoid process* (ensiform cartilage).

The upper border of the manubrium presents a curved notch known as
the *suprasternal (jugular) notch*. The manubrium ends by joining the body
at an angle called the *sternal angle* or *angle of Louis* (sometimes quite errone-
ously called the angle of Ludwig). This angle is an important bony landmark which is easily seen and felt in the living subject. It marks the level
of the plane of Louis to which reference will be made later and it also indicates
the level of the second costal cartilage.

The lateral border of the sternum articulates with the clavicle and the
upper seven costal cartilages.

Muscles attached to the sternum include the sternomastoid, pectoralis
major and rectus abdominis (xiphoid process) to its anterior surface; the

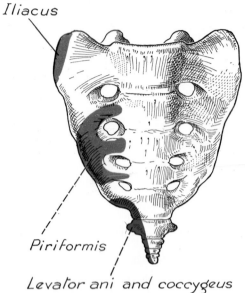

Iliacus

Piriformis

Levator ani and coccygeus

FIG. 44.—The sacrum and coccyx, anterior aspect.

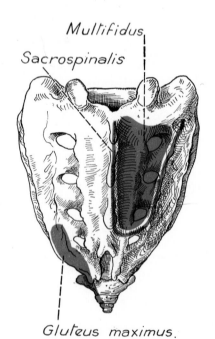

Multifidus

Sacrospinalis

Gluteus maximus.

FIG. 45.—The sacrum and coccyx, posterior aspect.

sternohyoid, sternothyroid, sternocostalis and diaphragm (xiphoid process) to its posterior surface.

The linea alba is attached to the extreme tip of the xiphoid process.

The Ribs (fig. 47). There are twelve pairs of ribs; the upper seven are attached through their costal cartilages to the sternum and are, therefore, known as *true* ribs, the lower five are not directly attached to the sternum and are known as *false* ribs, whilst the lower two ribs end in free extremities anteriorly and are known as *floating* ribs.

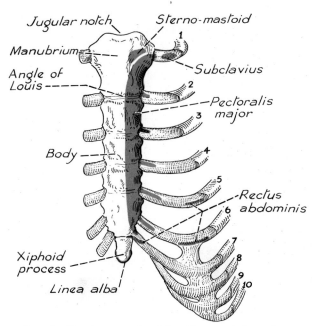

FIG. 46.—The sternum and costal cartilages, anterior surface.

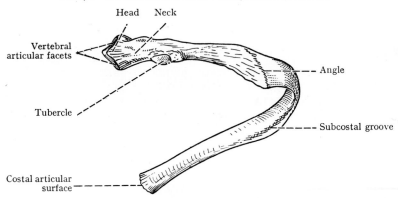

FIG. 47.—A typical rib seen from behind.

A *typical rib* (fig. 47) presents a head, neck, tubercle and a shaft which shows a deep groove on its under surface (the *subcostal groove*). The **head** is attached by a ligament to an intervertebral disc and articulates not only with the body of the corresponding vertebra but with the vertebra above. The *tubercle* articulates with the transverse process of the corresponding vertebra. The *subcostal groove* lodges the intercostal vessels and nerve and these structures lie in the order, vein, artery, nerve from above down (fig. 123). A typical rib is bent forwards at the *angle* and is also twisted.

The first, second, tenth, eleventh and twelfth ribs are atypical and are worthy of closer attention

The first rib (fig. 49) is short and flat and presents a superior and an inferior surface. It is more sharply curved than any of its fellows. Its head presents one articular facet which articulates with the body of the first thoracic vertebra. A landmark on this rib is the *scalene tubercle* on its medial border which gives attachment to the scalenus anterior. In front of this tubercle there is a shallow groove for the subclavian vein and behind it a deeper groove for the subclavian artery, behind which the scalenus medius is attached to a roughened area on the superior surface of the bone. Its lateral border gives origin to part of the first digitation of serratus anterior. The subclavius muscle is attached to the anterior extremity of the superior surface.

The second rib is markedly curved and presents a rough elevation on its lateral border to which part of the origin of serratus anterior is attached. The scalenus posterior muscle is attached to the second rib immediately behind the anterior.

The tenth rib usually has one facet only on the head.

The eleventh and twelfth ribs have neither tubercle nor neck. The twelfth rib has no angle and is very short.

The ribs give attachment to the intercostal muscles, and the lower ribs to all the muscles which form the abdominal wall. Certain important muscles which act upon the upper limb, notably the pectoralis major and minor, the latissimus dorsi and serratus anterior are also attached to the ribs (figs. 126 and 135).

It should be noted that the ribs not only protect the thoracic organs but also the upper abdominal organs, notably the liver, spleen and suprarenals, and to a less extent the stomach and kidneys.

Sometimes an extra rib is present, emerging from the seventh cervical vertebra, this is known as a *cervical rib*. It causes pressure on nerves with muscle wasting and vascular symptoms due to pressure on sympathetic nerve fibres which are passing to supply the arteries of the upper limb. The symptoms are not due to direct pressure on the subclavian artery as was once thought. Cervical rib is often bilateral.

THE BONES OF THE UPPER EXTREMITY

The Clavicle (figs. 50 and 51) lies horizontally and articulates with the sternum and first costal cartilage medially and with the acromion process of the scapula laterally. Its medial two-thirds are convex forwards and

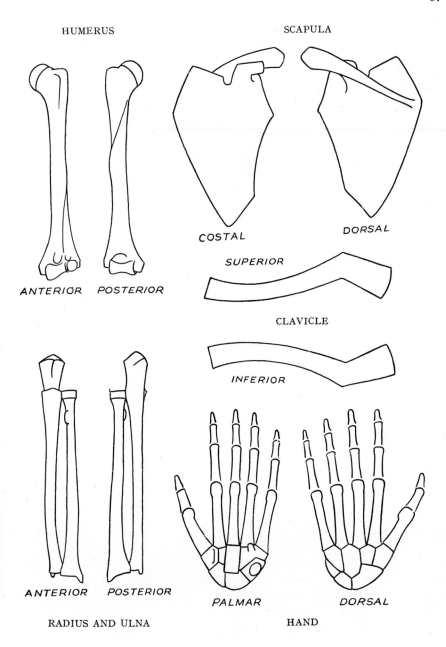

HUMERUS

SCAPULA

COSTAL

DORSAL

ANTERIOR POSTERIOR

SUPERIOR

CLAVICLE

INFERIOR

ANTERIOR POSTERIOR

RADIUS AND ULNA

PALMAR

DORSAL

HAND

FIG. 48.—The bones of the upper extremity are here produced in outline to encourage the student to draw the bones and insert the muscle markings.

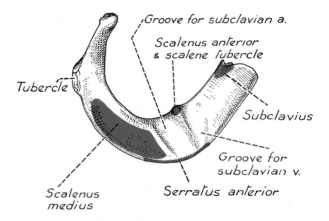

Groove for subclavian a.

*Scalenus anterior
& scalene tubercle*

Tubercle

Subclavius

*Groove for
subclavian v.*

*Scalenus
medius*

Serratus anterior

FIG. 49.—The right first rib superior aspect.

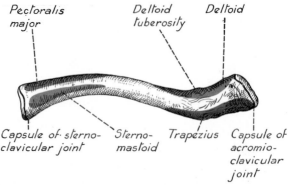

*Pectoralis
major*

*Deltoid
tuberosity*

Deltoid

*Capsule of sterno-
clavicular joint*

*Sterno-
mastoid*

Trapezius

*Capsule of
acromio-
clavicular
joint*

FIG. 50.—The right clavicle, superior aspect.

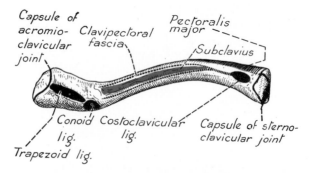

*Capsule of
acromio-
clavicular
joint*

*Clavipectoral
fascia*

*Pectoralis
major*

Subclavius

*Conoid
lig.*

*Costoclavicular
lig.*

*Capsule of sterno-
clavicular joint*

Trapezoid lig.

FIG. 51.—The right clavicle, inferior aspect.

round; its lateral third, concave forwards and flat and its inferior surface grooved and ridged. With this information it is possible to determine to which side of the body any given clavicle belongs.

The clavicle presents the following features: The *deltoid tuberosity* on the anterior border of its outer third (not constant), the **conoid tubercle**, **trapezoid ridge, subclavian groove** and the **rhomboid (costal) impression** on its inferior surface.

The clavicle gives attachment to the following structures: At its sternal end, to the interclavicular ligament, the articular disc and the capsule of the sternoclavicular joint; on its inner half, to the sternomastoid superiorly and the pectoralis major anteriorly, to a few fibres of the sternohyoid muscle posteriorly. The rhomboid or costoclavicular ligament is attached to the

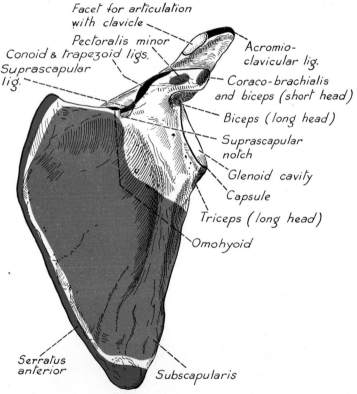

FIG. 52.—The left scapula, anterior (costal) surface.

rhomboid impression, and the subclavius muscle to the subclavian groove. To the margins of this groove, the clavipectoral fascia is attached. The clavicle gives attachment on its outer third to the deltoid muscle anteriorly and the trapezius posteriorly, while the conoid tubercle and trapezoid ridge give attachment to the conoid and trapezoid ligaments which together constitute the coracoclavicular ligament.

The capsule of the acromioclavicular joint is attached to the extremity of the acromion.

The Scapula (figs. 52 and 53) is a flat triangular bone which lies on the posterior thoracic wall between the 2nd and the 7th ribs. From its posterior surface the *spine of the scapula* projects backwards and can be palpated along its entire length. The spine ends in the flattened *acromion* the tip of which can be readily seen and felt. It marks the upper level of the shoulder joint. On the acromion there is a facet which articulates with the clavicle. The base of the spine presents a triangular smooth area over which the trapezius muscle glides.

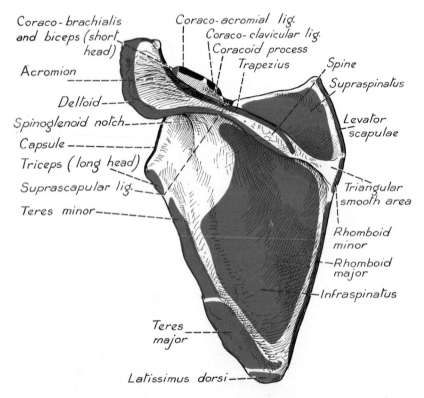

FIG. 53.—The left scapula, posterior surface.

The superolateral angle of the body of the bone is formed by the pear-shaped *glenoid cavity* which articulates with the head of the humerus.

Projecting upwards and forwards above the glenoid cavity is the *coracoid process*, the tip of which can be palpated in the infraclavicular fossa (delto-pectoral triangle) immediately beneath the junction of the middle and outer thirds of the clavicle. On the medial aspect of the base of the coracoid process is the *suprascapular notch* which transmits the suprascapular nerve.

The spine of the scapula divides the posterior surface of the bone into a *supraspinous fossa* above and an *infraspinous fossa* below.

Between the root of the spine and the glenoid cavity is the *spinoglenoid notch* which transmits the suprascapular nerve and vessels after their emergence from the supraspinous fossa.

The anterior or costal surface of the scapula presents a shallow fossa known as the *subscapular fossa*.

The scapula articulates with the head of the humerus at the glenoid cavity forming the shoulder joint and with the lateral end of the clavicle at the acromion forming the acromioclavicular joint.

The trapezius muscle is inserted into the superior border of the spine and the deltoid muscle takes origin from the inferior border of the spine extending on to the adjacent acromion.

The inferior angle of the bone can be located easily in the living subject. It marks the level of the 7th rib and the spine of the 7th thoracic vertebra.

The scapula gives attachment to the following structures: The suprascapular ligament bridges the suprascapular notch and from this and the adjacent superior border the inferior belly of the omohyoid muscle takes origin. The capsule of the shoulder joint and the glenoid labrum are attached to the margin of the glenoid cavity, the capsule of the acromioclavicular joint to the margin of the articular surface on the acromion.

The levator scapulae, rhomboideus minor and major muscles are inserted into the medial (vertebral) border.

The supraspinatus and infraspinatus muscles arise from the supra- and infraspinous fossae respectively. The teres minor and major muscles take origin from the lateral (axillary) border and a few fibres of the latissimus dorsi from the inferior angle.

The long head of biceps arises from a small tubercle above the glenoid cavity, and the long head of triceps from a small tubercle below the glenoid cavity.

The anterior or costal surface of the bone gives origin to the subscapularis muscle, while the serratus anterior is inserted into the vertebral border on this surface.

The coracoid process gives origin at its tip to the conjoined tendon of short head of biceps and coracobrachialis, and receives the insertion of pectoralis minor on its medial border. The coraco-acromial and coracohumeral ligaments are attached to its lateral border, while the conoid and trapezoid portions of the coracoclavicular ligaments are attached to its base.

The Humerus (figs. 54 and 55) articulates with the glenoid cavity of the scapula above, and with the radius and ulna below. It consists of a shaft, an upper and a lower end.

The humerus presents the following features: The *upper end* consists of a *hemispherical head*, at the margin of which is a slight constriction called the *anatomical neck*, the *greater* and *lesser tuberosities* below which is the *surgical neck*. Between the two tuberosities is the well-marked *bicipital groove*. The *shaft* presents, near the middle of its lateral border, a roughened elevation called the **deltoid tuberosity** and ehind and below this is the **spiral groove** which runs downwards, forwards d laterally and in its lower part accommodates the radial nerve.

The **lower end** of the bone presents the edial and **lateral epicondyles**, an articular surface laterally called the **capit m** and another medially called the **trochlea**, the latter extending on to t posterior surface. Above the

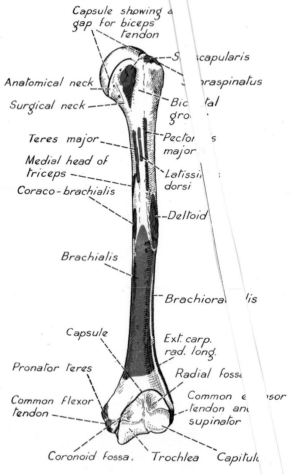

Capsule showing a
gap for biceps
tendon

S capularis

Anatomical neck

raspinatus

Surgical neck

Bic tal
gro

Teres major

Pector s
major

Medial head of
triceps

Latissi
dorsi

Coraco-brachialis

Deltoid

Brachialis

Brachiora lis

Capsule

Ext. carp.
rad. long.

Pronator teres

Radial foss

Common flexor
tendon

Common e sor
tendon an
supinator

Coronoid fossa.   Trochlea   Capitul

FIG. 54.—The left humerus, anterior surface.

capitulum is the shallow **radial fossa** which receives the hea   the radius when the forearm is flexed; above the trochlea anteriorly   the deeper **coronoid fossa** which in similar circumstances receives the coron   process of the ulna. Above the trochlea posteriorly is the **olecranon fossa**, v   h receives the olecranon process of the ulna when the forearm is extended

The humerus gives attachment to the following struct   s: At its

upper end, the capsule is attached to the anatomical neck and extends down the shaft for a short distance postero-medially. The supraspinatus, infraspinatus and teres minor muscles are inserted into the three facets on the greater tuberosity and the subscapularis to the facet on the lesser tuberosity. The transverse humeral ligament which retains the tendon of biceps in position is attached to the margins of the bicipital groove superiorly.

On *the shaft* the pectoralis major is inserted into the lateral lip of the bicipital groove, the teres major into the medial lip, while the tendon of

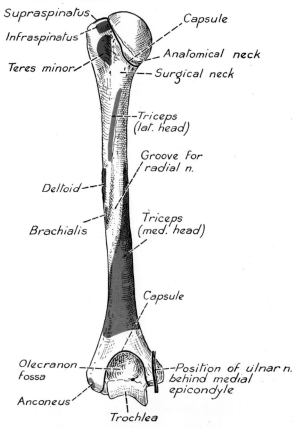

FIG. 55.—The left humerus, posterior surface.

latissimus dorsi is inserted into the floor of the groove. The deltoid muscle is inserted into the deltoid tuberosity, the coracobrachialis muscle is inserted on the medial surface of the shaft opposite this and the brachialis muscle takes a broad origin from the lower half of the front of the shaft. The upper half of the shaft posteriorly gives a linear origin to the lateral head of triceps, the lower half a broad origin to the medial head of triceps, the two heads being separated by the spiral groove.

The *lower end* gives attachment to the common flexor tendon and pronator teres from the medial epicondyle and the common extensor tendon and supinator from the lateral epicondyle. The posterior aspect of the lateral epicondyle gives origin to the anconeus muscle, while the posterior aspect of the medial epicondyle presents a groove which lodges the ulnar nerve.

Above the epicondyles, the *medial supracondylar ridge* gives attachment to the medial intermuscular septum and the *lateral supracondylar ridge* to the

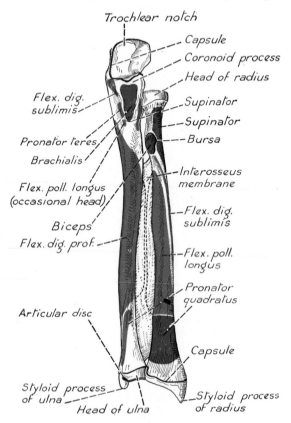

Fig. 56.—The left radius and ulna, anterior surface.

lateral intermuscular septum and also origin to the brachioradialis muscle above and the extensor carpi radialis longus muscle below.

The capsule of the elbow joint is attached to the lower end of the bone, above (sometimes across) the fossae previously described, extending on to the epicondyles.

The Radius (figs. 56 and 57) is the lateral bone of the forearm. Its upper end forms part of the elbow joint and its lower end part of the wrist joint.

The radius presents the following features: At the *upper end* of the bone is the small circular *head* which articulates with the radial notch on the ulna and with the capitulum on the humerus. Below the head is the constricted *neck*, and below this the *radial tuberosity*.

The *shaft* of the bone presents the *oblique line* anteriorly, which ends laterally in the prominent *pronator tubercle* and a sharp medial or *interosseous border*.

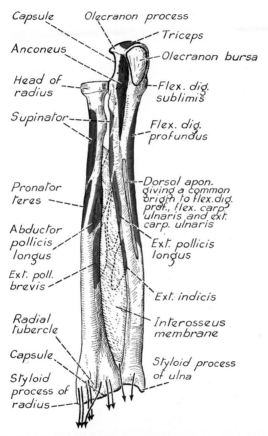

FIG. 57.—The left radius and ulna, posterior surface. The arrows indicate the position of tendons at the wrist (see p. 47 and fig. 58).

The bone in contradistinction to the ulna widens from above down and its *lower end* presents laterally the palpable *styloid process* and medially the *ulnar notch*, by which the bone articulates with the head of the ulna. Its articular surface is divided into two by a ridge; the lateral area articulates with the scaphoid bone and the medial area with the lunate bone (fig. 58).

On the posterior aspect of the distal end of the bone is the small but important dorsal (Lister's) tubercle which can be palpated on the back of the wrist and is a guide to the position of the tendons (figs. 57 and 58).

The radius gives attachment to the following structures: At the *proximal end*—the biceps is inserted into the posterior aspect of the tuberosity. The head of the radius is surrounded by the annular ligament within which it rotates in movements of pronation and supination.

On the anterior aspect of *the shaft*, the major part of the flexor digitorum sublimis arises from the oblique line and the origin of the flexor pollicis longus and the insertion of the pronator quadratus are attached to the shaft below this. The supinator is inserted into the neck and upper part of the shaft as far down as the oblique line. The pronator teres is inserted into the pronator tuberosity on the lateral aspect of the shaft. The abductor pollicis longus and extensor pollicis brevis take origin from the posterior aspect of the shaft. The interosseous membrane is attached to the sharp medial border.

At the *distal end* of the bone the capsule of the wrist joint is attached around the whole margin of the articular surface. The brachioradialis muscle is inserted into the base of the styloid process. The base of the articular disc of the wrist joint is attached to a ridge which divides the distal articular surface from the ulnar notch (fig. 90).

The distal end of the bone is grooved on its dorsal aspect. These grooves lodge the extensor tendons passing to the hand and will be described in detail with similar grooves on the ulna.

The Ulna is the medial bone of the forearm. Its upper end forms part of the elbow joint but its lower end is excluded from the wrist joint by the articular disc. It is longer than the radius although it does not extend down so far and it tapers markedly from above down.

The ulna presents the following features: The *upper end* is massive and is known as the *olecranon process*. This is hollowed out anteriorly to form the *trochlear notch* which articulates with the trochlea of the humerus. The triangular *coronoid process* below this presents the small *radial notch* on its lateral aspect which articulates with the head of the radius.

The *shaft* presents the deep *supinator fossa* below the radial notch which lodges but gives no attachment to the biceps tendon. Behind this fossa is the sharp *supinator crest*.

The shaft consists of three surfaces which are situated anteriorly, laterally and medially. The latter two surfaces are separated from each other by a prominent *posterior border* which can be readily palpated beneath the skin.

The *lower end* of the bone presents a small rounded *head* which terminates medially in a prominent *styloid process*.

The ulna gives attachment to the following structures: At the *upper end* the capsule of the elbow joint is attached to the margins of the trochlear and radial notches. The annular ligament is attached to the anterior and posterior borders of the radial notch.

The triceps is inserted into the posterior aspect of the superior surface of the olecranon; the anconeus into its lateral surface extending down on to the shaft; the ulnar head of flexor carpi ulnaris arises from its medial surface extending down to the aponeurosis on the posterior border.

The coronoid process receives the insertion of the brachialis, and its medial border presents three small tubercles which give origin from above down to the flexor digitorum sublimis, the pronator radii teres and the flexor pollicis longus.

The *shaft* gives part origin to the supinator from the supinator crest and the posterior part of the supinator fossa.

The anterior and medial surfaces and the posterior border of the shaft give origin to the flexor digitorum profundus. The lower part of the anterior surface gives origin to pronator quadratus. The sharp lateral border gives attachment to the interosseous membrane.

The posterior border gives attachment to an aponeurosis which is common to three muscles, viz., the flexor digitorum profundus, the flexor carpi ulnaris and the extensor carpi ulnaris.

The posterior surface of the shaft gives origin from above down to the abductor pollicis longus, extensor pollicis longus and extensor indicis.

The *lower end* forms the head of the bone and gives attachment to the

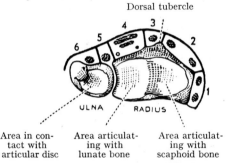

Dorsal tubercle

| Area in contact with articular disc | Area articulating with lunate bone | Area articulating with scaphoid bone |

FIG. 58.—The distal end of radius and ulna showing the extensor retinaculum and fascial compartments for tendons (see text below).

capsule of the wrist joint, while the lateral aspect of the base of the styloid process gives attachment to the apex of the articular disc of that joint (fig. 90).

The lower end of the bone is grooved on its dorsal aspect by the extensor carpi ulnaris tendon (fig. 58).

The dorsal aspect of the lower end of the radius and ulna presents a series of grooves which are converted into tunnels by fibrous septa extending down to the ridges from the extensor retinaculum. Six tunnels are formed in this way (fig. 58) and they contain the following structures from the lateral to the medial side:—

(1) The tendons of the abductor pollicis longus and extensor pollicis brevis.

(2) The tendons of extensor carpi radialis longus and brevis.

(3) The tendon of extensor pollicis longus bounded laterally by the dorsal (radial) tubercle.

(4) The tendons of extensors digitorum and indicis with the posterior interosseous nerve and the anterior interosseous artery.

(5) The tendon of extensor digiti minimi between the two bones.

(6) The tendon of extensor carpi ulnaris.

The Bones of the Wrist and Hand (figs. 59 and 60). There are eight carpal bones consisting of two rows of four. *The proximal row latero-medially* is made up of the scaphoid, lunate, triquetral and pisiform bones.

The distal row latero-medially is made up of the trapezium, trapezoid, capitate and hamate bones.

The features of the bones of the wrist and hand. It is necessary merely to identify the carpal bones on the articulated hand but the student's

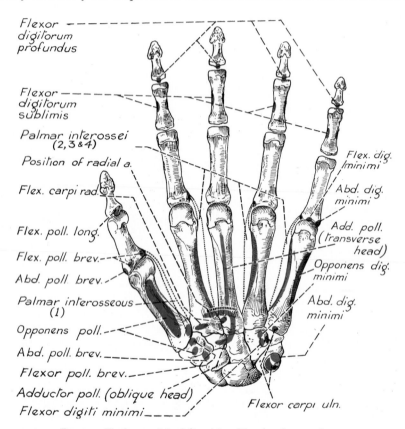

Flexor digitorum profundus

Flexor digitorum sublimis

Palmar interossei (2, 3 & 4)

Position of radial a.

Flex. carpi rad.

Flex. poll. long.

Flex. poll. brev.

Abd. poll. brev.

Palmar interosseous (1)

Opponens poll.

Abd. poll. brev.

Flexor poll. brev.

Adductor poll. (oblique head)

Flexor digiti minimi

Flex. dig. minimi

Abd. dig. minimi

Add. poll. (transverse head)

Opponens dig. minimi

Abd. dig. minimi

Flexor carpi uln.

FIG. 59.—The bones of the left wrist and hand, palmar surface.

attention is called particularly to the shape, size and position of the scaphoid bone since this is commonly the site of fracture, to the groove on the trapezium which lodges the tendon of flexor carpi radialis, to the hook-shaped process on the hamate and to the pea-like pisiform. Note the shape of the metacarpal bones and particularly the rounded heads of the four medial metacarpals which form the knuckles. Note that there are three phalanges for each of the fingers but two only for the thumb.

The bones of the wrist and hand give attachment to the following structures. On reference to figs. 59 and 60 it will be seen that the flexor carpi ulnaris is inserted (in part) into the pisiform bone and that the abductor digiti minimi takes origin (in part) from that bone. The abductor pollicis brevis takes origin (in part) from the scaphoid bone. The opponens pollicis and flexor pollicis brevis both arise from the trapezium. The adductor pollicis (oblique head) takes origin (in part) from the trapezoid and capitate and its C-shaped origin is extended on to the base of the second and third

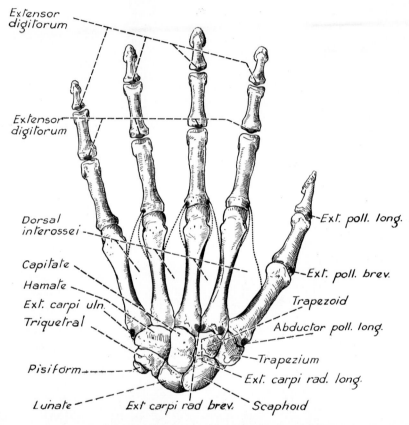

Extensor digitorum

Extensor digitorum

Dorsal interossei

Capitate

Hamate

Ext. carpi uln.

Triquetral

Pisiform

Lunate

Ext. carpi rad. brev.

Scaphoid

Ext. carpi rad. long.

Trapezium

Abductor poll. long.

Trapezoid

Ext. poll. brev.

Ext. poll. long.

FIG. 60.—The bones of the left wrist and hand, dorsal surface.

metacarpal bones. The opponens digiti minimi and flexor digiti minimi take origin from the hook of the hamate.

Opponens pollicis is inserted into the lateral border of the first metacarpal bone, the flexor carpi radialis tendon into the bases of the second and third metacarpals and the four palmar interossei arise from the first, second, fourth and fifth metacarpal bones. The adductor pollicis (transverse head) arises from the third metacarpal bone and the opponens digiti minimi is inserted into the medial border of the fifth metacarpal bone.

Abductor pollicis brevis, adductor pollicis and flexor pollicis brevis are

4 + A.PH.

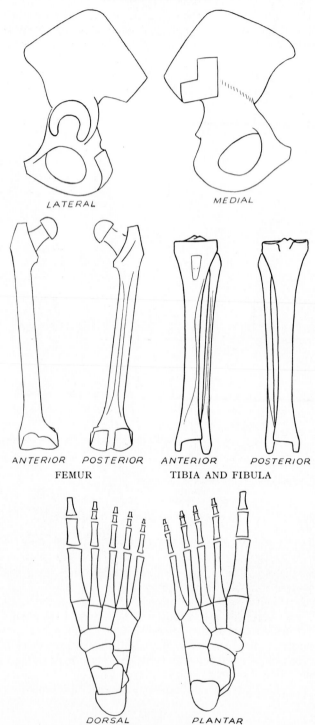

LATERAL   MEDIAL

ANTERIOR POSTERIOR ANTERIOR POSTERIOR

FEMUR   TIBIA AND FIBULA

DORSAL   PLANTAR

FOOT

FIG 61.—The bones of the lower extremity are here reproduced in outline to encourage the student to draw the bones and insert the muscle markings.

inserted into the base of the proximal phalanx of the thumb; the palmar, interossei are inserted (in part) into the proximal phalanges of the first, second fourth and fifth digits and also inserted into the base of the proximal phalanx of the fifth digit are the flexor and abductor digiti minimi.

The tendons of flexor digitorum sublimis are inserted into the borders of the middle phalanges and the tendons of flexor digitorum profundus into the bases of the distal phalanges of the fingers. The tendon of flexor pollicis longus is inserted into the base of the distal phalanx of the thumb.

On the dorsal aspect of the hand no muscles are attached to the carpal bones; the abductor pollicis longus is inserted into the base of the meta-carpal of the thumb; the tendons of extensor carpi radialis longus and brevis are inserted into the bases of the second and third metacarpal bones respec-tively, and the tendon of extensor carpi ulnaris is inserted into the base of the fifth metacarpal bone.

The four dorsal interossei arise by two heads from the contiguous sides of the first and second, second and third, third and fourth and fourth and fifth metacarpal bones and are inserted (in part) into the proximal phalanges of the second, third and fourth digits, the proximal phalanx of the middle finger having two interossei inserted into it. The extensor pollicis brevis is inserted into the base of the proximal phalanx of the thumb. The tendons of extensor digitorum are inserted into the middle of the distal phalanges of the fingers and give slips to the bases of the proximal phalanges. The tendon of extensor pollicis longus is inserted into the base of the distal phalanx of the thumb.

THE BONES OF THE LOWER EXTREMITY

The Innominate Bone (figs. 62 and 63) consists of three bones which fuse together about the time of puberty. They are called the ilium, the ischium and the pubis. The innominate bones articulate with the sacrum and form the anterolateral walls of the pelvis.

Important features are: The *anterior superior* and the *anterior inferior iliac spines*, the *iliac crest* which is described as presenting lateral, inter-mediate and medial lips with a *tubercle* on its lateral aspect about 5 cm. behind the anterior superior spine, the *posterior superior* and *posterior inferior iliac spines* bounding a flat mass of bone called the *ala* of the ilium, the *body* of the ilium lying below this and forming part of a cup-shaped socket called the *acetabulum* which articulates with the head of the femur.

Below and medial to the anterior inferior spine is the *iliopubic eminence* which marks the junction of the body of the ilium with the superior ramus of the pubis. The sharp upper border of the superior ramus is known as the *pectineal line*, medial to this is the *pubic tubercle* and more medially is the *pubic crest* which is the superior border of the body of the pubis. The inferior border of the superior ramus bounding the oval *obturator foramen* is known as the *obturator crest*. The *body* of the pubis lies below the pubic crest and the medial border of the body is called the *symphyseal surface*. The body is succeeded by the *inferior ramus of the pubis* and this in the adult

4*

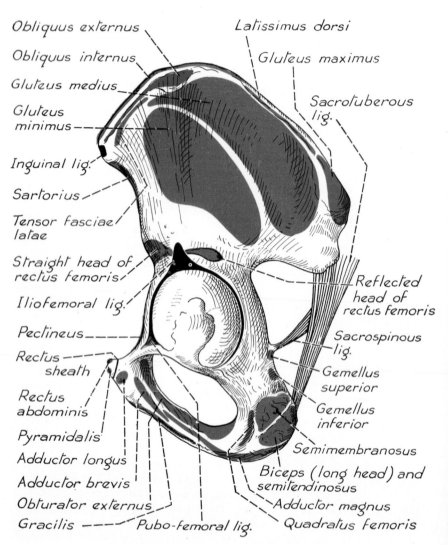

Obliquus externus

Obliquus internus

Gluteus medius

Gluteus minimus

Inguinal lig.

Sartorius

Tensor fasciae latae

Straight head of rectus femoris

Iliofemoral lig.

Pectineus

Rectus sheath

Rectus abdominis

Pyramidalis

Adductor longus

Adductor brevis

Obturator externus

Gracilis

Latissimus dorsi

Gluteus maximus

Sacrotuberous lig.

Reflected head of rectus femoris

Sacrospinous lig.

Gemellus superior

Gemellus inferior

Semimembranosus

Biceps (long head) and semitendinosus

Adductor magnus

Quadratus femoris

Pubo-femoral lig.

FIG. 62.—The left innominate bone, lateral aspect.

is demarcated from the *inferior ramus of the ischium* by a ridge. The inferior ramus of the ischium is succeeded by the **superior ramus** and the angle of union between these two parts of the bone forms the *ischial tuberosity*. The superior ramus of the ischium is succeeded by the **body** of that bone which forms a large part of the acetabulum.

The position of the **greater** and **lesser sciatic notches** should be noted and that of the *ischial spine* which is the division between them.

The medial or pelvic aspect of the bone presents similar features and in

addition shows the *auricular articular surface* by which the bone articulates
with the sacrum at the sacro-iliac joint, the *iliac part of the pectineal line*
(forming part of the pelvic brim), and the sharp *falciform margin* of the
ischial tuberosity.

The iliac crest gives attachment to the following structures (fig. 64):
The lateral lip of the iliac crest receives the insertion of the external oblique

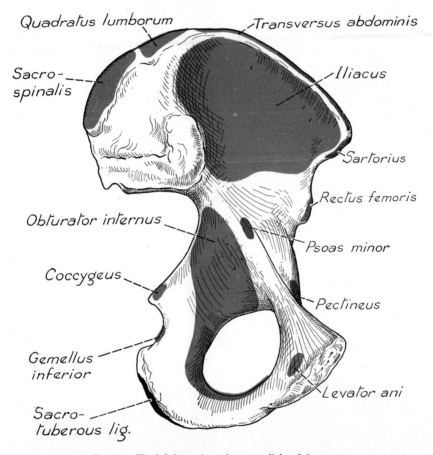

FIG. 63.—The left innominate bone, medial, pelvic aspect.

muscle (in part), gives origin to tensor fasciae latae and part origin to latissimus dorsi and gluteus maximus muscles in that order from before back.

The medial lip gives origin to transversus abdominis, quadratus lumborum
and sacrospinalis in that order from before back. The intermediate lip
anteriorly gives origin (in part) to the internal oblique muscle.

**The lateral aspect of the innominate bone gives attachment to the
following structures:** The inguinal ligament is attached to the anterior
superior spine. The sartorius muscle takes origin from this spine and from

the notch below. The straight head of rectus femoris arises from the anterior inferior spine and the reflected head from an adjacent rough area of bone above the acetabulum, the attachment of the apex of the iliofemoral ligament intervening between these two heads.

The gluteus minimus, medius and maximus are attached to the lateral aspect of the ala in that order from before back, minimus and medius being separated by the middle gluteal line and medius and maximus by the posterior gluteal line.

The capsule of the hip joint is attached to the margin of the acetabulum, while the base of the pubofemoral ligament is prolonged on to the obturator crest (fig. 62).

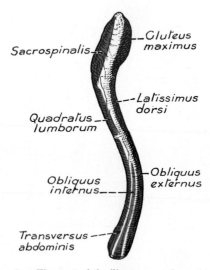

FIG. 64.—The crest of the ilium as seen from above.

The pectineal line gives origin to the pectineus muscle, the pubic crest gives origin to the rectus abdominis and pyramidalis muscles.

The angle between the superior and inferior rami gives origin to the adductor longus.

The inferior ramus of the pubis gives origin to adductors brevis and gracilis (at the border of the bone) while the origin of adductor magnus extends from the inferior ramus of the ischium on to the adjacent tuberosity.

The obturator externus takes origin from the obturator membrane (which fills in the obturator foramen) and adjacent border of bone, the quadratus femoris and inferior gemellus take origin from the body of the ischium, while the superior gemellus arises from the ischial spine.

The ischial tuberosity gives origin to the semimembranosus muscle on its superolateral aspect and to the conjoined tendon of biceps and semi-tendinosus on its superomedial aspect, to the hamstring portion of adductor magnus on its inferolateral aspect, while the falciform border of the tuberosity gives attachment to the sacrotuberous ligament. The sacrospinous and sacrotuberous ligaments convert the sciatic notches into the greater and lesser sciatic foramina.

The *greater sciatic foramen* transmits the piriformis muscle which almost fills the space with the superior gluteal vessels and nerve emerging above it, and the sciatic nerve, the posterior cutaneous nerve of the thigh, the nerve to quadratus femoris, the nerve to obturator internus, the internal pudendal vessels and nerve and the inferior gluteal vessels and nerve below it.

The *lesser sciatic foramen* transmits the tendon of obturator internus, and its nerve, and the internal pudendal vessels and nerve. The latter structures have emerged from the pelvic cavity and are passing to the perineum.

The medial aspect of the bone gives attachment to the following structures: The iliacus muscle arises from the iliac fossa on the pelvic aspect of the ala, the psoas minor is inserted into the pectineal line. The obturator internus arises from the obturator membrane and the adjacent bone extending as far back as the greater sciatic notch and the levator ani muscle, forming the pelvic floor, takes origin from the body of the pubis and from the ischial spine.

The falciform margin of the ischial tuberosity which gives attachment to the sacrotuberous ligament is well seen on this surface.

The Femur (figs. 65, 66 and 67) presents an upper end comprising a *head, neck, greater* and *lesser trochanters*; a *shaft* and a lower end comprising two *condyles*.

It articulates with the acetabulum of the innominate bone above and with the patella and tibia below. It is the longest and strongest bone in the body.

The femur presents the following features: The *head* forms two-thirds of a sphere. In its centre there is a depression called the *fovea capitis*.

The *neck* connects the head with the shaft forming an angle of about 120° in the male and rather less in the female. Knowledge of the size of this angle is of great importance, since it is altered in certain diseases.

The trochanters lie at the junction of the neck with the shaft.

The *greater trochanter* is quadrate and easily palpable in the upper part of the lateral aspect of the thigh. On its medial aspect is the well marked *trochanteric fossa.* The *lesser trochanter* is much smaller and is deeply placed on the medial aspect of the thigh. Between the two trochanters are the *intertrochanteric line* anteriorly and the much bolder *intertrochanteric crest* posteriorly, on which is the *quadrate tubercle.*

The *shaft* is smooth and round and presents posteriorly a ridge called the *linea aspera*, the margins of which diverge above and below. The lower divergencies form the *supracondylar ridges.* On the upper lateral border of the linea aspera is the *gluteal tuberosity.*

The *distal end* presents the lateral and medial condyles which are separated by the *intercondylar notch.* Surmounting these condyles are the epicondyles. On the medial epicondyle is the prominent *adductor tubercle.* On the lateral aspect of the lateral condyle is the *groove for the tendon of the popliteus muscle.* A small area of bone between the condyles in front articulates with the patella. Between the supracondylar ridges on the posterior aspect of the bone there is a smooth triangular area known as the *popliteal surface* of the femur.

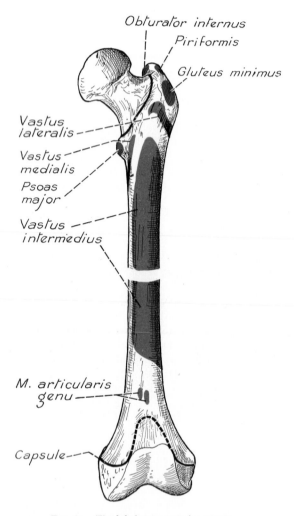

FIG. 65.—The left femur, anterior aspect.

The femur gives attachment to the following structures: On the head of the bone the ligamentum teres of the hip joint is attached to the fovea capitis.

On the greater trochanter the gluteus medius is inserted along an oblique line on its lateral aspect; the gluteus minimus on its anterior aspect; the obturator internus and gemelli and the piriformis are inserted into facets of the superior border. The obturator externus is inserted into the trochanteric fossa on the medial surface of this trochanter.

The capsule of the hip joint and the capsular ligaments are attached anteriorly to the intertrochanteric line and posteriorly to the neck of the

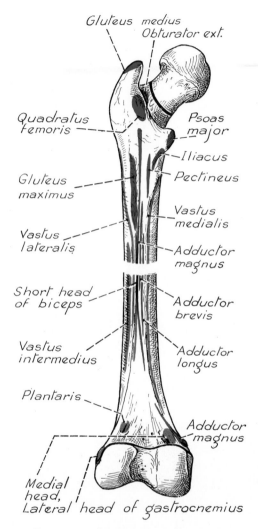

Gluteus medius
Obturator ext.
Quadratus femoris
Psoas major
Iliacus
Gluteus maximus
Pectineus
Vastus medialis
Vastus lateralis
Adductor magnus
Short head of biceps
Adductor brevis
Vastus intermedius
Adductor longus
Plantaris
Adductor magnus
Medial head,
Lateral head of gastrocnemius

FIG. 66.—The left femur, posterior aspect.

femur 1·5 cm. above the intertrochanteric crest. On this crest the quadratus femoris is inserted into the quadrate tubercle.

The iliopsoas muscle is inserted on the lesser trochanter.

The shaft of the bone anteriorly gives an extensive origin to the vastus intermedius, and below this muscle to the articularis genu, while the upper part of this surface receives extensions from the vastus medialis and the vastus lateralis muscles. The middle lip of the linea aspera and the medial supracondylar ridge give an extensive insertion to the adductor magnus extending from the quadrate tubercle to the adductor tubercle. From the medial lip of the linea aspera, vastus medialis takes origin, and between this muscle and adductor magnus, the linea aspera receives the insertions of

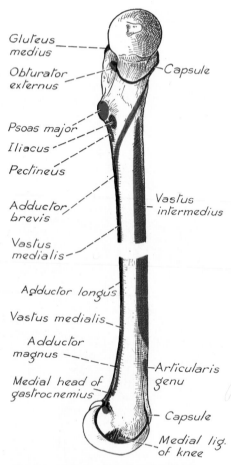

Gluteus medius

Obturator externus

Capsule

Psoas major

Iliacus

Pectineus

Adductor brevis

Vastus intermedius

Vastus medialis

Adductor longus

Vastus medialis

Adductor magnus

Articularis genu

Medial head of gastrocnemius

Capsule

Medial lig. of knee

FIG. 67.—Medial surface of the left femur.

pectineus, adductor brevis and adductor longus (fig. 66). From the lateral lip of the linea aspera, vastus lateralis takes origin; between this and the middle lip, gluteus maximus is inserted (in part) into the gluteal tuberosity, whilst the short head of biceps arises lower down.

The attachment of the capsule of the knee joint to the femur should be noted; it is attached to the margin of the articular surface posteriorly, but is entirely absent anteriorly. Through this gap in the capsule the synovial membrane of the knee joint herniates to form a pouch beneath the tendon, the suprapatellar bursa (fig. 107). The capsule is attache medial condyle well below the adductor tubercle and to the lateral c above the popliteal groove.

The two heads of gastrocnemius arise from the posterior aspect of the con dyles, and the small plantaris immediately above the lateral head of gastroc- nemius. The popliteus muscle arises from the anterior aspect of the popliteal groove on the lateral condyle.

Two ligaments of the knee joint, the anterior and posterior cruciate and the infrapatellar synovial fold, are attached to the intercondyloid fossa.

The Patella is a sesamoid bone (i.e. a seed-like bone developed in a tendon) lying within the quadriceps tendon. It is triangular in shape with an apex which is directed downwards and which gives attachment to the ligamentum patellae. Its posterior surface articulates with the femur and this part of the bone presents a vertical ridge which fits into the groove on the patellar surface of the femur., The articular surface of the patella is thus divided into a larger lateral part which articulates with the lateral condyle of the femur and a small medial part which articulates with the medial condyle of the femur.

The patella causes the quadriceps to pull on the tibia at an angle and thus increases its power considerably.

The Tibia (figs. 68, 69 and 70) sustains the whole weight of the body which is transmitted from the femur. It is the medial bone of the leg, a large part of it being subcutaneous and easily palpable. It articulates with the condyles of the femur and head of the fibula above and with the distal end of the fibula and the talus below.

The tibia presents the following features: Its *upper end* is divided into two *condyles*, the upper surfaces of which articulate with the condyles of the femur, the medial and lateral semilunar cartilages intervening. Lying between these articular surfaces is the intercondylar eminence separating the anterior from the posterior intercondylar areas.

The lateral condyle presents on its lateral aspect the round *fibular articular surface* and on the posterior aspect of the medial condyle a groove for the insertion of the semimembranosus muscle.

The *shaft* presents the easily palpable *tubercle* above. It has a prominent anterior border which with the adjacent medial surface is subcutaneous and forms the shin. The posterior surface presents the oblique *soleal line* above, from which a faint vertical line passes downwards to divide the posterior part of the middle of the shaft into two areas. The interosseous, or lateral border gives attachment to the interosseous membrane.

The *distal end* of the bone articulates with the talus and the fibula, and is prolonged downwards medially, to form the *medial malleolus*.

The tibia gives attachment to the following structures: To the superior articular surface, the medial and lateral semilunar cartilages and the anterior and posterior cruciate ligaments of the knee joint are attached as indicated in fig. 71.

The capsule of the knee joint is attached to the margins of the articular surface except anteriorly where it passes down to blend with the ligamentum patellae.

The iliotibial tract is attached to the lateral condyle as are a few fibres of certain muscles reflected from the fibula, viz., the biceps femoris, extensor

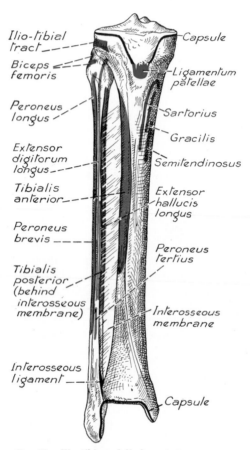

FIG. 68.—The tibia and fibula, anterior aspect.

digitorum longus and peroneus longus (sometimes). The semimembranosus is inserted into the groove on the posterior aspect of the medial condyle.

The upper part of the medial subcutaneous surface of the shaft receives the insertion of three muscles of the thigh, viz., the sartorius, gracilis and semitendinosus. The lateral surface of the shaft gives an extensive origin to the tibialis anterior. The posterior surface receives the insertion of the popliteus above, the soleus originates partly from the soleal line, while the area of bone below this gives origin to tibialis posterior laterally and flexor digitorum longus medially.

The tubercle gives attachment to the ligamentum patellae.

The lower end of the bone gives attachment to the capsule of the ankle joint at the margin of the articular surface.

The deltoid ligament is attached to the medial malleolus. The groove behind the medial malleolus lodges the tendon of tibialis posterior which at this level usually separates flexor digitorum longus from the bone. More

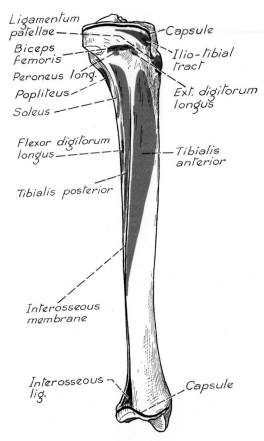

FIG. 69.—The right tibia, lateral aspect.

laterally the flexor hallucis longus and posterior tibial vessels and nerve lie in contact with the bone.

The Fibula (figs. 68, 70 and 72) lies on the lateral aspect of the tibia and while it forms the lateral malleolus of the ankle joint, it is excluded from the knee joint.

The fibula presents the following features: The *proximal end,* or *head,* is quadrate and is surmounted by a styloid process.

The *shaft* in a typical specimen presents *four borders* and *four surfaces* but the *anterior surface* does not extend throughout the length of the shaft for in the upper third of the bone the anterolateral and anteromedial borders are fused.

The *anteromedial border* gives attachment to the interosseous membrane.

The *distal end* of the bone presents the triangular *lateral malleolus* which is subcutaneous.   On the posteromedial aspect of this malleolus is the well-

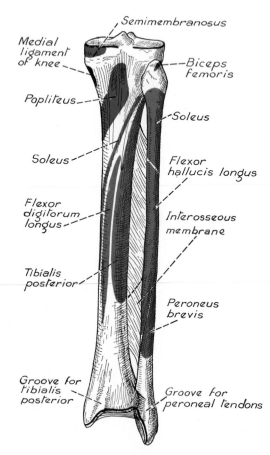

FIG. 70.—The tibia and fibula, posterior aspect.

marked *malleolar fossa*, a very useful landmark in distinguishing the lower from the upper end of the bone and if it is remembered that this fossa lies posteriorly, there is no difficulty in assigning the fibula to its correct side in the body.

The fibula gives attachment to the following structures: The lateral ligaments of the knee joint are attached to the styloid process and a feature of the long lateral ligament is that it divides the insertion of biceps femoris which is attached to the head into two parts. The shaft gives origin to the extensor digitorum longus, extensor hallucis longus and peroneus tertius from the anterior surface, the peroneus longus and brevis from the

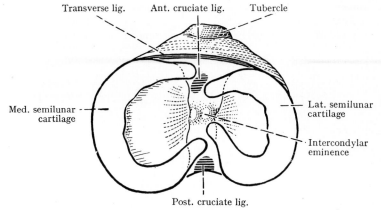

Fig. 71.—The condyles of the right tibia as seen from above.

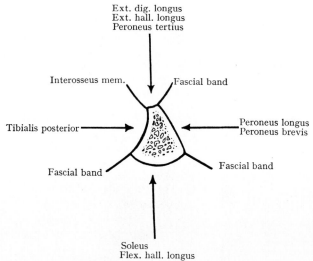

Fig. 72.—Transverse section through the right fibula, the muscles attached to each surface are indicated.

lateral surface the soleus and flexor hallucis longus from the posterior surface and tibialis posterior from the medial surface.

The capsule of the ankle joint is attached to the margins of the distal articular surface, the lateral ligament of that joint being attached to the lateral malleolus. A groove behind the lateral malleolus lodges peroneii brevis et longus, the brevis lying nearer the bone.

The Bones of the Foot

The *bones of the foot* comprise the tarsal bones, the metatarsals and pha-langes.

The *tarsal bones* comprise the calcaneum, talus, navicular, cuboid and the three cuneiform bones.

The Calcaneum articulates above with the talus and in front with the cuboid.

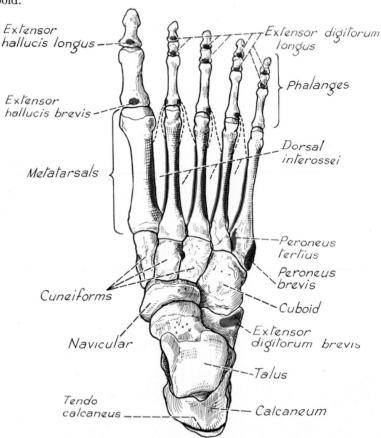

FIG. 73.—The right foot, dorsal surface.

The calcaneum presents the following features: The *posterior surface* forms the prominence of the heel and is divided by a *transverse ridge*; the smooth area above the ridge is in contact with a bursa which separates it from the tendo calcaneus.

The lateral surface presents the small **peroneal tubercle** which separates the peroneus brevis above from the peroneus longus below.

The medial surface presents a well-marked shelf of bone known as the *sustentaculum tali,* on which part of the talus lies.

The superior surface is largely articular. It presents two articular facets for the talus, an anterior and a posterior separated by the *sulcus calcanei*. A rough area on its anterolateral aspect marks the origin of extensor digitorum brevis. This can be palpated on the dorsum of the foot and should be located.

The inferior or plantar surface presents an *anterior tubercle* in the mid-line and *medial* and *lateral tubercles* at the junction of the posterior and plantar surfaces.

The calcaneum gives attachment to the following structures: The extensor digitorum brevis arises from its superior surface, and the interosseous

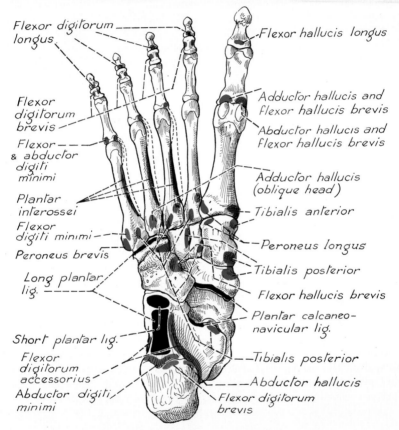

FIG. 74.—The right foot, plantar surface.

talocalcanean ligament is attached to the sulcus calcanei; the tendo calcaneus and the plantaris muscle are inserted into the transverse ridge on the posterior surface. The flexor accessorius arises by two heads, one from the medial surface and the other in front of the lateral tubercle; abductor digiti minimi arises from the medial and lateral tubercles; abductor hallucis and flexor digitorum brevis from the medial tubercle only; the long plantar ligament arises from the plantar surface in front of the medial and lateral tubercles and the short plantar ligament from the anterior tubercle.

The anterior border of the sustentaculum tali gives attachment to a slip from the tibialis posterior muscle and also to the plantar calcaneonavicular and deltoid ligaments.

The Talus articulates with the tibia and fibula above, with the calcaneum and plantar calcaneonavicular ligament below and with the navicular bone in front. It consists of a *head, neck* and *body*.

The talus presents the following features: On the body there is a superior articular surface which is wider in front than behind, a large triangular lateral articular facet for articulation with the lower end of the fibula, a smaller lunate medial articular facet for articulation with the lower end of the tibia. The small posterior surface presents a deep groove for the tendon of flexor hallucis longus. On the anterior surface of the head there is an articular facet for the navicular bone and on its plantar surface anterior and middle facets for the calcaneum and a medial facet for the plantar calcaneonavicular ligament. These two surfaces are separated from the larger posterior articular facet which also articulates with the calcaneum by a deep groove called the *sulcus tali*.

There are no muscles attached to the talus but numerous ligaments are attached to the bone and the interosseous talocalcanean ligament is attached to the sulcus tali.

The remaining tarsal bones need only be identified: The characteristic feature of the *cuboid* is the deep groove on its plantar surface lodging the tendon of peroneus longus. The feature of the *navicular bone* is its important medial tuberosity which can be seen and felt in the foot and to which the main tendon of the tibialis posterior is attached. The plantar calcaneo-navicular ligament is attached to its plantar surface. The position of the three wedge-shaped *cuneiform bones* should be noted lying immediately in front of the navicular bone and are usually referred to as the medial, inter-mediate and lateral cuneiform bones.

The tendons of tibialis anterior and tibialis posterior are inserted into the medial side of the inferior aspect of the medial cuneiform bone; the flexor hallucis brevis arises from the lateral cuneiform and adjacent cuboid; fascial slips from the tendon of tibialis posterior are attached to the intermediate and lateral cuneiforms and adjacent metatarsal bones and to the cuboid. The peroneus longus tendon is inserted into the lateral side of the inferior aspect of the medial cuneiform and adjacent base of the first metatarsal bone.

The metatarsals and phalanges are arranged in a manner similar to those of the hand. The base of the 5th metatarsal forms a prominent landmark on the dorsum of the foot.

The position of the structures attached to the bones of the foot is indicated in figs. 73 and 74 and needs no further elaboration here, since reference will be made to the subject when dealing with the individual muscles.

CHAPTER III

JOINTS

GENERAL CLASSIFICATION OF JOINTS

A joint is formed when two or more skeletal structures meet. Bones are united to form joints in three different ways and all the joints of the body fall into one of these categories:

(1) *Fibrous Joints:* the bones are united by intervening fibrous tissue.

(2) *Cartilaginous Joints:* the bones are united by intervening cartilage.

(3) *Synovial Joints:* the bones are separated by a joint cavity and are united by a sheath of fibrous tissue (the capsule) and lined by synovial membrane which secretes a lubricant called the synovial fluid.

These three varieties of joints must now be considered in further detail.

(1) Fibrous Joints are of two types:

(*i*) *Sutures* (fig. 75) are immovable joints found only in the skull. The bones are united by a thin strip of fibrous tissue which is continuous with

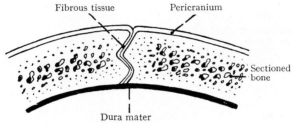

Fibrous tissue   Pericranium

Sectioned bone

Dura mater

Fig. 75.—A sutural joint.

the pericranium (i.e., the periosteum which covers the skull bones) and with the endosteal layer of dura mater lining the interior of the skull.

(*ii*) *Syndesmoses.*—In these joints the bones are united by bands of fibrous tissue which are often appreciable in size. Examples of such joints are found in the vertebral column, e.g., the ligamenta flava and ligamentum nuchae; also in the leg and forearm, e.g., the interosseous membranes and ligaments. Limited movement is permitted at these joints.

(2) Cartilaginous Joints (synchondroses) are of two types:

(*i*) *Primary.* The feature of these joints is that they are quite fixed and usually temporary. Each consists of a bar of hyaline cartilage which eventually becomes ossified. They disappear when growth is completed. Examples are seen in the epiphyseal plates which separate epiphyses from diaphyses in the long bones, in the bar of cartilage which separates the basiocciput from the basisphenoid, while the first sternocostal joint is an even more striking primary synchondrosis (fig. 82).

(*ii*) *Secondary.* In this type the bony surfaces are separated by a disc of fibrocartilage. There is no capsule but the bones are united by ligaments.

These joints are situated in the mid-line of the body and examples are seen in the symphysis pubis and in the joints between the bodies of the vertebrae. There is limited movement at these joints.

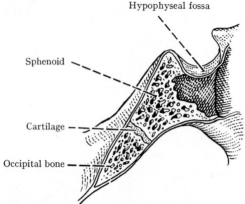

Fig. 76.—A primary cartilaginous joint—joint between the basi-occiput and the basi-sphenoid.   (This disappears between the 18/25 year.)

(**3**) **Synovial Joints** (diarthroses).   The feature of a synovial joint is its mobility and *a typical synovial joint* has certain common characteristics: **A typical synovial joint** (fig. 77) presents the following features:

(*i*) *The bony articular surfaces* are covered with hyaline cartilage which forms a smooth, white shiny mass on the surface.   It is important to note that while the synovial membrane is usually described as lining the joint it does not extend over the articular cartilage.

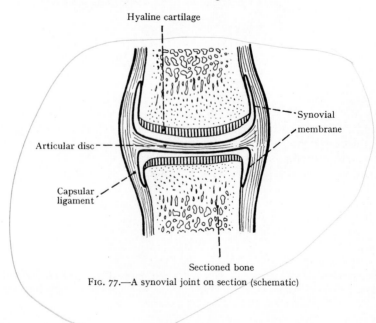

Fig. 77.—A synovial joint on section (schematic)

(*ii*) *The articular capsule* is attached to the bones at or near the margin of the articular surfaces and forms a fibrous tissue envelope for the joint. It blends with the periosteum covering the bones and is perforated by blood vessels and nerves. It is sometimes deficient over certain areas.

The capsule is frequently reinforced by thickened bands. These are called the *ligaments* of the joint. Further fibrous bands may be present which lie outside the capsule, and these are known as *accessory ligaments* of the joint.

(*iii*) *The synovial membrane* lines the capsule and covers the intracapsular structures with certain notable exceptions, e.g., the semilunar cartilages of the knee joint. It does not extend over the articular cartilage (fig. 77). The synovial membrane may form fringe-like processes filled with fat which are packed into the spaces in the joint cavity. Should the capsule be deficient in any part, the synovial membrane forms a pouch (bursa) beneath the structures covering the joint (muscles or tendons).

The synovial membrane is responsible for the secretion of *synovial fluid* which is formed in the same way as lymph, from the blood plasma. It is a mucinous fluid looking something like egg-white and is present in a minimal amount not only in synovial joints but also in synovial tendon-sheaths and bursae. Its function is threefold, it lubricates, it nourishes and it absorbs. It lubricates the articulating surfaces and it acts as a nutrient medium for the articular cartilage which is an avascular structure. Synovial fluid also contains phagocytic cells which absorb the debris produced by friction between joint surfaces as well as micro-organisms which may have migrated into the joint cavity. Should the synovial membrane become inflamed (synovitis) as the result of injury or disease its capillaries become more permeable and an effusion of fluid is likely to occur into the joint. There is very rapid absorption from joints where the synovial membrane is extensive, e.g., the knee, so that a septic joint may be associated with severe constitutional disturbances.

(*iv*) *Intracapsular structures* are sometimes present, viz., *ligaments* which unite articular surfaces, e.g., the cruciate ligaments of the knee joint and the ligamentum teres of the hip joint; *articular discs* which are usually attached to the capsule and may or may not completely separate the articular surfaces, e.g., the semilunar cartilages of the knee joint, the discs in the mandibular and sternoclavicular joints; the *glenoid ligaments* which serve to deepen the cup-shaped cavities in the hip and shoulder joints and the subsynovial *pads of fat* already referred to which fill the crevices in the interior of a joint.

The tendon of long head of biceps lies within the capsule of the shoulder joint and the tendon of popliteus within the capsule of the knee joint.

There are six varieties of Synovial Joints:

(*i*) *Plane Joint.* The articular surfaces are flat and permit of gliding movements with very limited rotation of one bone upon another—examples are seen in the joints between the carpal bones at the wrist and the tarsal bones in the foot.

(*ii*) *Saddle Joint.* This joint may be likened to the inversion of one saddle upon another at right angles. Movements permitted are triaxial, viz.,

5—A.PH.

flexion, extension, abduction, adduction with some degree of circumduction which is a combination of these movements. The only true saddle joint in the body is the carpometacarpal joint of the thumb.

(*iii*) *Hinge Joint* (ginglymus). In this type of joint, movement is permitted around a single transverse axis. The capsule is notably weak in front and behind, but is strengthened laterally by powerful ligaments. Movements taking place are limited to flexion and extension. Examples are the elbow, ankle and interphalangeal joints.

(*iv*) *Pivot Joint* (trochoid). In this type of joint movement is permitted around a single longitudinal axis. This may take the form of a ring rotating around a pivot, e.g., the atlas rotating around the odontoid process of the axis or a pivot rotating within a ring, e.g., the head of the radius rotating within the annular ligament and the radial notch on the ulna. Rotary movements only are permitted at this type of joint.

(*v*) *Ball and Socket Joint* (cotyloid). In this type of joint a globular head of bone fits into a cup-shaped cavity. Extensive polyaxial movements are permitted including flexion, extension, abduction, adduction, rotation and circumduction. The latter movement is one in which the head of the bone circumscribes the cup-shaped cavity around a number of axes and should be distinguished from rotation in which the bone moves around a single longitudinal axis. The capsule is characteristically lax in order to facilitate this wide range of movement. Examples are the hip and shoulder joints.

(*vi*) *Condyloid Joint* is a modified ball and socket joint wherein the articular surfaces are oval with a convexity articulating with a concavity. Movements permitted are triaxial, viz.:—flexion, extension, abduction and adduction with some degree of circumduction. An example is the radiocarpal joint.

The Temperomandibular (Jaw) Joint

Articulation between the head of the mandible and the mandibular fossa on the temporal bone. The mandibular joint is composed of two parts. The articulation between the articular disc and the mandibular fossa is a synovial plane joint, permitting gliding movement; the articulation between the head of the mandible and the articular disc is a hinge joint where the movements of elevation and depression mainly take place through a transverse axis. It should be understood that the two components of this joint never act independently.

Capsule is thin and lax. It is attached to the margins of the articular surfaces and is reinforced laterally by the *temperomandibular ligament* (fig. 78) which is attached to the tubercle on the zygoma and to the posterior border of the neck of the mandible.

An *articular disc* lies within the joint cavity and divides it into two separate compartments. The margin of the disc is attached to the capsule (fig. 79) and in front to the lateral pterygoid muscle.

Synovial membrane lines the capsule and is reflected on to the surfaces of the articular disc. It is thus also divided into two separate parts.

Accessory ligaments are the *sphenomandibular ligament* which is attached above to the spine of the sphenoid, and below to the lingula on the mandible (fig. 37) and the *stylomandibular ligament* which is attached above to the styloid process and below to the posterior border of the ramus of the mandible (figs. 78 and 79).

Movements of the Joint. In all movements of the mandible both compartments of each joint and both joints are involved. The movements of opening and closing the mouth are due to a rotation through a horizontal axis of the head of the mandible on the articular disc. Opening the mouth is accompanied by protrusion of the jaw and this is done by the lateral ptery-goid muscle pulling the condyle and disc forwards over the articular eminence. The mouth is opened by gravity but if it is to be widely opened, then the mylohyoid, anterior belly of digastric, geniohyoid and platysma come into play. For the mouth to close, the lateral pterygoids must first relax and then the temporales, masseters and medial pterygoids contract. It is the special duty of the posterior fibres of the temporalis muscle to retract the jaw during this movement. The medial and lateral pterygoids are responsible for the chewing movements and these movements are due to the head and disc of each side alternately rotating around a vertical axis within the articular fossa, thus moving the mandible from side to side.

Nerve supply to joint. Masseteric and auriculotemporal nerves.

Chief relations. The parotid gland lies superficial and posterior to the joint and separates it from the external ear. The lateral pterygoid muscle is inserted into the capsule and articular disc. Above the joint is the middle ear cavity; medial to it is the tympanic plate of the temporal bone upon which a portion of the parotid gland may rest; the bony part of the pharyngo-tympanic tube and the auriculotemporal nerve.

JOINTS OF THE VERTEBRAL COLUMN

These consist of a series of articulations between the bodies and arches of the vertebrae.

The *articulations between the bodies of the vertebrae* consist of a series of secondary cartilaginous joints with pads of fibrocartilage (intervertebral discs) between the articulating surfaces (fig. 80). The bodies of the vertebrae are bound together by the *anterior and posterior longitudinal ligaments*, the former extending from the atlas and the latter from the axis, to the sacrum. Both ligaments are attached to the intervertebral discs as well as the bodies of the vertebrae and it is important to note that the posterior longitudinal ligament, attached to the posterior aspect of the bodies, lies within the vertebral canal.

Exceptions to this simple arrangement are found in the cervical region where in addition to the cartilaginous joints a synovial joint is found on each of the lateral aspects of the vertebral body.

An *intervertebral disc* is composed of a ring of fibrocartilage called the *annulus fibrosus* with a central core of spongy, elastic material, which acts as a buffer and is known as the *nucleus pulposus*. The discs are firmly attached to the articulating surfaces of the bodies of the vertebrae and to the longi-tudinal ligaments. They act as shock absorbers and enable movements to be performed freely without damage or discomfort. They are thickest in

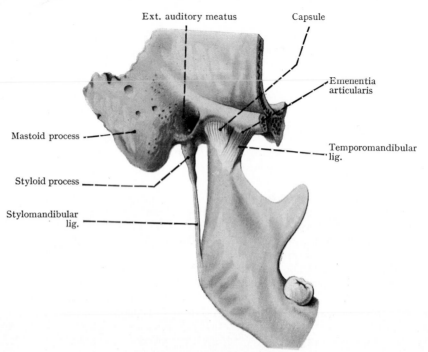

Ext. auditory meatus   Capsule

Emenentia
articularis

Mastoid process

Temporomandibular
lig.

Styloid process

Stylomandibular
lig.

Fig. 78.—The mandibular joint.

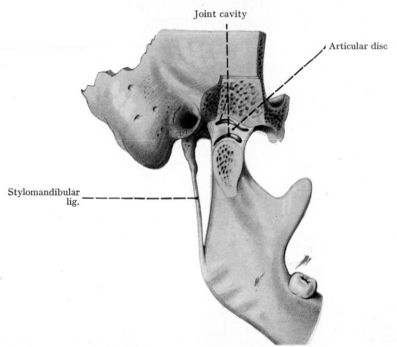

Joint cavity

Articular disc

Stylomandibular
lig.

Fig. 79.—The mandibular joint opened to show the articular disc.

the lumbar region and are an important factor in contributing to the curvature of the vertebral column. They have a tendency to become displaced backwards into the neural canal and then pressing on the cord or spinal nerves cause considerable pain. A "slipped disc" can be completely crippling.

The articulations between the arches of the vertebrae consist of a series of synovial plane joints between the articular processes presenting the usual features and permitting of some gliding movement. These joints are strengthened by the following ligaments, (fig. 80) :—

The *ligamenta flava* powerful ligaments extending between adjacent laminae.

Interspinous ligaments extending between adjacent spines.

Supraspinous ligaments attached to the tips of adjacent spines.

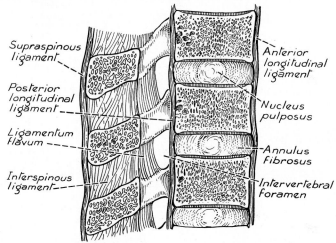

Fig. 80.—Part of the vertebral column showing in sagittal section ligaments and intervertebral discs.

Ligamentum nuchae lying in the nape of the neck and comparable to the supraspinous ligaments in other regions. It is attached to the external occipital protuberance and external occipital crest and to the tips of the spines of all the cervical vertebrae. Its posterior free border gives origin to the trapezius, splenius capitis and rhomboideus minor.

Intertransverse ligaments, weak bands extending between adjacent transverse processes. The intertransverse ligament between the transverse process of L.5 and the ala of the sacrum is known as the *lumbosacral ligament*.

Movements permitted by the vertebral column as a whole are: Flexion forwards, extension, flexion laterally and rotation.

Flexion (bending forwards) is performed by rectus capitis anterior, rectus capitis lateralis, longus capitis et cervicis and sternomastoid in the neck region; by gravity and rectus abdominis in the thoracic region; and by that muscle and quadratus lumborum in the lumbar region.

Flexion of the trunk upon the hip joint is performed initially by iliopsoas and then by gravity when the subject is standing or sitting with both feet on the ground. Rectus abdominis assists in this movement when rising from the supine position. It should be noted that almost all the true flexors of the vertebral column are confined to the cervical region and thus flexion is greatest in this region. If the hip joint be fixed, flexion of the vertebral column in the thoracic and lumbar regions is extremely limited and is actually less than the amount of extension possible. This limitation of flexion is due to the unyielding inter-vertebral discs and to the ligamentous action of the extensors of the spine. Gravity has a constant tendency to flex the vertebral column, and the art of balancing in the upright position consists in educating the extensors of the spine to counteract this. In old age, when probably as a result of deficient blood supply, the muscles tire easily, a characteristic stoop is assumed.

Thus the extensors of the vertebral column are constantly in action and we rest them either by lying down or by sitting in a chair, the back of which is built to slope backwards and thus to counteract the action of gravity. Further relief is obtained by resting the elbows on the arms of a chair or the chin upon the hand.

Extension (*bending backwards*) is greatest in the cervical and least in the thoracic region. It is performed in the cervical region by splenius capitis et cervicis, semispinalis, rectus capitis posterior major and minor, and the superior and inferior oblique capitis muscles. In the thoracic and lumbar regions extension is performed chiefly by sacrospinalis and its derivatives, viz., the spinalis, longissimus and iliocostalis groups and these are assisted by the multifidus, interspinales, rotatores and inter-transversales groups.

Lateral flexion (*bending sideways*) is accompanied by rotation of the bodies of the vertebrae to the opposite side and is freest in the cervical and lumbar regions. It is produced by the vertebral muscles acting on one side only and is performed by the scalenes, semispinalis and splenius capitis in the neck region and by the sacrospinalis, quadratus lumborum and abdominal muscles in the lumbar region. In the thoracic region it is checked by the ribs and sternum.

Rotation accompanies lateral flexion, but is almost absent in the lumbar region. Like lateral flexion it is produced by muscles acting on one side only. It is performed by the multifidus, rotatores, sternomastoid, scalenes, splenius capitis and semispinalis muscles.

Rotation of the trunk is performed by internal oblique of the side to which rotation takes place working with external oblique of the opposite side.

JOINTS OF THE RIBS AND STERNUM

The *head of a typical rib* articulates with the body of the corresponding thoracic vertebra, with the body of the vertebra above and with the articular disc between these two vertebrae. Each joint is of the synovial plane type with a capsule which is strengthened anteriorly by the *radiate ligament* (fig. 81).

This ligament consists of three bands which pass to the bodies of the adjacent vertebrae and to the intervertebral disc. There is also an *intra-articular* ligament (fig. 81) which lies within the joint cavity. It is attached to the ridge on the head of the rib which separates the articular surfaces and to the intervertebral disc.

The *neck of the rib* is attached to the corresponding transverse process and to the transverse process of the vertebra above by the *superior* (consisting of anterior and posterior layers) and *inferior costotransverse ligaments* (fig. 81).

The *tubercle of a rib* articulates with the transverse process of the corresponding thoracic vertebra to which it is attached by the *lateral costotransverse ligament*.

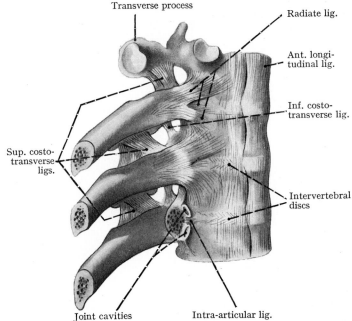

Transverse process

Radiate lig.

Ant. longitudinal lig.

Inf. costotransverse lig.

Sup. costotransverse ligs.

Intervertebral discs

Joint cavities   Intra-articular lig.

FIG. 81.—The right costovertebral joints. (Redrawn from Gray's "Anatomy.")

The *sternal end of each rib* presents a concavity into which the corresponding costal cartilage fits. It is held there by a fusion between the periosteum and perichondrium.

The sternocostal articulations. The cartilages of the true ribs (except the first) articulate with the sternum by synovial joints. Each joint has a *capsule* which is reinforced by *anterior* and *posterior sternocostal ligaments*. In addition there is an *intra-articular ligament* within the joint cavity between the second costal cartilage and the sternum, but this is usually absent in the others. A small *costoxiphoid ligament* connects the 7th costal cartilage with the xiphoid process of the sternum (fig. 82).

The junction of the first costal cartilage with the sternum is a primary cartilaginous joint which eventually ossifies.

Movements of the ribs and the mechanism of respiration. In normal respiration the transverse diameter of the thorax is increased by contraction of the external and internal intercostal muscles, which elevate the bodies of the ribs and carry them upwards and outwards (comparable to raising a bucket handle). The anteroposterior diameter of the thorax is increased by the ribs simultaneously pushing the sternum forwards. At

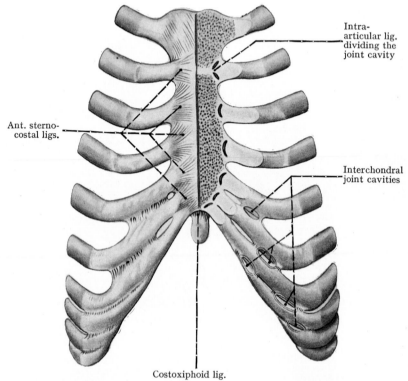

Intra-articular lig. dividing the joint cavity

Ant. sterno-costal ligs.

Interchondral joint cavities

Costoxiphoid lig.

FIG. 82.—Sternocostal and interchondral articulations seen from the front; the first sternocostal joint has no cavity since it is a primary cartilaginous joint.

the same time the vertical diameter of the chest is increased by the contraction and consequent flattening of the diaphragm. Thus the increase in the capacity of the chest is brought about by the excursions of the ribs, but the first and second ribs are not normally affected since these are fixed by their attachments to the neck muscles (scalenes), nor the 12th rib which is fixed by the quadratus lumborum. In quiet respiration, movement is confined chiefly to the lower ribs but in deep breathing all the ribs are brought into action.

As a result of the flattening of the diaphragm there is an increase in intra-abdominal pressure which is countered by the relaxation of the muscles of the anterior abdominal wall, especially the upper fibres of transversus abdominis so that a bulge appears in the epigastrium.

Expiration is brought about by the flattening of this bulge by transversus abdominis but is chiefly due to the elastic recoil of the lungs and the relaxation of the diaphragm and intercostal muscles. The subcostales and sterno-costalis are concerned with depressing the ribs and therefore they, like the transversus abdominis are muscles of expiration. Strong contraction of the anterior abdominal wall causes forced expiration.

If for any reason respiration becomes difficult, then all the muscles which are attached to the thoracic cage are called upon to act as auxiliary elevators of the ribs, notably pectorales major and minor, sternomastoid, the scalenes and subclavius, while the extensors of the spine act as synergists by fixing the head in the extended position and by arching the thoracic vertebrae.

It is important to understand that the lungs play a purely passive role during respiration. The pressure of the air within the thoracic cavity is normally below that of the atmospheric air and during inspiration when the capacity of the thorax is increased, this pressure becomes more sub-atmospheric or negative; consequently the alveoli dilate, the lungs expand and air is sucked in. During expiration intrathoracic pressure is raised, and so air is driven out of the alveoli.

JOINTS OF THE UPPER EXTREMITY

Sternoclavicular Joint

Articulation between the sternal end of the clavicle, the manubrium sterni and the first costal cartilage.

Type. Synovial, double plane joint.

Capsule surrounds the joint and is attached to the margins of the articular surfaces. It is reinforced anteriorly and posteriorly by the strong *sterno-clavicular ligaments*.

Articular disc (fig. 83) is a flat circular fibrocartilaginous disc within the joint cavity. It is attached above to the superior articular surface of the clavicle and below to the cartilage of the first rib, and divides the joint into two compartments. Its circumference is attached to the articular capsule, and the disc is covered by synovial membrane. It prevents the medial displacement of the clavicle.

Accessory ligaments. The weak *interclavicular ligament* is attached to the sternal ends of the clavicles where it blends with the capsule and running across the jugular notch is attached to the upper border of the sternum.

The *costoclavicular ligament* is a strong band which is attached to the junction of the first rib with the first costal cartilage and to the rhomboid impression on the inferior surface of the clavicle. It tethers the clavicle medially.

Movements. This joint, together with the acromioclavicular joint, are known as the joints of the shoulder girdle. Movement of the scapula automatically means movement of the clavicle also. In forward and backward movements of the shoulder girdle the articular disc and clavicle move upon the manubrium. Forward movement is produced by serratus anterior. Backward movement is produced by trapezius and the rhomboids.

In elevation and depression of the shoulder girdle, movement takes place between the clavicle and the articular disc. Elevation is produced by sternomastoid, the upper fibres of trapezius, the levator scapulae and the rhomboids, and is limited by the costoclavicular ligament. Depression is produced by the lower fibres of trapezius, subclavius, pectoralis minor and by gravity, and is checked by the first rib, the sternoclavicular ligaments and the articular disc.

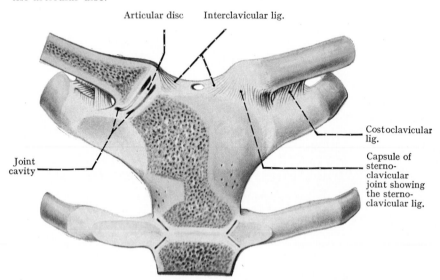

Fig. 83.—The sternoclavicular joint (opened on the right side). (Redrawn from Gray's "Anatomy.")

Compare the sternocostal joint of the first rib (primary cartilaginous joint) with that of the second rib (synovial joint).

Nerve supply. Nerve to subclavius muscle and the medial supraclavicular nerve.

Chief Relations. The joint is subcutaneous above. Anteriorly it is covered by some fibres from sternomastoid and pectoralis major. Posteriorly it is covered by the sternohyoid and is related to the innominate artery on the right, the left innominate vein and left common carotid artery on the left and to the trachea behind these vessels.

Acromioclavicular Joint

Articulation between the lateral end of the clavicle and the acromion of the scapula.

Type. Synovial, plane joint.

Capsule surrounds the joint and is attached to the margins of the articular surfaces. It is reinforced above by the *acromioclavicular ligament* and anteriorly and posteriorly respectively by aponeuroses from the deltoid and trapezius muscles.

Articular disc, often absent or may be incomplete, is attached to the capsule.

Accessory ligaments. The *coracoclavicular ligament* is made up of the strong conoid and trapezoid ligaments.

The *conoid ligament* (fig. 85) is attached above to the conoid tubercle on the inferior surface of the clavicle and below to the base of the coracoid process of the scapula. The *trapezoid ligament* (fig. 85) is attached above to the trapezoid ridge on the inferior surface of the clavicle and below to the superior surface of the coracoid process of the scapula.

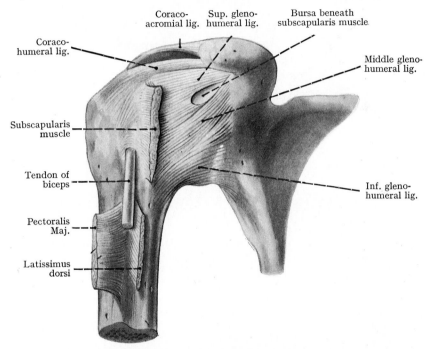

FIG. 84.—The capsule of the shoulder joint.

The *coraco-acromial ligament* (figs. 84 and 85) may be regarded as an accessory ligament of this joint since it helps to keep the acromion process of the scapula in contact with the lateral end of the clavicle. It is triangular in shape, attached by its apex to the tip of the acromion and by its base to the lateral border of the coracoid process of the scapula. It also protects the shoulder joint and helps to prevent upward displacement of the humerus.

Movements. The function of the acromioclavicular joint is to allow gliding movement of the scapula on the clavicle when the scapula rotates as the arm is thrust forward or when it is elevated above the head (fig. 270.) The acromioclavicular joint also comes into play in elevation and depression of the shoulder and enables the scapula to maintain close contact with the chest wall as it moves up and down on a vertical axis.

Nerve supply.   Suprascapular nerve.

Chief Relations.   Deltoid in front, trapezius behind; the joint is subcutaneous above.

The Shoulder Joint

Articulation between the globular head of the humerus articulating with the shallow glenoid cavity of the scapula.

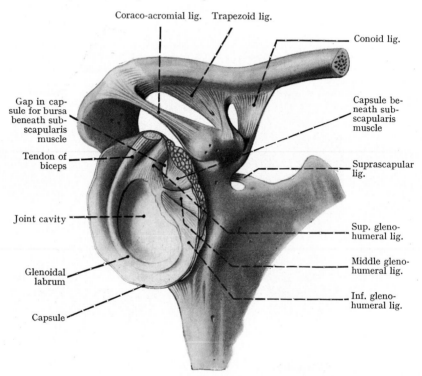

FIG. 85.—The interior of the shoulder joint.

Type.   Synovial, ball-and-socket joint.

Capsule surrounds the joint and is attached to the margin of the glenoid cavity of the scapula outside the labrum, and to the anatomical neck of the humerus extending on to the shaft of the bone for a short distance medially. A feature of the shoulder joint is its wide range of movement and to this end the capsule is notably thin and lax.   The shoulder joint is the most unstable joint in the body and is dislocated more frequently than all the other joints in the body put together.   It relies for its stability upon muscles and not upon its capsule or ligaments.   The capsule is reinforced by fibrous slips from the adjacent muscles, notably supraspinatus, infraspinatus, teres minor, subscapularis, latissimus dorsi, pectoralis major and triceps so that it is subjected to some degree of tension when the muscles moving the joint are in action. The capsule is poorly supported inferiorly and is subjected to great strain when the arm is abducted.

The capsule is further strengthened by ligaments. The glenohumeral ligaments (figs. 84 and 85), consist of three weak bands attached to the medial margin of the glenoid labrum. The *superior glenohumeral ligament* passes to the upper border of the bicipital groove on the humerus, the

Coracoid process   Clavicle

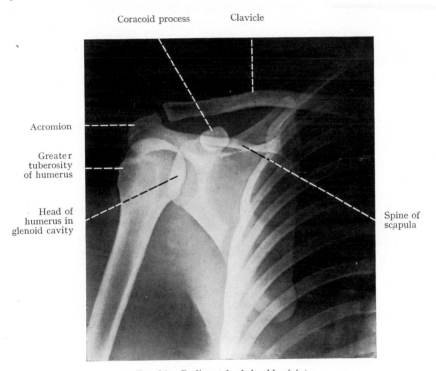

Acromion

Greater
tuberosity
of humerus

Head of
humerus in
glenoid cavity

Spine of
scapula

FIG. 86.—Radiograph of shoulder joint.

middle glenohumeral ligament to the lesser tuberosity and the *inferior glenohumeral ligament* to the lower part of the anatomical neck.

The *coracohumeral ligament* (fig. 84) is more important and more powerful. It strengthens the capsule superiorly and is attached to the lateral aspect of the root of the coracoid process and to the greater tuberosity of the humerus and is believed to be the divorced tendon of pectoralis minor. This ligament limits both adduction and lateral rotation. Successful reduction of a dislocated shoulder by Kocher's method (the easiest method and the one usually applied) is dependent upon the integrity of the coracohumeral ligament.

The capsule is perforated by the long head of biceps which traverses the joint and is also deficient beneath the tendon of subscapularis and sometimes beneath the tendon of infraspinatus allowing the synovial membrane to herniate in the form of bursae. It should be noted that the tendon of biceps though intracapsular is extrasynovial.

Synovial membrane lines the capsule and forms bursae where the capsule is deficient, viz., beneath the subscapularis (fig. 84 and 85) and infraspinatus muscles (sometimes). It covers the outer surface of the glenoid labrum, ensheaths the tendon of long head of biceps and is prolonged on that tendon for a short distance outside the joint extending down as far as the surgical neck of the humerus.

The *transverse humeral ligament* is a small band which stretches across the bicipital groove and so holds the long tendon of biceps in position.

The *glenoid labrum* is a thick rim of fibrocartilage which is attached to the

Tuberosity of radius　　　Head of radius

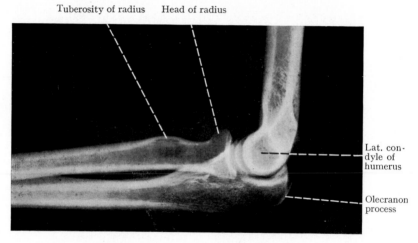

Lat. condyle of humerus

Olecranon process

FIG. 87.—Radiograph of elbow joint.

margin of the glenoid cavity, serving to deepen it. It gives part origin to the long heads of both biceps and triceps.

Movements. The joint moves in conjunction with the joints of the shoulder girdle.

Flexion (forwards) is performed by coracobrachialis, biceps, pectoralis major and the anterior fibres of deltoid.

Extension (backwards) is performed by teres major, latissimus dorsi and the posterior fibres of deltoid.

Abduction is performed chiefly by the middle fibres of deltoid assisted by supraspinatus (*q.v.*).

Adduction is performed by pectoralis major and latissimus dorsi assisted by teres major, teres minor and coracobrachialis.

Lateral rotation is performed by infraspinatus and teres minor.

Medial rotation is performed by latissimus dorsi, subscapularis and teres major.

Circumduction is a combination of these movements.

In wide movements of the shoulder joint the four short muscles inserted around the head of the humerus, viz.: the supraspinatus, infraspinatus, teres minor and subscapularis, are probably engaged in maintaining the integrity of the joint. Their main function would appear to be to keep the head of the humerus in apposition with the glenoid cavity of the scapula, while the larger and more powerful muscles perform the movements. These muscles also make tense the loose capsule and so prevent its insinuation between the articular surfaces.

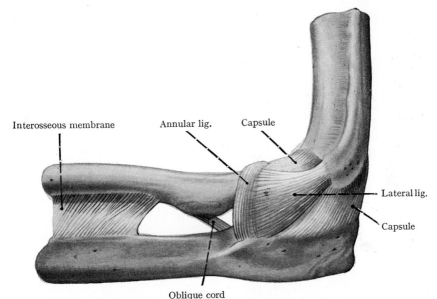

FIG. 88.—The left elbow joint—lateral aspect.

Nerve Supply. Circumflex, suprascapular and lateral pectoral nerves.

Chief Relations. Subscapularis muscle anteriorly, infraspinatus and teres minor posteriorly, supraspinatus superiorly, long head of triceps and circumflex nerve inferiorly. The tendon of long head of biceps passes through the joint (fig. 84).

Elbow Joint

Articulation between the trochlea and capitulum of the humerus above and the trochlear notch of the ulna and head of the radius below.

Type. Synovial, hinge joint.

Capsule surrounds the joint and is attached above and anteriorly to the lower end of the humerus above the radial and coronoid fossae and extends on to the medial epicondyle; above and posteriorly to margins of the olecranon fossa. It is attached below to the upper margin of the coronoid process of the ulna and the upper and lateral margins of the olecranon process. It is not attached to the radius but it blends with the annular ligament which surrounds the head of that bone so the elbow and superior radio-ulnar joints have a common capsule.

The capsule is reinforced by the *lateral ligament* which is attached to the lateral epicondyle of the humerus and to the annular ligament (fig. 88) and by the *medial ligament*, consisting of three bands which have a common attachment to the medial epicondyle of the humerus. The anterior band passes to the medial margin of the coronoid process, the posterior to the

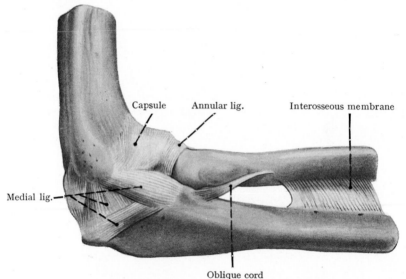

Capsule Annular lig. Interosseous membrane

Medial lig.—

Oblique cord

FIG. 89.—The left elbow joint—medial aspect.

medial margin of the olecranon process, while a weak central band passes to some transverse fibres which connect the two preceding bands (fig. 89).

Synovial membrane is extensive, for in addition to lining the capsule it is reflected on to the coronoid, radial and olecranon fossae and on to the medial surface of the trochlea. It also lines the annular ligament and so is common to the elbow and proximal radio-ulnar joints which therefore have a common joint cavity.

Movements. The elbow joint is a hinge joint and is thus capable of two movements, viz., flexion and extension.

Flexion is performed by brachialis, biceps brachii, brachioradialis and pronator teres. When great resistance is to be overcome the muscles arising from the common flexor and common extensor tendons may be called upon to assist in flexing the joint.

Extension is performed by triceps and to a small extent by anconeus.

The flexors are nearly twice as powerful as the extensors and thus in hemiplegia the forearm is flexed.

When the elbow is fully flexed the head of the radius and the coronoid process of the ulna lie in the radial and coronoid fossae on the humerus respectively. Flexion is checked by the tension of the muscles and ligaments on the back of the joint and by the forearm impinging upon the arm.

When the elbow is fully extended the olecranon process of the ulna fits into the olecranon fossa on the humerus, but usually this is not driven right home owing to the tension of the anterior part of the capsule.

Nerve supply. Median, ulnar, radial and musculocutaneous nerves.

Chief Relations. Brachialis covers nearly the whole of the joint in front, but the brachioradialis and extensor carpi radialis longus cover the joint to a small extent laterally. The brachialis separates the joint from the structures which lie within the cubital fossa, viz., the median nerve, tendon of biceps, and the brachial artery dividing into radial and ulnar arteries.

Lateral to the joint are the common extensor tendon and supinator; medial to it are the common flexor tendon and ulnar nerve; posterior to it are the triceps (a bursa intervening) anconeus (laterally) and the ulnar nerve (medially).

The Carrying Angle. It should be noted that the medial aspect of the trochlear process of the humerus extends below the lateral aspect and that this has the effect of pushing the ulna, and with it the forearm, laterally, when the forearm is fully extended. In these circumstances the arm and forearm are not in the same straight line but form an angle, more prominent in women than men, called "the carrying angle." The size of this angle varies in different individuals but average measurements are given as 167° in the female and 173° in the male (Gray). The angle disappears when the forearm is fully flexed and is likely to be altered in fractures of the lower end of the humerus or when the internal lateral ligaments of the elbow joint are torn.

Proximal Radio-Ulnar Joint

Articulation between the head of the radius within the annular ligament and the radial notch on the ulna.

Type. Synovial, pivot joint.

Capsule and synovial membrane common to it and the elbow joint.

Annular ligament (figs. 88 and 89) is attached to the anterior and posterior margins of the radial notch on the ulna and so forms a ring which holds the head of the radius in position and enables it to rotate around a vertical axis. The small *quadrate ligament* forms a floor for this ring and is attached to the distal margins of the annular ligament and to the adjacent bones.

The Middle Radio-Ulnar Joint

The middle radio-ulnar joint is a syndesmosis and consists of a fibrous interosseous membrane and an oblique cord when present which hold the radius and ulna together.

The interosseous membrane (figs. 88 and 89) is a thin but strong membrane uniting the bones of the forearm and is attached to their interosseous borders.

It commences 2 cm. below the tuberosity of the radius and ends by blending with the capsule of the wrist joint. Its fibres run obliquely downwards and medially so that shocks resulting from a fall on the outstretched hand are transmitted from the radius to the ulna and thence to the humerus and clavicle.

An *oblique tendinous cord* (figs. 88 and 89) is sometimes present which stretches from the radius just below the tuberosity to the apex of the coronoid process of the ulna. It is supposed to be a detached tendon of flexor pollicis longus.

Distal Radio-Ulnar Joint

Articulation between the head of the ulna and the ulnar notch on the radius.

Type. Synovial, pivot joint. Its movements are complementary to the superior radio-ulnar joint.

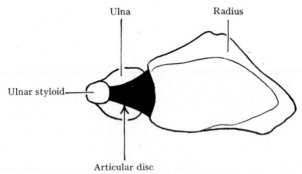

Fig. 90.—The articular disc of the distal radio-ulnar joint.
The distal articular surfaces of the radius and ulna are shown.

Capsule spans the joint in front and behind, but is deficient above allowing a pouch of synovial membrane to herniate upwards for a variable distance in front of the interosseous membrane (recessus sacciformis) (fig. 91).

Articular disc (figs. 90 and 91) is a triangular fibrocartilaginous plate; its apex is attached to the lateral aspect of the base of the styloid process of the ulna and its base to the ridge between the carpal and ulnar articular surfaces at the lower end of the radius. Its upper surface articulates with the head of the ulna and thus excludes that bone from the wrist joint; its lower surface articulates with the lunate bone or with the triquetral bone when the hand is adducted. Its upper surface is covered with the synovial membrane of the inferior radio-ulnar joint and its lower surface with the synovial membrane of the radiocarpal joint. The margins of the disc are attached to the capsules of the radio-ulnar and radiocarpal joints, so that it can be regarded as dividing the wrist joint into two separate parts.

Movements permitted at the radio-ulnar joints are:

Pronation (palm of hand facing backwards) is performed by pronator teres and pronator quadratus.

Supination (palm of hand facing forwards) is a much more powerful movement than pronation and is performed by biceps and supinator.

Brachioradialis is considered to be a flexor of the forearm but may assist in either pronation or supination.

In performing the movements of pronation, the head of the radius rotates within the annular ligament, while the distal end of the radius with the articular disc and hand, rotates around the head of the ulna.

The nerve supply to the distal radio-ulnar joint is the same as that to the wrist joint *q.v.*

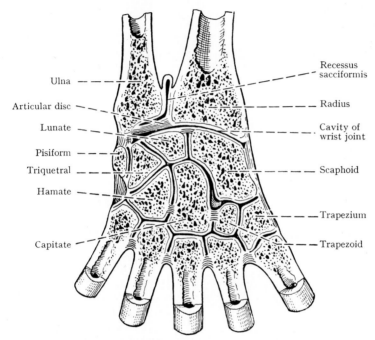

FIG. 91.—The wrist and intercarpal joints, in section.

The Radiocarpal (Wrist) Joint

Articulation between the distal end of the radius and articular disc; and the scaphoid, lunate and triquetral bones.

Type. Synovial, condyloid joint.

Capsule is attached to the margins of the articular surfaces. It is reinforced anteriorly by a strong *anterior radiocarpal ligament* (fig. 92) which is attached to the distal ends of the radius and ulna and to the proximal row of carpal bones and also to the capitate. A weaker band, the *posterior radiocarpal ligament* (fig. 93) reinforces the capsule posteriorly and is attached to the radius and proximal row of carpal bones. Laterally, the capsule is strengthened by the *lateral ligament* (figs. 92 and 93) which is attached to the styloid process of the radius and to the scaphoid and trapezium, while medially it is similarly strengthened by the *medial ligament* (fig. 92) which is attached to the styloid process of the ulna and to the triquetral and pisiform bones.

Movements permitted at this biaxial joint are:

Flexion, which is a much more powerful movement than extension and

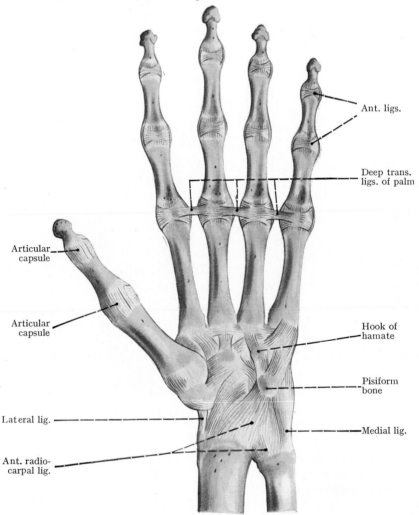

Ant. ligs.

Deep trans. ligs. of palm

Articular capsule

Articular capsule

Hook of hamate

Pisiform bone

Lateral lig.

Medial lig.

Ant. radio-carpal lig.

FIG. 92.—The ligaments of the wrist and hand, anterior aspect.

is performed by the flexor carpi radialis, palmaris longus and flexor carpi ulnaris, assisted by the flexors of the fingers.

Extension is performed by the extensores carpi radialis et ulnaris assisted by the extensors of the fingers.

Abduction is performed by the extensores carpi radialis longus et brevis, flexor carpi radialis, abductor pollicis longus and extensores pollicis longus et brevis.

Adduction is performed by the extensor and the flexor carpi ulnaris.

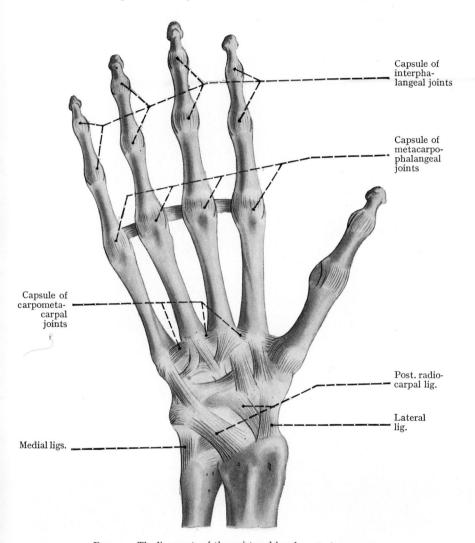

Capsule of interphalangeal joints

Capsule of metacarpophalangeal joints

Capsule of carpometacarpal joints

Post. radiocarpal lig.

Lateral lig.

Medial ligs.

FIG. 93.—The ligaments of the wrist and hand, posterior aspect.

Nerve Supply. Anterior and posterior interosseous nerves and the deep branch of the ulnar nerve.

Chief Relations. Flexor tendons and the median and ulnar nerves anteriorly, extensor tendons posteriorly, radial artery laterally, dorsal branch of the ulnar nerve and artery medially.

Intercarpal Joints

The intercarpal joints are synovial, plane joints united by anterior, posterior and transverse ligaments.

Movement is slight and consists of gliding and rotating.

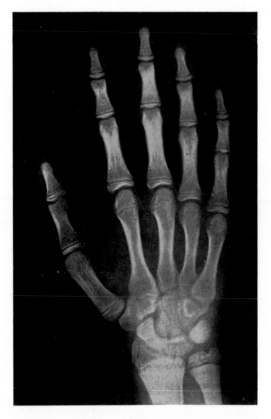

Fig. 94.—Radiograph of wrist and hand from a child aged 14 years.

Carpometacarpal and Intermetacarpal Joints of Fingers

The carpometacarpal and intermetacarpal joints of the fingers are synovial, plane joints united by anterior, posterior and interosseous transverse ligaments. They have a common joint cavity and synovial membrane.

Movement is slight and confined to gliding.

Carpometacarpal Joint of Thumb

Articulation between the trapezium and the base of the first metacarpal bone.

Type. Synovial, saddle joint. This is the only joint of its kind in the body except for a small joint between the ossicles of the ear.

Capsule surrounds the joint and is attached to the margins of the articular surfaces.

Synovial membrane lines the joint and forms a separate cavity.

Movements permitted are:

Abduction. By adbuctores pollicis longus et brevis.

Adduction. By adductor pollicis.

Flexion. So that the digit lies at right angles to the palm, by flexor pollicis brevis and opponens pollicis.

Extension. By extensores pollicis longus et brevis.

Opposition. Thumb medially rotated by opponens and then adducted and the phalanges flexed so that the thumb comes into opposition with the fingers. This is one of the most important of the finer movements of the hand for it is responsible for the pincer action between the thumb and fingers.

Metacarpophalangeal Joints

Articulations between the heads of the metacarpal bones and the bases of the proximal phalanges.

Type. Synovial, condyloid joints.

Capsule attached to the margins of the articular surfaces and is reinforced anteriorly by the thick fibrocartilaginous *palmar ligaments* and on each side by the strong *collateral ligaments* which run obliquely from the side of the metacarpal head to the base of the phalanx. Posteriorly the capsule is separated from the overlying extensor expansion by a bursa which facilitates the free movement of the latter.

Accessory ligaments are the *deep transverse ligaments of the palm* which connect together the palmar ligaments of the second, third, fourth and fifth metacarpophalangeal joints (fig. 92) which lie between the heads of the metacarpal bones.

Movements permitted are:

Flexion by the flexores digitorum sublimis et profundus the lumbricals and interossei.

Extension by extensor digitorum assisted by extensor indicis and extensor digiti minimi.

Abduction and *Adduction* of the fingers to and from the mid-line (third digit) by the interossei and the short muscles of the little finger. At the metacarpophalangeal joint of the thumb, flexion is produced by flexores pollicis longus et brevis and extension by extensores pollicis longus et brevis. Abduction and adduction of the thumb are carried out at the carpometacarpal joint.

Interphalangeal Joints

These are synovial, hinge joints.

Each has a capsule reinforced by ligaments similar to those of the metacarpophalangeal joints.

Movements permitted are:

Flexion by the flexores digitorum sublimis et profundus.
Extension by the extensor digitorum.

JOINTS OF THE PELVIS AND LOWER EXTREMITY

Two pelvic joints may be said to concern the student of physiotherapy, viz., the lumbosacral and sacro-iliac joints.

Lumbosacral Joint

Articulation between the 5th lumbar vertebra and the sacrum. This joint presents the usual features of an intervertebral joint but the inter-transverse ligament is unusually strong and extends from the transverse process of the 5th lumbar vertebra to the ala of the sacrum and is known

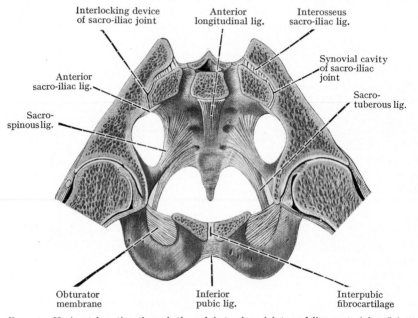

Fig. 95.—Horizontal section through the pelvis to show joints and ligaments (after Sobotta). (From " Gynaecological and Obstetrical Anatomy" by Smout and Jacoby.)

as the *lumbosacral ligament*. A characteristic of this joint is its obliquity for when standing in the upright position the sacrum is almost horizontal. The 5th lumbar vertebra is prevented from falling forwards into the pelvis by the articulating surfaces and by a powerful accessory ligament called the *iliolumbar ligament*, which is attached to the transverse process of the 5th lumbar vertebra to the iliac crest and the iliac fossa.

Sacro-iliac Joint

Articulation between the auricular articular surface on the ilium and a similar surface on the sacrum.

Type. Primarily a synovial hinge joint, but some gliding movement also occurs.

Capsule is reinforced by the *anterior sacro-iliac ligament* which stretches between the articular surfaces on the antero-inferior aspect of the joint; by the *short posterior sacro-iliac ligament* which runs transversely behind the interosseous ligaments and is attached to the tuberosity on the ilium and to the tubercles on the 1st and 2nd sacral vertebrae and by the *long posterior*

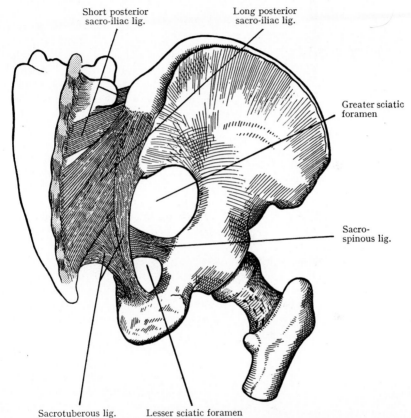

Short posterior
sacro-iliac lig.

Long posterior
sacro-iliac lig.

Greater sciatic
foramen

Sacro-
spinous lig.

Sacrotuberous lig.   Lesser sciatic foramen

FIG. 96.—The posterior aspect of the sacro-iliac joint.
(From " Gynaecological and Obstetrical Anatomy" by Smout and Jacoby.)

The short posterior sacro-iliac ligaments run transversely. The long posterior sacro-iliac ligaments run obliquely and blend with the sacrotuberous ligament. The sacrospinous ligament lies in front of the sacro-tuberous ligament.

sacro-iliac ligament which passes obliquely downwards from the posterior superior iliac spine to the tubercles on the 3rd and 4th sacral vertebrae blending with the sacrotuberous ligament (fig. 96). In addition the articulating surfaces are united by *the interosseous sacro-iliac ligaments* which are strong bands running between the bones on the postero-superior aspect of the joint.

Accessory ligaments are the *iliolumbar ligament* previously described, the *sacrotuberous ligament* which is attached to the posterior superior spine of the ilium, to the tubercles on the 3rd, 4th and 5th sacral vertebrae and to the lateral border of the coccyx above and to the falciform margin of the ischial tuberosity below; and the *sacrospinous ligament* which is attached to the ischial spine and the lower part of the lateral margin of the sacrum and to the coccyx.

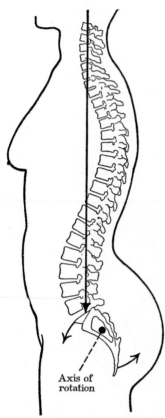

Movements. Very little movement takes place at this joint under normal circumstances. Such movement as there is is due to the superincumbent body weight being transmitted through the joint and is not due to muscular action. There is a tendency for the sacrum to rotate through a horizontal axis which passes through the centre of the articulating surfaces (fig. 97) and to glide between the two innominate bones through a vertical axis, but these movements are nothing more than a little interplay between the bones in order to counteract the shocks and jars which might otherwise follow common movements. Stability at this joint is essential, and in order to ensure this, the muscles which span the joint anteriorly and posteriorly, viz., iliacus, piriformis, the deep muscles of the back and gluteus maximus, together with biceps femoris when it arises from the sacro-tuberous ligament are used as ligaments in limiting movement. In addition, there are powerful restraining ligaments, which can be grouped as the ligaments which run transversely, viz., the anterior, interosseous, and short posterior sacro-iliac ligaments, all of which are attached to the upper half of the sacrum and the ligaments which run

Axis of rotation

Fig. 97.—Rotation of sacrum through a transverse axis.

obliquely, viz., the long posterior, the sacro-spinous, and sacrotuberous ligaments, all of which are attached to the lower half of the sacrum. The transverse ligaments are therefore concerned in preventing the upper half of the sacrum from rotating forwards and the oblique ligaments in preventing the lower half of the sacrum from rotating backwards. Thus, the sacrum is said to be suspended between the innominate bones by guy ropes. In addition the sacro-iliac joint is provided with a unique interlocking device for the articular surfaces are irregular, and when an extraordinary movement is to be performed such as jumping from a height the muscles spanning the joint draw the bones into closer apposition so that elevations on one bone fit into depressions on the other and the joint is momentarily locked. The range of movement at this joint is considerably increased during the later stages of pregnancy and at parturition. It is decreased as age advances and tends to ossify in middle life.

Nerve Supply. From the sacral plexus, the superior gluteal and obturator nerves.

Chief Relations. *Anterior:* psoas, iliacus, obturator nerve, lumbosacral trunk and common iliac vessels above; upper part of sacral plexus and piriformis below. *Posterior:* sacrospinalis, multifidus and gluteus maximus muscles.

Hip Joint

Articulation between the hemispherical head of the femur and the cup-shaped acetabular cavity on the innominate bone.

Type. Synovial, ball and socket.

Capsule surrounds the joint and is attached to the margin of the acetabulum outside the acetabular labrum, to the transverse acetabular ligament on the innominate bone, to the intertrochanteric line, to the medial aspect of the

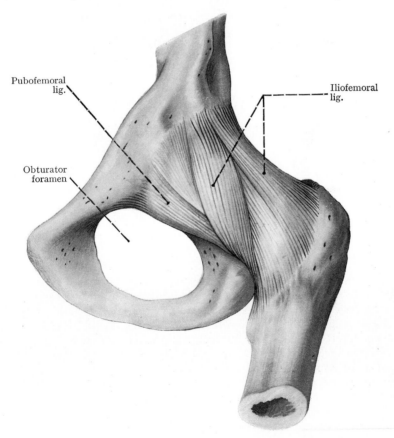

Pubofemoral
lig.

Iliofemoral
lig.

Obturator
foramen

Fig. 98.—The capsule of the left hip joint, anterior aspect.

base of the greater trochanter, to the neck of the femur, 2 cm. above the intertrochanteric crest, and to the base of the lesser trochanter.

The capsule is reinforced by the *iliofemoral ligament* (fig. 98) which is triangular in shape. Its apex is attached to the lateral aspect of the anterior inferior spine directly between the two heads of rectus femoris (fig. 62) and as it descends it divides into two bands; one passes to the base of the greater trochanter and the other to the base of the lesser trochanter, where it blends with the pubofemoral ligament. The *pubofemoral ligament* (fig. 98) also

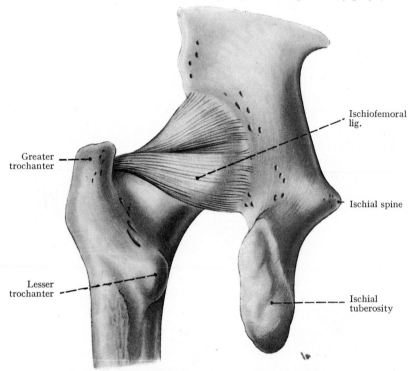

Greater trochanter

Lesser trochanter

Ischiofemoral lig.

Ischial spine

Ischial tuberosity

FIG. 99.—The capsule of the left hip joint, posterior aspect.

strengthens the capsule and is triangular. The base of this ligament is attached to the superior ramus of the pubis (fig. 62), while its apex is attached to the lesser trochanter. The capsule is strengthened posteriorly by a weaker band called the *ischiofemoral ligament* (fig. 99) which is attached to the body of the ischium near the acetabular margin and sweeps upwards and laterally over the back of the neck of the femur in a spiral manner.

There is usually a gap in the capsule between the pubofemoral and ilio-femoral ligaments through which a pouch of synovial membrane herniates to form the *psoas bursa* (fig. 149).

Synovial membrane lines the capsule, covers both surfaces of the acetabular labrum and the fat which lies in the acetabular fossa ensheaths the liga-mentum teres and also forms the psoas bursa.

Acetabular labrum is a ring of fibrocartilage which is attached to the margins of the acetabulum and to the transverse acetabular ligament. It serves to deepen the acetabular fossa.

Transverse acetabular ligament is continuous with the acetabular labrum and is attached to the margins of the acetabular notch, converting it into a tunnel through which the blood vessels and nerves enter the joint.

Ligamentum teres is attached to the fossa on the head of the femur (fovea capitis), to the margins of the acetabular notch on the innominate bone and

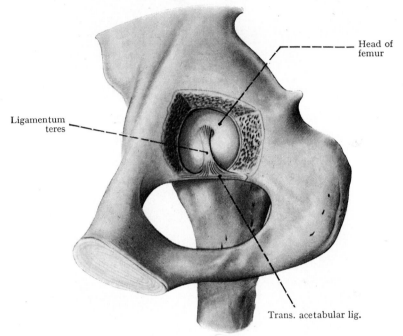

FIG. 100.—The right hip joint as seen from within the pelvic cavity after a portion of bone has been removed.

to the transverse acetabular ligament (fig. 100). It lies within the cavity of the joint and is ensheathed by synovial membrane.

Movements permitted are:

Flexion (thigh bent forwards) by iliopsoas chiefly, assisted by rectus femoris, sartorius and the adductors. This movement is limited by the hamstrings when the leg is extended.

Extension (thigh bent backwards) by the gluteus maximus chiefly, assisted by all the hamstring muscles. The extensor muscles are rather more powerful than the flexors.

Abduction by gluteus medius and minimus chiefly, assisted by tensor fasciae latae, piriformis and sartorius.

Adduction by the adductors magnus, longus and brevis chiefly, assisted by gracilis, pectineus and the lower fibres of gluteus maximus.

Lateral rotation by gluteus maximus, quadratus femoris, piriformis, obturator internus, obturator externus and to some extent by the adductor muscles also. This movement is much more powerful than medial rotation.

Medial rotation by gluteus minimus and medius, tensor fasciae latae, iliopsoas, pectineus and the lower fibres of adductor magnus.

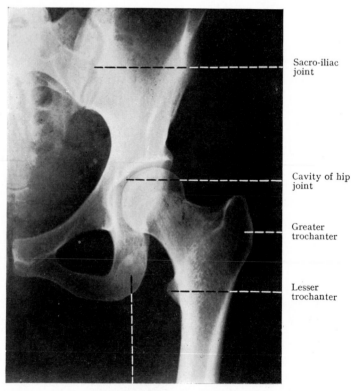

Sacro-iliac joint

Cavity of hip joint

Greater trochanter

Lesser trochanter

Ischial tuberosity

FIG. 101.—Radiograph of the left hip and sacro-iliac joints.

Nerve supply. Femoral, obturator, accessory obturator, and sciatic nerves, nerve to quadratus femoris and branches from the sacral plexus direct.

Chief Relations. *Anterior:* iliopsoas, pectineus, rectus femoris. *Posterior:* piriformis, obturator internus et gemelli, and quadratus femoris, separate the joint from the sciatic nerve. *Superior:* gluteus minimus. *Inferior:* obturator externus and the tendon of insertion of iliopsoas.

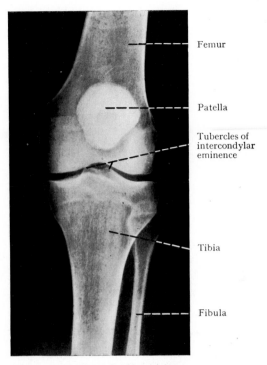

Femur

Patella

Tubercles of
intercondylar
eminence

Tibia

Fibula

FIG. 102.—Radiograph of knee joint.

Knee Joint

Articulation between the condyles of the femur and the condyles of the tibia and their semilunar cartilages on the one hand and between the lower end of the femur and the patella on the other.

Type. Synovial. The joint between the femur and the tibia is an atypical hinge joint since some degree of rotation occurs; that between the femur and patella is an atypical plane joint since the articular surfaces are somewhat irregular and the movement which takes place there is not merely gliding.

The articular surfaces on the femur are confined chiefly to the inferior and posterior aspects of the condyles but ascend also on to the anterior aspect, especially of the lateral condyle. In this connection it will be seen that the lateral articular surface on the patella is larger than the medial one. The superior surfaces of the condyles of the tibia are articular and are separated by the centrally situated anterior and posterior intercondylar areas and the intercondylar eminence. These articular surfaces support the fibrocartilaginous semilunar cartilages which separate the condyles of the tibia from the femur.

Capsule ensheaths the joint and may be said to be attached to the margins of the articular surfaces, with certain important reservations. On the front of the femur the capsule is entirely absent, allowing the synovial membrane to pouch beneath the quadriceps tendon forming the suprapatellar bursa (fig. 107). On the lateral epicondyle of the femur the capsule is attached above the popliteal groove, on the medial epicondyle it is attached below the adductor tubercle. Anteriorly the capsular attachment extends to the tibial tubercle (fig. 68). There is a gap in the tibial attachment of the capsule behind the lateral condyle which allows the tendon of the popliteus to

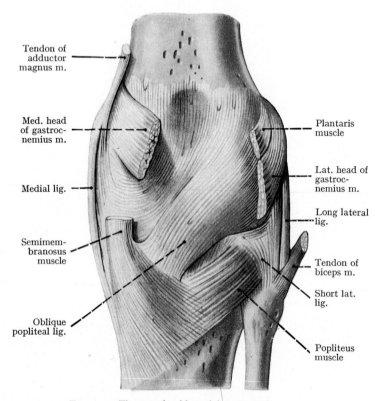

Tendon of
adductor
magnus m.

Med. head
of gastroc-
nemius m.

Medial lig.

Semimem-
branosus
muscle

Oblique
popliteal lig.

Plantaris
muscle

Lat. head of
gastroc-
nemius m.

Long lateral
lig.

Tendon of
biceps m.

Short lat.
lig.

Popliteus
muscle

FIG. 103.—The capsule of knee joint—posterior aspect.

emerge (fig. 70), and a further gap may be present beneath the medial head of gastrocnemius.

The capsule is reinforced by the following ligaments:

Ligamentum patellae (fig. 107) is part of the quadriceps extensor tendon and extends from the apex of the patella to the tibial tubercle. It is separated from the synovial membrane by the large infrapatellar pad of fat and from the upper end of the tibia by the small, isolated infrapatellar bursa. The capsule is also reinforced in this region by the patellar retinacula formed by fascial expansions from the vasti, the fascia lata and the iliotibial tract which form an interlacing aponeurosis on the front of the capsule.

Long lateral ligament (fig. 103) is attached to the lateral condyle of the femur above the popliteal groove and to the head of the fibula, where it splits the insertion of the biceps tendon into two parts (figs. 103, 104 and 106). It is believed to be the divorced tendon of peroneus longus and is separated from the capsule.

Short lateral ligament (fig. 103) lies behind the long ligament, is adherent to the capsule and consists of arching fibres which extend from the capsule to the head of the fibula. Beneath these arching fibres the tendon of popliteus emerges. This ligament blends with the fascia over popliteus and is attached by its base to the lateral semilunar cartilage.

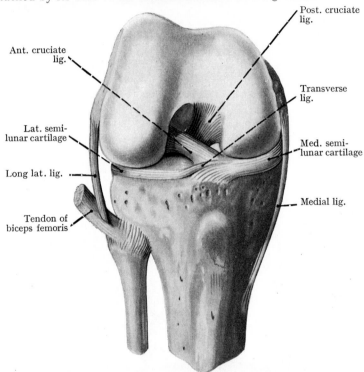

Post. cruciate lig.

Ant. cruciate lig.

Transverse lig.

Lat. semi-lunar cartilage

Med. semi-lunar cartilage

Long lat. lig.

Medial lig.

Tendon of biceps femoris

FIG. 104.—The interior of the knee joint—anterior aspect.

Medial ligament (fig. 103) is attached above to the medial condyle of the femur below the adductor tubercle. Inferiorly, it splits into two bands, both of which are attached to the medial condyle of the tibia, the semimembranosus muscle intervening between them (fig. 106). The superficial band (long medial ligament) is wide and flat thus contrasting with the lateral ligament and the deeper band (short-medial ligament) is firmly attached to the medial semilunar cartilage. The medial ligaments are more liable to be torn than the lateral ligaments.

Oblique popliteal ligament (*of Winslow*) (fig. 103) reinforces the capsule posteriorly and is formed by a fascial slip from the semimembranosus muscle which passes upwards and laterally.

7—A.PH.

The synovial membrane lines the capsule to a limited extent only. It is attached to the intracapsular portions of the articulating bones as far as their articular surfaces. On the anterior aspect of the joint it forms a pouch superiorly which herniates beneath the quadriceps muscle and extends for three fingers breadth above the upper border of the patella forming the important *suprapatellar bursa* which is retained in position by the articularis genu muscle. Below this herniation it is absent from the articular surface of the patella and below this it lines the infrapatellar pad of fat which separates

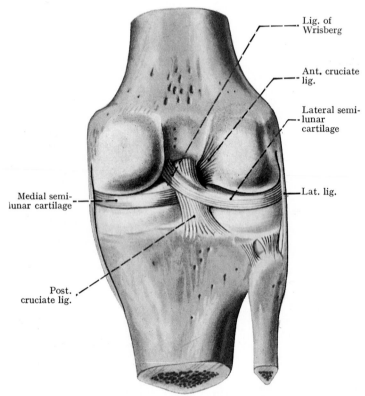

Lig. of Wrisberg

Ant. cruciate lig.

Lateral semi-lunar cartilage

Lat. lig.

Medial semi-lunar cartilage

Post. cruciate lig.

Fig. 105.—The interior of the knee joint—posterior aspect.

it from the capsule and the ligamentum patellae (fig. 107). From this point it is reflected into the interior of the joint as *the infrapatellar fold* which has a free edge on each side and is attached above to the intercondylar notch on the femur. The lower fringed margins of this fold are filled with fat and are called *the alar folds*. From the margins of the patella the synovial membrane lines the medial and lateral surfaces of the capsule. Just behind the lateral ligament and below the lateral semilunar cartilage there is a gap in the capsule through which the synovial membrane herniates between the tendon of popliteus and the posterior edge of the lateral condyle of the tibia, forming the *popliteal bursa* which may extend as far as the superior tibiofibular joint and communicate with it.   Similarly, behind the posteromedial aspect of the capsule there is a further gap in the capsule beneath the medial head of gastrocnemius where the synovial membrane herniates, often extending beneath the semimembranosus muscle, forming the *semimembranosus bursa*. Passing backwards the synovial membrane lines the capsule covering the femoral condyles, but on reaching the intercondyloid notch posteriorly the synovium is carried in front of the cruciate ligaments so that the front and sides of these ligaments only are covered.   The synovial membrane is

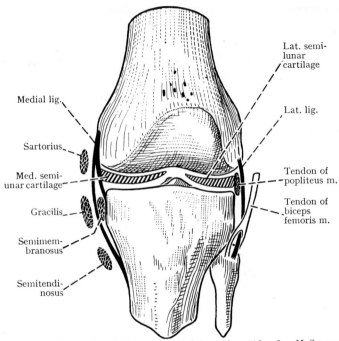

Medial lig.

Sartorius

Med. semi-
unar cartilage

Gracilis

Semimem-
branosus

Semitendi-
nosus

Lat. semi-
lunar
cartilage

Lat. lig.

Tendon of
popliteus m.

Tendon of
biceps
femoris m.

FIG. 106.—The interior of the knee joint—Schematic.   (After Lee McGregor.)

separated from the posterior part of the capsule by these ligaments and a pad of fat.

The *cruciate ligaments* (figs. 71, 104 and 105) are two powerful intracapsular ligaments named anterior and posterior according to their tibial attachments, which cross each other within the joint cavity.   The *anterior cruciate ligament* is attached to the anterior intercondyloid area of the tibia and passes upwards and backwards to be attached to the posterior part of the medial surface of the lateral condyle of the femur.   The *posterior cruciate ligament* is attached to the posterior intercondyloid area of the tibia and passes upwards and forwards to be attached to the anterior part of the lateral surface of the medial condyle of the femur.   The anterior cruciate ligament limits hyper-extension, the posterior cruciate ligament keeps the tibia applied to the femur in full flexion.   Rupture of one or both of these ligaments results in a flail joint.

The *semilunar cartilages* (figs. 71, 104, 105 and 106) lie on the surface of the tibia to which they are attached at their periphery by the *coronary ligaments* which are portions of the capsule and are sufficiently lax to allow some movement of the periphery of the semilunar cartilages relative to the tibial condyles. The tibial surface of each semilunar cartilage is flat; the femoral surface is concave. The cartilages are triangular on section, the base of the triangle being situated at the periphery. They are attached at

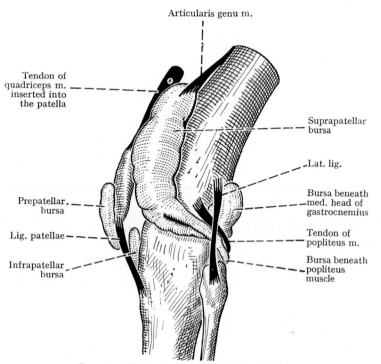

FIG. 107.—Bursae in relation to the knee joint.

their anterior margins by a band of fibrous tissue called the *transverse ligament*. It is believed that they are concerned with the lubrication of the joint and act like sponges in absorbing the synovial fluid.

The *lateral semilunar cartilage* is attached by its anterior horn to the anterior intercondylar area on the tibia immediately in front of the intercondylar eminence, and by its posterior horn to the posterior intercondylar area immediately behind this eminence; it is thus almost a complete circle (fig. 71). Some fibres of popliteus are attached to the posterior border of the lateral semilunar cartilage either directly or through the arcuate ligament and its tendon grooves it and separates it from the capsule (fig. 106).

The posterior border of the lateral semilunar cartilage is attached to the medial femoral condyle by two slips called the *lateral meniscal ligaments*, viz., a weak anterior band lies in front of the posterior cruciate ligament called the *ligament of Humphry* and a strong posterior band lies behind that ligament called the *ligament of Wrisberg.*

The *medial semilunar cartilage* is attached by its anterior horn to the anterior intercondylar area on the tibia in front of the anterior cruciate ligament and by its posterior horn to the posterior intercondylar area in front of the posterior ligament.

It is important to realise that the semilunar cartilages are firmly attached to the tibia and must move with it but the periphery of the medial semilunar cartilage is also attached to the medial ligament and so to the femur and therefore the periphery of this cartilage must move with the femur also. Should the femur and tibia fail to move synchronously, as may sometimes happen when with the knee flexed and the tibia fixed, the femur is suddenly medially rotated; the cartilage may be torn across. This condition is variously known as "slipped cartilage" or "torn cartilage" and may be classed as a form of "internal derangement of the knee joint." The medial cartilage is damaged far more frequently than the lateral (six to eight times more frequently—Watson Jones) because it is more fixed, while the lateral semilunar cartilage is not attached firmly to the femur at its periphery and is drawn back during flexion of the knee by the contraction of popliteus which is attached to it. The lateral meniscal ligaments facilitate this movement as the semilunar cartilage swings on them.

Movements permitted are:

Flexion. Only one flexor of the knee acts exclusively on that joint, viz., the short head of biceps. Others also function as extensors of the hip, viz., the long head of biceps, semimembranosus and semitendinosus, others as flexors of the hip, viz., the sartorius and gracilis, while others plantarflex the ankle, viz., gastrocnemius. Popliteus may act as a flexor but only after flexion has been initiated. Flexion is checked by contact of the leg with the thigh. Although it might appear otherwise, the extensors are more powerful than the flexors, for the position of extension is usually more difficult to maintain than that of flexion.

Extension is performed by the quadriceps muscles, of which one—the rectus femoris— is also a flexor of the hip. Extension is checked by the anterior cruciate ligament and by the tension of the posterior part of the capsule.

Medial rotation of the tibia on the femur initiates flexion and is known as "unlocking the knee joint." It is performed by the popliteus.

Lateral rotation of the tibia on the femur accompanies extension and is known as "locking the knee joint." It is to some extent passive due to the shape of the femoral articular surfaces but is also due to the pull on the tibia of the lowest fibres of vastus lateralis (Last).

When the joint is flexed and thus the medial and lateral ligaments are relaxed slight medial rotation can be performed by semitendinosus and to a less extent by semimembranosus, gracilis and sartorius and lateral rotation by biceps. In flexion and extension the semilunar cartilages move with the tibia, but when the tibia is rotated with the knee flexed the semilunar cartilages move with the femur on the tibia (Last).

The gluteus maximus by its insertion into the iliotibial band steadies the extended knee.

The articularis genu muscle makes tense the suprapatellar bursa when the knee is extended thus preventing the synovial membrane being nipped between the femur and the patella (fig. 107).

Nerve supply. Femoral, obturator, medial and lateral popliteal nerves.

It should be noted that the knee joint is innervated by the same spinal segments as the hip joint and it is not uncommon for an affection of the hip, e.g., tuberculosis, to give rise to pain in the knee and vice versa.

Chief Relations. *Anterior:* prepatellar bursa and patellar nerve plexus. *Posterior:* popliteal vessels and other structures in the popliteal fossa. *Lateral:* biceps tendon. *Medial:* semimembranosus, sartorius, gracilis and semitendinosus.

Bursae in relation to the Knee Joint are numerous and are to be found wherever a muscle or tendon crosses a bone. The suprapatellar, semi-membranosus and popliteal bursae which communicate with the interior of the joint have already been described and these with the prepatellar bursa are the only ones worthy of special mention.

Prepatellar bursa lies in front of the lower half of the patella and the upper part of the ligamentum patellae. It does not communicate with the knee joint. It is liable to become inflamed by constant friction when frequently kneeling "on all fours." Prepatellar bursitis is known, therefore, as "house-maid's knee." Because the inflammation is so very localised the disability is of a minor nature.

Proximal Tibiofibular Joint

Articulation between the head of the fibula and the lateral condyle of the tibia.

Capsule is attached to the margins of the articular surfaces. It is lined by synovial membrane which may be continuous with that of the knee joint. This is a synovial plane joint at which a limited amount of gliding may take place.

Middle Tibiofibular Joint

This joint consists of an interosseous membrane uniting the bones of the leg.

Interosseous membrane is a strong band connecting the bones of the leg and attached to their interosseous borders. Its fibres run downwards and laterally.

Distal Tibiofibular Joint

Articulation between the lower end of the fibula and a notch on the tibia. The bones are bound tightly together by ligaments which are of importance because the ankle joint is dependent upon them for its stability.

The *anterior and posterior inferior tibiofibular ligaments* bind the malleoli anteriorly and posteriorly, while the posterior ligament is further reinforced by the *inferior transverse ligament* which articulates with the talus and is attached to the posterior border of the medial malleolus and to the malleolar fossa on the medial aspect of the lateral malleolus.

The *interosseous ligament* is a strong, thick band which lies deep to the above ligaments and is the thickened distal border of the interosseous membrane.

The distal tibiofibular joint is an integral part of the ankle joint.

Ankle Joint

Articulation between the distal end of the tibia, the two malleoli, and the talus.

Type. Synovial, hinge joint.

Capsule is attached to the margins of the articular surfaces and is reinforced by the *deltoid ligament* (fig. 108) medially, which is triangular in shape and is attached by its apex to the tip of the medial malleolus while its base,

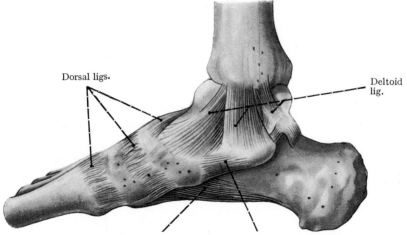

Dorsal ligs.

Deltoid lig.

Long plantar lig.   Plantar calcaneonavicular lig.

FIG. 108.—The ankle joint—medial aspect. (Redrawn from Gray's "Anatomy.")

consisting of three bands, is attached to the tuberosity of the navicular bone, the plantar calcaneonavicular or spring ligament, the sustentaculum tali and the body of the talus. In addition its deeper fibres are attached to the neck of the talus. The capsule is reinforced laterally by the *lateral ligament* (fig. 109) which is attached to the medial aspect of the lateral malleolus and like the internal ligament, divides into three bands, one passing horizontally forwards to the neck of the talus and is called the anterior talofibular ligament, a middle band passing downwards to the calcaneum and is called the calcaneofibular ligament and a posterior band called the posterior talofibular ligament which arises from the malleolar fossa on the lateral malleolus and passes horizontally to the talus. The lateral ligament is important clinically for it is the anterior talofibular ligament which is usually torn in sprained ankle.

Synovial membrane lines the capsule and may extend upwards to the base of the interosseous membrane as the *recessus sacciformis* (cf. wrist).

Movements permitted are:

Dorsiflexion (toes pointing upwards) performed by tibialis anterior, peroneus tertius, extensor digitorum longus and extensor hallucis longus and is checked by the posterior ligaments of the ankle joint.

Plantar flexion (toes pointing downwards) performed by gastrocnemius, plantaris, soleus, tibialis posterior, peroneus longus and brevis, flexor digitorum longus and flexor hallucis longus, and is checked by the anterior ligaments of the ankle joint.

It is important to note that the movements of inversion and eversion do not occur at this joint.

The superior articular surface of the talus is wedge-shaped, the wide end of the wedge being directed forwards. This arrangement prevents the

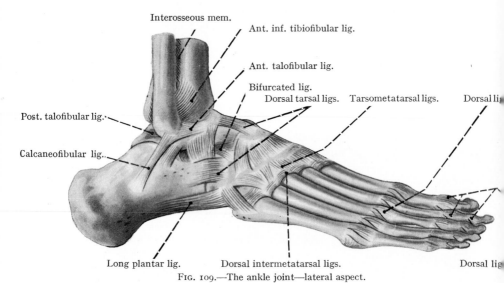

Interosseous mem.
Ant. inf. tibiofibular lig.
Ant. talofibular lig.
Bifurcated lig.
Dorsal tarsal ligs.   Tarsometatarsal ligs.   Dorsal li
Post. talofibular lig.
Calcaneofibular lig.
Long plantar lig.   Dorsal intermetatarsal ligs.   Dorsal lig

FIG. 109.—The ankle joint—lateral aspect.

leg moving too far forwards on the foot and may also be a limiting factor in dorsi-flexion.

Nerve supply. Anterior and posterior tibial nerves.

Chief Relations. Tibialis anterior, extensor hallucis longus, extensor digitorum longus and peroneus tertius with the anterior tibial vessels and nerve lying between the extensores hallucis et digitorum anteriorly; the peroneus brevis and longus laterally in that order behind the lateral malleolus; the tendo calcaneus and plantaris posteriorly; the tibialis posterior, flexor digitorum longus, posterior tibial vessels and nerve and flexor hallucis longus medially.

Tarsal Joints

These can be classified as synovial, plane joints, allowing limited gliding movements and some degree of rotation.

The *subtaloid joint*, or posterior talocalcanean joint, is an articulation between the posterior concave, articular facet on the talus and the convex facet on the posterior aspect of the superior articular surface of the calcaneum. It has a capsule reinforced by lateral, medial and posterior ligaments but union is maintained chiefly by the *interosseous ligament*, which is thick and strong at its lateral end, and lies within the sinus tarsi. This ligament separates the talocalcanean joint posteriorly from the talocalcaneonavicular joint anteriorly and is common to both.

The *talocalcaneonavicular joint* includes the anterior part of the talocalcanean joint and is a form of ball-and-socket joint in which the hemispherical head of the talus articulates with the posterior concave articular surface on the navicular bone, with the anterior articular facet on the superior surface of the calcaneum, with the medial limb of the bifurcated ligament and with the dorsal surface of the plantar calcaneonavicular ligament. It has a thin capsule which is strengthened posteriorly by the interosseous ligament. The joint allows considerable rotatory and gliding movements.

The *calcaneocuboid joint* is a synovial plane joint between the anterior surface of the calcaneum and the posterior surface of the cuboid. The articular capsule is strengthened by the lateral limb of the bifurcated ligament dorsally and by the long and short plantar ligaments on the plantar surface of the foot. The joint allows limited rotatory and gliding movements.

The talocalcaneonavicular joint and the calcaneocuboid joint together constitute the *mid-tarsal*, or *transverse tarsal joint*, the position of which can be determined by drawing a line transversely across the foot from immediately behind the tuberosity of the navicular bone to a point 2 cm. behind the base of the fifth metatarsal bone. It is at the mid-tarsal and subtaloid joints that the important movements of *inversion and eversion* of the foot take place, when the foot rotates around the head of the talus and turns inwards (inversion) or outwards (eversion). Normally inversion is accompanied by adduction of the foot and plantar flexion of the ankle joint, and eversion by abduction and dorsiflexion. Adduction and abduction occur as a result of gliding between the talus and calcaneum at the subtaloid joint. Inversion is limited by the interosseous ligament and eversion by the plantar calcaneonavicular and deltoid ligaments. Slight gliding movements may take place at the other intertarsal joints but these are of importance only in so far as they increase the suppleness of the foot.

The muscles responsible for inversion are tibialis posterior, tibialis anterior and, to a lesser extent, flexor digitorum longus and flexor hallucis longus. *The muscles responsible for eversion* are the peronei longus et brevis and, to a lesser extent, extensor digitorum longus and peroneus tertius.

The remaining joints need not be described in detail. Each joint is united by dorsal and plantar ligaments and by strong interosseous ligaments which fill the spaces between the bones and blend with the ligaments on the dorsal and plantar surfaces of the foot. Only those ligaments of outstanding importance will be described.

The *bifurcated ligament* (fig. 109) lies on the dorsum of the foot. It is a strong Y-shaped band attached by its base to the calcaneum and by its limbs to the cuboid and navicular bones.   Not only does it act as a dorsal ligament but its medial limb forms part of the socket for the talus in the talocalcaneonavicular joint and in that respect is comparable to the plantar calcaneonavicular ligament.

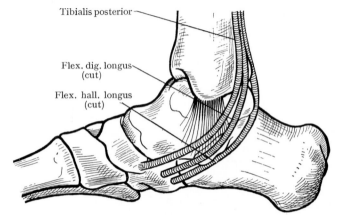

Tibialis posterior

Flex. dig. longus (cut)

Flex. hall. longus (cut)

FIG. 110.—The tendons in relation to the medial malleolus.
Note also their relation to the sustentaculum tali.

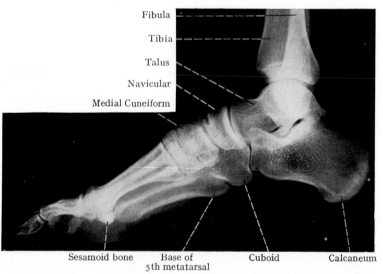

Fibula

Tibia

Talus

Navicular

Medial Cuneiform

Sesamoid bone   Base of   Cuboid   Calcaneum
                      5th metatarsal
FIG. 111.—Medial Aspect of right foot.

The *plantar calcaneonavicular or spring ligament* (figs. 108 and 112) is the most important ligament in the foot for it supports the head of the talus which carries the main weight of the body.   It is attached to the sustentaculum tali and to the plantar surface of the navicular bone and blends medially with the deltoid ligament.   The tendons of tibialis posterior, flexor digitorum longus and flexor hallucis longus are all related to its plantar surface and help to support it.   It plays an important part in maintaining the arches of the foot by supporting the head of the talus and by limiting eversion.   The fact that the deltoid ligament blends with its medial border is an important factor in this respect.

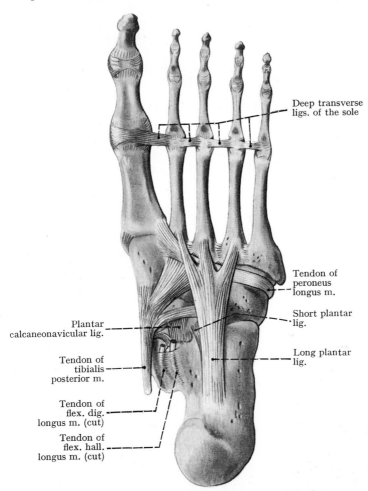

FIG. 112.—The ligaments on the plantar surface of the foot.

Note slips from the tibialis posterior passing backwards to the sustentaculum tali, laterally to the cuboid and forwards to the cuneiforms and bases of the metatarsal bones.

The long plantar ligament (fig. 112) is attached to the plantar surface of the calcaneum between the two heads of flexor accessorius and extends on to the edge of the groove on the cuboid and thence to the bases of the 2nd, 3rd and 4th metatarsal bones.   It converts the groove on the cuboid into a tunnel through which the peroneus longus tendon passes.

lantar ligament is attached to the anterior tubercle on the plantar
.he calcaneum, whence it passes forwards and medially to the
.t lies deep to the long plantar ligament (fig. 112).

Metatarsal and Phalangeal Joints (fig. 109)

1. *tarsometatarsal joints* are of the synovial, plane variety. The joint
between the first cuneiform and the first metatarsal has a capsule, the rest
are united only by dorsal, plantar and transverse ligaments.

Of the *intermetatarsal joints* only the first is separate. The lateral four
metatarsal bones are united at their bases by dorsal, plantar and interosseous
ligaments. The heads of all the metatarsal bones are united by the deep
transverse ligaments of the sole.

The *metatarsophalangeal joints* and *interphalangeal joints of the foot* correspond with those of the hand, except that the deep transverse ligaments of
the sole are extended to the great toe (fig. 112).

The movements of adduction and abduction of the toes are very limited
and take place to and from the mid-line of the 2nd digit and not the 3rd as
in the hand.

The Arches of the Foot

A reference to the imprint of a normal foot (fig. 114) will show that the
weight of the body is sustained by the outer part of the foot only. The
outer part is, therefore, concerned with weight-bearing and balance, but the
inner part is an arched spring which by postural muscle tone can adjust itself
to circumstances and is chiefly concerned with propulsion. The arching of
the foot is a characteristic peculiar to man and is present in the foetus before
birth. Further "the internal arrangement of the trabeculae of the cancellous
tissue in the bones of the foot is laid down in accordance with the stresses
and strains essential to arch formation" (Wood-Jones). The integrity of the
arch is dependent upon muscles chiefly since they alone exhibit tone and can
accommodate themselves to circumstances. To an important but less
extent it is dependent upon ligaments and the shape of the individual
bones. The arch is to some extent static in races accustomed to wearing
shoes.

The arches of the foot consist of a longitudinal and a transverse arch.

The longitudinal arch, for the purposes of description, is divided into
medial and lateral arches.

The medial longitudinal arch is made up of the following bones: the
calcaneum, talus, navicular, the three cuneiforms and the three medial
metatarsal bones.

The arch has an anterior pillar formed by the **heads** of the metatarsal
bones and a posterior pillar formed by the calcaneum.

The **weak point of the arch** is the gap between the sustentaculum tali and
the navicular bone (fig. 113) and this is bridged by the plantar calcaneonavicular ligament on which the head of the talus rests. This is also the
highest point of the arch and is, therefore, subject to the greatest strain.

The **arch is maintained by** the ligaments which span the individual bones on the plantar surface of the foot (those on the dorsal surface cannot in any way prevent the collapse of the arch); the plantar fascia; the short muscles of the foot, particularly those which span the arch, such as the abductor hallucis, and also the flexor hallucis longus and flexor digitorum longus. These might be classed as accessory factors in maintaining the arch for the main factor concerned is the maintenance of the balance of power between the invertors and evertors.

The medial longitudinal arch is flattened when the foot is everted. The plantar calcaneonavicular ligament is concerned with limiting eversion and is called into play when the invertors of the foot, viz., the tibiales anterior et posterior, weaken and fail to counter effectively the pull of the evertors, viz., the peronei longus et brevis.

The condition of flat foot commences when the tibialis posterior tires by reason of overstrain. The tibialis posterior tires before the tibialis anterior because it is subject to much greater strain, for not only is this muscle an invertor, it is also a plantar flexor. The plantar flexors raise the heel in walking and are called upon to perform this task by overcoming the weight of the body. The task of tibialis posterior is thus much greater than that of its collaborator tibialis anterior.

The lateral longitudinal arch is composed of the following bones: the calcaneum, the cuboid and the 4th and 5th metatarsals. The anterior pillar

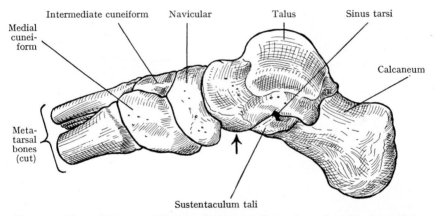

FIG. 113.—The medial aspect of the foot—the arrow indicates the weak spot in the medial longitudinal arch.

of the arch is formed by the *heads* of these metatarsals, and the posterior pillar by the calcaneum.

The *arch is supported by* the plantar ligaments, particularly the long and short plantar ligaments; by the plantar fascia and the short muscles of the foot, particularly the abductor digiti minimi. The most powerful support is, however, given by the peroneus longus which acts as a lever at the centre of the arch (cuboid bone) (fig. 112) and to a less extent by the peroneus brevis.

The transverse arch consists of a series of arches running transversely across the foot. Each foot makes a half dome so that it is not until the feet are approximated that the transverse arch is complete. The pillars of the arch are then formed by the lateral margins of the feet. The anterior part of the transverse arch of each foot flattens under the weight of the body but recoils when pressure is released. A dropping of this part of the arch results in metatarsalgia.

The *arch is supported by* the transverse plantar ligaments, the transverse head of adductor hallucis, but more especially by the tendon of peroneus longus which spans the arch (fig. 112).

Although the arches of the foot are described as consisting of three parts it should be borne in mind that for all practical purposes the foot consists of one arch since the failure of any part of the arch leads to the collapse of the foot as a whole.

When the arch falls the head of the talus falls between the sustentaculum tali and the navicular bone, early evidence of which is suggested by tenderness in the overlying area. It will be evident, therefore, that the condition of flat foot commences with a failure of the medial longitudinal arch. The first line of defence is muscular and much more powerful than the second, which is ligamentous. With the weakening of the invertors and the stretching of the plantar calcaneonavicular ligament, the powerful peronei pull against

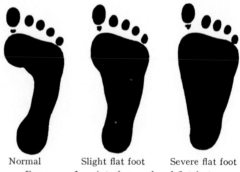

Normal   Slight flat foot   Severe flat foot
Fig. 114.—Imprint of normal and flat feet.

weakened antagonists and, therefore, the foot becomes everted and the forepart abducted, amounting to as much as 30° in advanced cases (Lake); the patient then walks on the inner side of the foot and becomes "splayfooted" in order to get greater leverage for the "take off."

With the fall of the head of the talus, the inner side of the foot is lengthened. This results in a cramping of the big toe which becomes adducted in an attempt to accommodate itself to the shoe. Extensor hallucis longus now pulls the big toe "like a bow string," adducting it still further but not extending it and not controlling effectively the action of the flexor hallucis. The final stage in flat foot is, therefore, seen as first an adduction and finally a flexion of the great toe. The second digit becomes cramped and is con verted into a hammer toe.

It should not be imagined that all these effects appear immediately or even in a short time. They serve to show the trend of complications which may ultimately ensue and they emphasise the importance of patience and perseverance in endeavouring to counter this painful and crippling disability.

Hammertoe is due to overcrowding of the toes in too small a shoe. There is a hyper-extension of the proximal phalanx, flexion of the middle phalanx and either extension or flexion of the distal phalanx.

CHAPTER IV

FASCIA AND MUSCLES

⌐...   ⌐ of the body is in two layers and is known as the superficial and deep fascia.

The superficial fascia lies immediately beneath the skin and consists of areolar tissue impregnated with fat. It forms a continuous layer over the whole body; but is absent in certain regions such as the eyelids, the auricle, the male external genitalia and parts of the female external genitalia (labia minora). It forms a protective covering, prevents heat loss and it also acts as padding, shielding the more delicate structures which lie beneath it. By virtue of its mobility and elasticity the superficial fascia enables the skin to move over the deep fascia. In certain parts of the body it may contain muscle fibres, e.g., the muscles of facial expression.

The cutaneous blood vessels and nerves, having emerged through the deep fascia, break up into their terminal branches in the superficial fascia before passing to supply the skin.

The deep fascia lies beneath the superficial fascia and is a dense membrane of fibrous tissue. It ensheaths the muscles and thus forms a strong band against which the muscle fibres contract. The deep fascia dips in between the muscles to form fibrous septa which blend with the periosteum of the underlying bone. Muscles frequently originate from or are inserted into the deep fascia, while in the regions of the ankle, the foot, the wrist and the hand, the deep fascia forms tunnels and pullies (retinacula) which bind the tendons to the bones.

Besides ensheathing the muscles, the deep fascia also surrounds the blood vessels and nerves and it is along the great fascial planes that these structures travel to their destination.

MUSCLES IN GENERAL

The muscles constitute the red meat of the body. Each is described as having an *origin* and an *insertion*. The origin is the part of the muscle that under normal circumstances remains fixed during movement; the insertion is the part that moves. As a rule, therefore, muscular movements take place from the origin of a muscle towards its insertion, but muscles often work in reverse, namely, from their insertions towards their origins.* In

---

* Arvedson applies the terms "concentric" and "eccentric" to certain movements which are accompanied by resistance either by the patient or the operator. He states that concentric movements are performed when "both ends of the working muscles are brought nearer to their respective centres and the muscles become shorter. This movement is performed by the patient against the resistance of the operator or some other outside source." He states that "in eccentric movements the muscles become longer *while working*, i.e., the ends move further from their centres. This takes place when a movement is performed by the operator or other outside force while the patient resists the movement."

order to understand the action of a muscle a precise knowledge of its attachments is, therefore, essential.

Muscles usually have their main attachment to bone. Sometimes, however, they are attached to the tendons of other muscles (e.g., flexor digitorum accessorius, extensor indicis and the lumbricals) or they may be attached to ligaments, the deep fascia or the skin. Muscles are sometimes directed obliquely, this speeds their action and increases their power, thereby effecting a considerable saving of energy.

The shape of a muscle depends on the arrangement of its fibres; thus some muscles are *quadrate* (e.g., pronator quadratus), others *fusiform* (e.g., semitendinosus), while others are *strap-like* (e.g., sartorius). Muscle fibres may be limited to one side of a tendon like the plumes of a pen—these are known as *unipennate muscles* (e.g. flexor pollicis longus); they may, however, lie on both sides of a central tendon when they are known as *bipennate muscles* (e.g. rectus femoris), and when great strength is necessary numerous small tendons lie within the muscle substance and these converge on to the tendon of insertion. These are known as *multipennate muscles* of which the deltoid is a striking example, but most of the triangular muscles have the same arrangement and in these cases the power of the muscle is further increased by the muscle fibres converging on to a relatively small insertion area.

A muscle may have a tendinous origin and frequently has a tendinous insertion. A tendon may be round or it may be flat. A broad, flat, tendinous sheet is known as an *aponeurosis*. Each muscle consists of a large number of muscle fibres which are bound together in bundles. Even when a muscle is firmly contracted, all the muscle fibres are not in action at any one time; a considerable number are held in reserve ready to take the strain and relieve their fellows when fatigued, although those fibres which are in action are always working at full capacity. It is doubtful whether a muscle is ever completely at rest; some of its fibres are probably in action under all circumstances, producing the condition known as "*muscle tone.*"

Muscles act on joints and the muscles performing any particular movement are grouped as protagonists, antagonists, synergists and fixation muscles. It should be understood that when any particular movement is performed, all muscles taking part in that movement, in whatever group they may be classed, act synchronously for they are all reciprocally innervated.

The protagonists are the prime movers in any muscular action.

The antagonists are generally considered to exercise a controlling influence on the action of the protagonists and, although under certain circumstances they may slow down the rate of movement, they facilitate it rather than impede it. Their function has been likened to that of "paying out the slack" in the same way that one might control a moving object by exercising a graduated relaxation of a cord attached to it, e.g., when the flexors of the wrist contract the movement is controlled by the graduated relaxation of the extensors. The antagonists also perform a useful function in controlling movements initiated by gravity.

8—A.PH.

During infancy we are occupied with the task of teaching the antagonists to control the protagonists and until co-ordination between these two groups is perfected we are unable to hold the body erect, to stand or to walk. This controlled relaxation is, therefore, a function acquired by practice and training. In the average untrained individual the antagonists limit all movements beyond those necessary to perform the ordinary routine duties of daily life. One might cite as an example the limiting action of the hamstrings when attempting to touch the toes. This limiting action is known as the "ligamentous action of muscles" and is so called because under these circumstances the antagonists are collaborating with ligaments whose function is to confine movement at any joint within a certain range.

The object of physical training is to produce a co-ordinated and controlled muscular relaxation which is the key to balance, poise and posture.

The synergists collaborate with the protagonists and their function is to facilitate and localise a particular movement. Not infrequently a protagonist may be capable of moving more than one joint and it is the duty of the synergist to fix the joint which is not involved. Thus, unlike the antagonists, they do not act on the same joint as the protagonists but they fix an adjacent joint in order that the protagonists may perform under the most favourable conditions possible. The action of "making a fist" might be quoted as an example. We are able only to make a very feeble fist when the wrist is flexed, and to make a firm fist we must not only flex the fingers but at the same time extend the wrist. Under these circumstances, therefore, the extensors of the wrist act as collaborators or synergists in the movement and by first extending and then fixing the wrist they enable the flexors of the fingers to act more powerfully.

The fixation muscles collaborate with the protagonists by steadying or fixing the bone or bones from which the protagonist originates or into which it is inserted. To quote an example—the biceps could take no part in flexing the elbow joint when the forearm is pronated, since the muscle is naturally a supinator, were it not for the fact that the pronators fix the radius.

Muscles always work in groups, never singly, and no group of muscles acts alone. Thus while we attempt to define the action of individual muscles we should remember always that they come into action only as part of a team, and that team may consist not only of fellow protagonists but also of antagonists, synergists and fixationists. Thus it becomes exceedingly difficult to describe with certainty the action of any particular muscle, and in view of all the circumstances it is not especially profitable to do so. It is probably true to say that each muscle has one principal action but most muscles take part in numerous subsidiary actions; indeed different parts of the same muscle may produce different movements, e.g., the deltoid is primarily an abductor of the arm, but its anterior fibres may help to flex and its posterior fibres to extend the arm.

Under certain circumstances a muscle may find itself in alliance with its antagonist, e.g., the antagonists of the flexor carpi radialis are the extensors longus and brevis, but when the hand is abducted these three muscles are fellow protagonists.

⎰Muscular action is controlled from the central nervous system b⎱ which pass along motor nerves, but it should be understood that all ⎰ are also supplied with sensory nerves by which afferent impulses pass ⎰ brain. Nerves, therefore, not only cause muscles to contract but prese⎰ their normal tone and at the same time convey important messages from the muscles to the higher centres of the brain giving information which is essential for co-ordination and sense of position.

It should be borne in mind that the stimulus which causes the protagonists to contract also causes the synergists and fixationists to contract and the antagonists to relax, for we should realise that movements, not muscles, are represented in the cerebral cortex. Thus we cannot consciously cause any individual muscle to contract unless we know its action. We could not, for instance, contract the deltoid if we did not know that the deltoid was an abductor of the arm.

All muscles have a rich blood supply, but this is not true of tendons. In tendons, lymphatic vessels predominate and are largely responsible for their nutrition.

Sometimes tendons, in order to avoid friction, are contained within *synovial sheaths*. In these circumstances there is an outer sheath of fibrous tissue in which are two layers of synovial membrane. One of these layers lines the fibrous tissue and the other covers the tendon. The synovial membrane secretes a synovial fluid which acts as a lubricant for the tendon and facilitates movement. As the result of a "strain" these synovial sheaths may become inflamed giving rise to a "tenosynovitis" a condition which is not uncommon at the wrist and ankle.

Sometimes friction is lessened by *bursae*, which are pouches formed of fibrous tissue and lined by synovial membrane. They contain a small amount of synovial fluid and are sometimes connected with the synovial cavity of a joint, e.g., the bursa beneath the psoas muscle; on the other hand they may be completely isolated, e.g., the bursa beneath the deltoid muscle.

THE MUSCLES OF THE HEAD AND NECK

The Scalp

The layers of the scalp may be conveniently tabulated thus:

Skin.
Connective tissue (dense).
*A*poneurosis (epicranial aponeurosis).
*L*oose connective tissue.
*P*ericranium (comparable to the periosteum elsewhere).

The *skin* is very thick and dense. It contains hair follicles and also sebaceous and sweat glands. The *dense connective tissue* contains numerous blood vessels and nerves. The *epicranial aponeurosis* is a flattened tendon common to two muscles, the frontalis and occipitalis. The former is not attached to bone but mingles with the skin of the forehead and the orbicularis oculi; the latter arises from the lateral two-thirds of the superior nuchal line on the occipital bone. The three outer layers of the scalp are intimately blended together and the *loose connective tissue* beneath them facilitates their movement over the skull. The *pericranium* covers the outer surface of the skull and is comparable to the periosteum which covers the remainder of the skeleton. It dips into the sutures to blend with the endosteal layer of dura mater which lines the interior of the skull.

The scalp can be stripped off the surface of the skull easily by tearing through the loose connective tissue layer, such an accident occurs occasionally as the result of the hair being caught in machinery.

The Muscles of Expression have only a small attachment to the bones of the face and skull and all are inserted into the skin. They are all supplied by the facial nerve and the student should note the effects of paralysis of these muscles in cases of facial palsy (fig. 171).

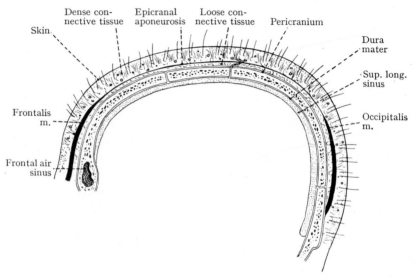

FIG. 115.—Sagittal section through the scalp.

It will not be necessary to describe the precise attachments of all the muscles of expression but the student should locate them by referring to fig. 116.

They are:

The extrinsic muscles of the ear (the auricularis group).

The muscles of the eyelids (orbicularis oculi, levator palpebrae superioris, and corrugator).

The muscles of the nose (nares, procerus and levator labii superioris alaeque nasi).

The muscles of the mouth (orbicularis oris, levator labii superioris, levator anguli oris, zygomaticus, risorius, buccinator, depressor anguli oris, depressor labii inferioris, mentalis, platysma).

Two of these muscles of expression are sufficiently important to justify a more detailed description, viz., the buccinator (fig. 116) and the platysma (fig. 117).

Buccinator
Origin. From the pterygomandibular ligament* and the outer surfaces of the alveolar processes of the maxilla and mandible extending as far forward as the first molar teeth.

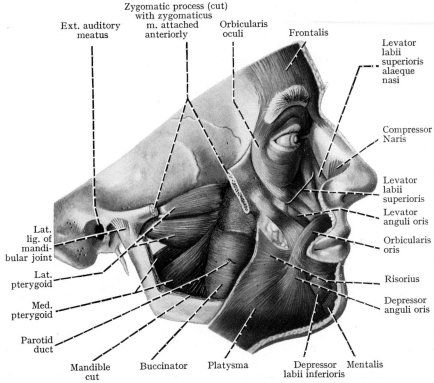

FIG. 116.—The muscles of expression and the deeper muscles of mastication.

Insertion. Into the angle of the mouth where the muscle mingles with others in this region.   Its fibres decussate so that the lower fibres pass to the upper lip and the upper fibres to the lower lip.

Nerve supply. Facial nerve.

Action. Besides being a muscle of expression it also flattens the cheek against the gums and prevents food accumulating in that region.

Platysma
Origin. From the fascia on the front of the chest.

* The pterygomandibular ligament is a tendinous band which is attached to the pterygoid hamulus on the medial pterygoid plate and to the medial surface of the mandible just behind the last molar tooth.   It gives attachment anteriorly to the buccinator and posteriorly to the superior constrictor muscle of the pharynx.

Insertion.   The muscle ascends over the clavicle in the superficial fascia. Its posterior fibres are inserted into the inferior border of the body of the mandible and then pass to the angle of the mouth, blending with the muscles in that region.   Its anterior fibres blend with their fellows of the opposite side behind and below the chin.

Nerve supply.   Cervical branch of the facial nerve.

Action.   Depresses the lower jaw and to that extent is a muscle of expression, but in hard physical exercise (e.g., running) it not infrequently acts in

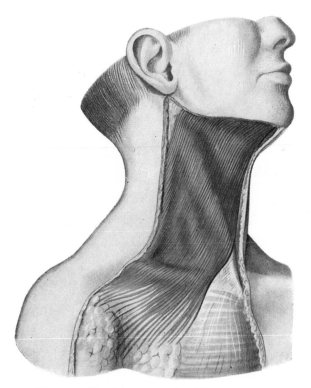

Fig. 117.—The platysma muscle.   (After Sobotta).

reverse.   In these circumstances the jaw is firmly fixed and the platysma tightens the skin and subcutaneous structures in the neck, thus facilitating the blood supply to and from the vital centres in the brain by preventing a kinking of the great vessels in the carotid sheath.

The Muscles of Mastication (figs. 116 and 118) include the masseter, the temporalis and the two pterygoids.   All are inserted into the lower jaw and all are supplied by the mandibular division of the trigeminal nerve.

Masseter

Origin. By two heads, a superficial head from the lower border and a deep head from the medial surface of the zygomatic process.

Insertion. Its fibres run downwards and slightly backwards to be inserted into the lateral aspect of the ramus of the mandible.

Nerve supply. Mandibular division of the trigeminal nerve.

Action. Raises the mandible and clenches the teeth.

Temporalis.

Origin. From the temporal fossa and the deep surface of the temporal fascia.

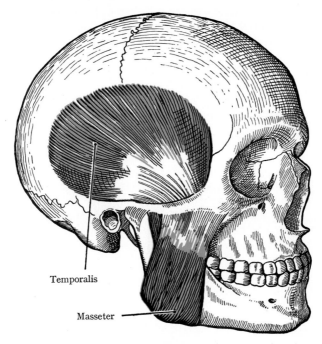

Temporalis

Masseter

FIG. 118.—The superficial muscles of mastication.

Insertion. The muscle is fan-shaped and its tendon passes deep to the zygomatic process to be inserted into the anterior border and medial surface of the coronoid process of the mandible.

Nerve supply. Mandibular division of the trigeminal nerve.

Action. Raises the mandible and clenches the teeth and its posterior fibres draw back the mandible when it is protruded.

Lateral Pterygoid (fig. 116)

Origin. The muscle arises by two heads—an upper head from the infratemporal fossa and a lower head from the lateral aspect of lateral pterygoid plate of the sphenoid bone.

Insertion. Its fibres are directed horizontally backwards and outwards to be inserted into the pterygoid fossa on the anterior aspect of the condyle of the mandible and into the articular disc and capsule of the jaw joint.

Nerve supply. Mandibular division of the trigeminal nerve.

Action. Pulls forward the condyle of the mandible and the articular disc and thus facilitates the opening of the mouth. When the mouth is to be closed the lateral pterygoid muscle is relaxed.

Medial Pterygoid (fig. 116)

Origin. The muscle arises by two heads, an upper head from the medial aspect of lateral pterygoid plate, and a lower head from the pyramidal process of the palatine bone and the tuberosity of maxilla. The lower head is small, and superficial to the lateral pterygoid muscle.

Insertion. Its fibres are directed downwards and backwards to be inserted into a rough area of bone on the inner aspect of the angle of the jaw.

Nerve supply. Mandibular division of the trigeminal nerve.

Action. Raises and protrudes the mandible.

The mouth is opened by gravity and by the relaxation of the muscles of mastication, although such muscles as the mylohyoid, anterior belly of digastric and the platysma are brought into play when it is necessary to open the mouth against resistance. Chewing movements are brought about by the co-ordination of the muscles of mastication but it should be borne in mind that the pterygoids working alternately are alone responsible for the lateral movements of the jaw which are so necessary in this connection.

The Muscles of the Neck include the large and prominent sterno-mastoid, the scalene muscles and a number of smaller muscles, details of which will not concern the student of physiotherapy, e.g., the infrahyoid group anteriorly, which are passing upwards to their insertion into the laryngeal cartilages. The levator scapulae and trapezius muscles will be considered with those of the upper limb.

Sternomastoid (fig. 228)

Origin. The muscle arises by two heads—a smaller sternal head which is attached to the anterior surface of the manubrium and a larger clavicular head which is attached to the superior border and anterior surface of the medial third of the clavicle.

Insertion. The muscle is inserted by two heads, one passing into the mastoid process of the temporal bone and the other into the adjacent superior nuchal line on the occipital bone.

Nerve supply. From the accessory (XIth cranial) nerve which pierces the medial surface of the muscle and from the 2nd and 3rd cervical nerves. The latter branches are probably afferent (special sensory branches) since the muscle is paralysed when the accessory nerve alone is cut.

Action. Its fibres pass upwards, backwards and laterally. The muscle, acting with its fellow on the opposite side, flexes the head against resistance, e.g. it can be seen and felt to contract firmly when rising from the supine position, for then the muscle is raising the head against gravity. It side-flexes the head to its own side and rotates it to the opposite side. In the condition of torticollis (wry neck), when the muscle is shortened due to a cicatrix (scar tissue) replacing muscle fibres following a tearing of the fibres at birth, the head is characteristically rotated and side flexed.

Like all the muscles attached to the thoracic cage, it is sometimes called upon to act as an accessory muscle of respiration. In these circumstances the head is fixed and the muscle acts towards its origin.

The Scalene Muscles

Origin. The scalene muscles consist of anterior, middle (scalenus medius) and posterior muscles. They arise from the transverse processes of the cervical vertebrae extending from the 2nd to the 6th segments. The middle scalene has the most extensive origin usually.

Insertion. The anterior and middle scalenes are inserted into the first rib, while the posterior scalene is inserted into the second rib.

Nerve supply. They are innervated by direct branches from the cervical plexus.

Action. They may either fix or elevate the 1st and 2nd ribs but frequently they act in reverse flexing the neck either forwards or laterally.

Scalenus anterior is almost entirely covered by sternomastoid. On it lie the phrenic nerve and carotid sheath, while near its insertion the muscle crosses the subclavian artery and separates the artery from the vein. The brachial plexus emerges between the scalenus anterior and scalenus medius.

The Axial Muscles

The Prevertebral Muscles. In this group we include muscles which arise from the vertebral column and are inserted either into another part of the column or into the skull. These muscles extend down as far as the upper thoracic region only, for they are all concerned with flexing the neck or the head.

They are the *longus capitis, rectus capitis anticus, rectus capitis lateralis* and *longus cervicis*, and were referred to when the movements of the vertebral column were discussed. While it is not necessary for the student of physiotherapy to know their precise attachments, their position in the body should be noted (fig. 119).

The Postvertebral Muscles. In this group we include the deep muscles of the back. These muscles include the *splenius capitis et cervicis, serratus posterior superior et inferior, sacrospinalis* and its derivatives, viz., *iliocostalis, longissimus* and *spinalis; semispinalis; multifidus* and a number of small muscles lying deeply, viz., *interspinales, intertransversarii, rotatores, superior* and *inferior oblique capitis, rectus capitis posterior major* and *minor*.

While these muscles are not included in the curriculum of the Chartered Society, a general idea of their disposition must be given if the student is to understand and appreciate the movements of the vertebral column (figs. 120 and 121).

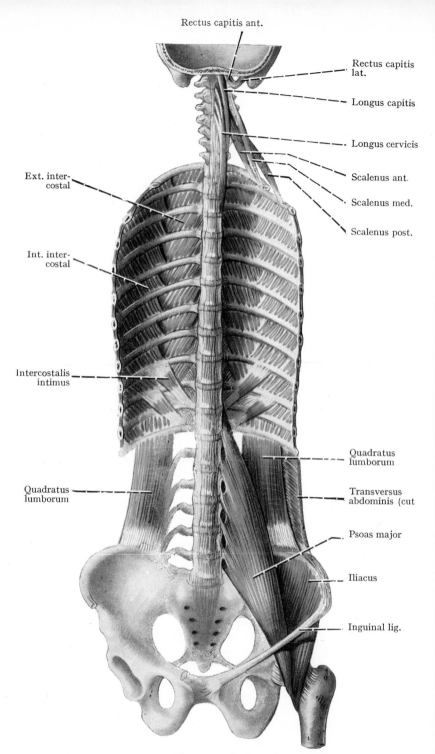

Rectus capitis ant.

Rectus capitis lat.

Longus capitis

Longus cervicis

Scalenus ant.

Scalenus med.

Scalenus post.

Ext. inter-costal

Int. inter-costal

Intercostalis intimus

Quadratus lumborum

Quadratus lumborum

Transversus abdominis (cut

Psoas major

Iliacus

Inguinal lig.

FIG. 119.—The prevertebral muscles.

126

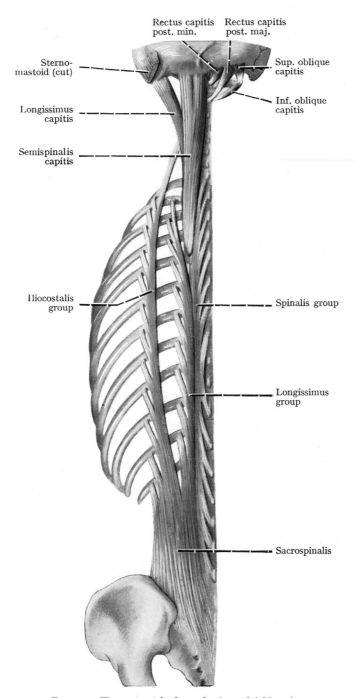

Rectus capitis
post. min.

Rectus capitis
post. maj.

Sterno-
mastoid (cut)

Sup. oblique
capitis

Inf. oblique
capitis

Longissimus
capitis

Semispinalis
capitis

Iliocostalis
group

Spinalis group

Longissimus
group

Sacrospinalis

FIG. 120.—The postvertebral muscles (superficial layer).

In general, it may be said that they are extensors of the spine and play an important part in maintaining the body in the erect position and in raising it from the stooping position. They counter the action of gravity which is always tending to cause the trunk to fall forwards and, therefore, they are never at rest unless the subject is lying perfectly flat in the supine position.

Splenius arises from the spines of the lower cervical and upper thoracic vertebrae and is inserted into the mastoid process and adjacent occipital bone (capitis) and into the upper cervical vertebrae (cervicis).

Serratus Posterior Superior arises from the lower cervical and upper thoracic spines and is inserted into the upper ribs near their angles.

Serratus Posterior Inferior (much smaller) (fig. 135) arises from the lower thoracic and upper lumbar spines and is inserted into the lower ribs near their angles.

Sacrospinalis (fig. 120) arises from the posterior aspect of the sacrum, the posterior part of the medial lip of the iliac crest and from the spines of all the lumbar vertebrae. As it passes upwards it divides into three groups, named from without in, the *iliocostalis* (attached to the ribs), *longissimus* (attached to the transverse processes of all the vertebrae in the lumbar, thoracic and cervical regions—except the atlas—and to the adjacent ribs), *spinalis* (attached to the spines in one region of the vertebral column and extending upwards is attached to spines a few vertebrae above).

An extension of the longissimus group passes to the mastoid process and is known as the *longissimus capitis*.

Lying under cover of the spinalis group are the *semispinalis muscles*. They are limited to the cervical and thoracic regions and extend between the transverse processes in one region and the spinous processes of a few vertebrae above.

An extension of the semispinalis group passes to the squamous portion of the occipital bone and is known as the semispinalis capitis. It is a muscle of some size and forms almost the whole of the roof of the sub-occipital triangle.

Multifidus (fig. 121) consists of a series of muscles which lie on the laminae of the vertebrae, extending from sacrum to axis. They arise for the most part from transverse processes and are inserted into the spines of adjacent vertebrae.

Rotatores (fig. 121) arise from the transverse processes in the thoracic region and are inserted into the laminae of the vertebrae above.

Interspinales and **Intertransversarii** (fig. 121) are attached to adjacent spines and transverse processes respectively.

The Rectus capitis posterior and **Obliquus capitis** (fig. 120) muscles are attached to the atlas or axis and to the adjacent squamous portion of the occipital bone.

The Lumbar fascia (fig. 122) consists of anterior, middle and posterior lamellae, of which the latter is by far the strongest. The anterior and middle lamellae form a sheath for quadratus lumborum and fuse laterally

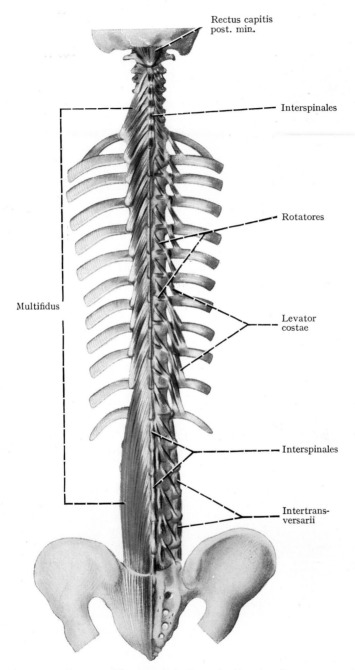

Rectus capitis
post. min.

Interspinales

Rotatores

Levator
costae

Interspinales

Intertrans-
versarii

Multifidus

FIG. 121.—The postvertebral muscles (deep layer).

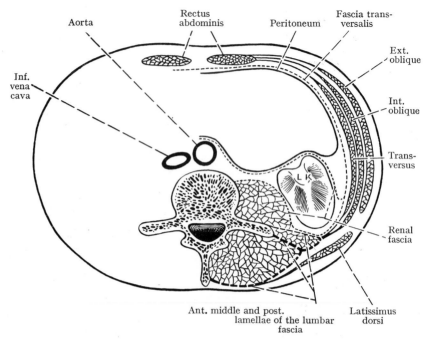

Aorta   Rectus abdominis   Peritoneum   Fascia transversalis

Ext. oblique

Inf. vena cava

Int. oblique

Transversus

Renal fascia

Ant. middle and post. lamellae of the lumbar fascia   Latissimus dorsi

FIG. 122.—Transverse section through the abdomen to show the arrangement of the lumbar fascia.

Note how the fascia transversalis blends with the renal fascia. In this figure the student is looking at the section from below. L.K.=left kidney.

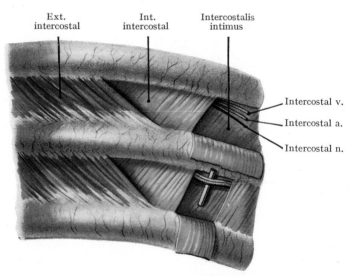

Ext. intercostal   Int. intercostal   Intercostalis intimus

Intercostal v.

Intercostal a.

Intercostal n.

FIG. 123.—A dissection of the lateral thoracic wall showing the intercostal muscles. The intercostal vessels and nerve have been displaced from the subcostal groove.

130

to blend with the tendon of origin of the transversus abdominis muscle. The posterior layer covers the sacrospinalis muscle and its derivatives and is carried with these muscles into the thoracic region.

The Intercostal muscles lie in three layers and are thus comparable to the three layers of muscles on the abdominal wall. The outermost layer is made up of the *intercostales externi*, the middle layer the *intercostales interni*, while the innermost layer consists of scattered groups of muscles called the *intercostales intimi* and *transversus thoracis*. The muscle forming the outer and middle layers pass from one rib to the next but the deep layer of muscles tends to skip a rib (fig. 119), while the *transversus thoracis* arises from the lower part of the sternum and is inserted into the costal cartilages of the upper ribs.

The external intercostals are deficient in front and are completed by the *anterior intercostal membrane*, the internal intercostals are deficient behind and are completed by the *posterior intercostal membrane* (fig. 181).

Nerve supply. All these muscles are supplied by the intercostal nerves.

Action. Elevate the ribs and so facilitate respiration by increasing the capacity of the thorax. The intercostales intimi and transversus thoracis depress the ribs (see the mechanism of respiration, p. 76).

The Diaphragm (fig. 124)

The diaphragm is a large dome-shaped muscle separating the thoracic and abdominal cavities.

Origin. From the posterior aspect of the xiphoid process, from the inner surface of the lower six costal cartilages interdigitating with the transversus abdominis, from the medial and lateral arcuate ligaments and from two crura. The right crus is attached to the bodies of the upper three and the left crus to the bodies of the upper two lumbar vertebrae. The splanchnic nerves pierce the crura to enter the abdomen, and the left crus is also pierced by the inferior hemiazygos vein and the right crus sometimes by the azygos vein.

Insertion into the central tendon which is shaped like a clover leaf with an anterior and two lateral lobes.

Nerve supply. Phrenic and the lower six intercostal nerves; the latter are probably sensory.

Action. The diaphragm is the chief muscle of respiration. During inspiration the crura and peripheral fibres contract and draw down the central tendon. The heart and abdominal viscera are pulled down and intra-abdominal pressure is raised. To compensate for this, the abdominal muscles relax and bulge outwards (abdominal respiration). Expiration is brought about by the elastic recoil of the lungs and diaphragm, assisted by the abdominal muscles especially transversus abdominis which with trans-versus thoracis are the antagonists of the diaphragm. The diaphragm is thus elevated and by increasing the intrathoracic pressure, drives the air from the lungs.

The regulation of the passage of air through the larynx in speech and singing is due to the ability to control the movements of the diaphragm.

The diaphragm is highest when lying flat, is lower when standing and lowest when sitting.

By raising intra-abdominal pressure the diaphragm assists in all expulsive efforts, particularly defaecation and parturition.

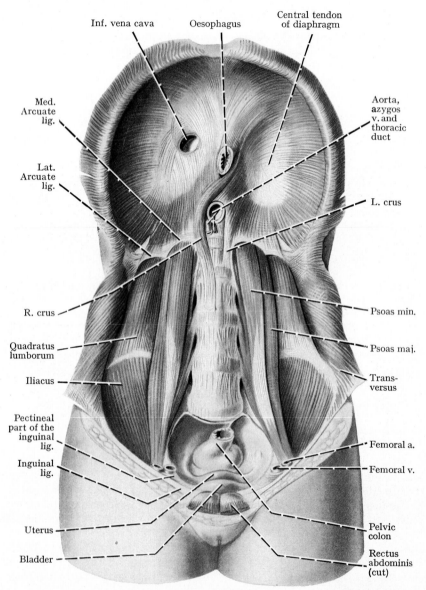

Inf. vena cava   Oesophagus   Central tendon of diaphragm

Med. Arcuate lig.

Lat. Arcuate lig.

Aorta, azygos v. and thoracic duct

L. crus

R. crus

Quadratus lumborum

Iliacus

Pectineal part of the inguinal lig.

Inguinal lig.

Uterus

Bladder

Psoas min.

Psoas maj.

Trans-versus

Femoral a.

Femoral v.

Pelvic colon

Rectus abdominis (cut)

FIG. 124.—The under-surface of the diaphragm and the muscles on the posterior abdominal wall. (After Sobotta.)

The lower part of the thorax has been pulled upwards and backwards to display the diaphragm.

There is little doubt that the diaphragm acts as a sphincter for the oesophagus. Also by its excursions it considerably augments the venous and lymphatic flow towards the thorax.

The *medial arcuate ligament* extends from the 1st or 2nd lumbar vertebrae to the transverse process of the 1st lumbar vertebra and is formed by the upper border of the sheath of the psoas muscle. The sympathetic chain descends beneath this arch.

The *lateral arcuate ligament* extends from the transverse process of the 1st lumbar vertebra to the 12th rib and is the upper border of the fascia covering the quadratus lumborum muscle. The subcostal vessels and nerve (twelfth intercostal) descend beneath this arch.

The seventh to the eleventh intercostal nerves enter the abdominal wall by passing between the digitations of the diaphragm.

The heart lies on the central tendon of the diaphragm and the pericardium is adherent to it. The central tendon is pierced by the inferior vena cava and the right phrenic nerve at the level of the 8th thoracic vertebra; the musculature of the diaphragm is pierced on the left of the mid-line by the oesophagus and the vagi nerves at the level of the 10th thoracic vertebra, while the aorta, azygos vein and thoracic duct pass behind the decussating fibres of the two crura at the level of the 12th thoracic vertebra.

The Fascia of the Abdominal Wall

The superficial fascia consists of a single sheet above the umbilicus but below that level it is divided into two distinct layers—a superficial fatty layer and a deep membranous layer. These layers are continued downwards over the external genitalia into the perineum, and also into the thigh where the deep layer blends with the fascia lata. The superficial layer constitutes the fat of the abdominal wall and in obese subjects the fat may be inches thick.

The deep fascia is very thin since a tough unyielding membrane would hamper the movements of respiration.

On the deep aspect of the anterior abdominal wall is the *fascia transversalis* (figs. 122 and 125) which is separated from the peritoneum by the extraperitoneal fat. The fascia transversalis lines the abdominal cavity—anteriorly it forms an uninterrupted sheet, posteriorly it blends with the renal fascia, superiorly it blends with the fascia lining the under surface of the diaphragm, inferiorly it fuses with the inguinal ligament to form the posterior wall of the inguinal canal. It is carried down into the thigh with the femoral vessels where it forms the anterior wall of the femoral sheath (fig. 125). About 1 cm. above the middle of the inguinal ligament the transversalis fascia is invaginated at the deep inguinal ring by the spermatic cord in the male or the round ligament of the uterus in the female (fig. 132, facing p. 141) and a portion of the fascia is prolonged on to these structures to form a sheath called the internal spermatic fascia.

The Muscles of the Anterior Abdominal Wall are the rectus ab-

9—A.PH.

dominis, pyramidalis, obliquus externus, obliquus internus and transversus abdominis.

Rectus Abdominis (fig. 126)

Origin. The muscle arises by two heads, one from the pubic crest and the other from the anterior ligaments of the symphysis.

Insertion. The muscle is inserted by two heads, one into the xiphoid process of the sternum, and the other, larger head, into the 5th, 6th and 7th costal cartilages.

The muscle is enclosed in an aponeurotic sheath (*vide* rectus sheath, p. 138) and its anterior surface shows three of four tendinous intersections where the sheath is adherent to the muscle (fig. 126). One of these is situated at the level of the umbilicus, another at the level of the tip of the xiphoid process,

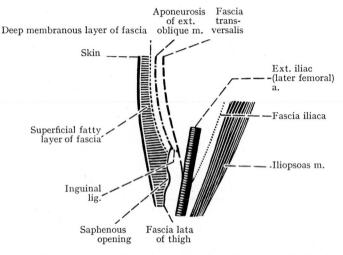

FIG. 125.—The arrangement of the fascial planes in the lower abdominal and upper thigh regions (diagrammatic).

while the others lie between these two. These intersections are known as the *lineae transversae*; they are said to be the homologues of the ribs which are carried into the abdomen in certain reptiles (crocodiles). They may be seen in the living subject, when the rectus is contracted.

Pyramidalis is a small vestigial triangular muscle, often absent. It lies in front of the rectus muscle but within the rectus sheath. It arises from the pubic crest and is inserted into the linea alba. It is well developed in marsupials (kangaroo), where it forms the anterior wall of the abdominal pouch.

It is supplied by the 12th thoracic nerve.

Obliquus externus abdominis (fig. 126)

The external oblique forms the anterolateral boundary of the abdominal wall.

Origin. By digitations from the lateral surfaces and inferior borders of the lower eight ribs blending with serratus anterior and latissimus dorsi muscles.

Insertion.   By fleshy fibres which pass downwards, forwards and medially into the anterior half of the lateral lip of the iliac crest and by a broad aponeurosis which lies medial to a line from the anterior spine to the ninth costal cartilage.   Below it is attached to the anterior superior spine and

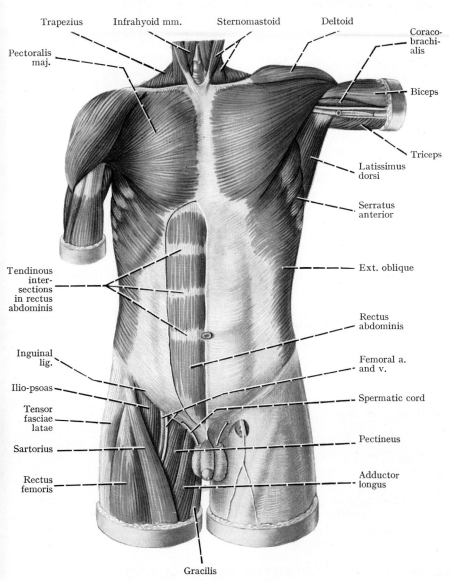

FIG. 126.—The superficial muscles on the anterior aspect of the trunk.

the pubic tubercle and between these two points its border turns back on itself in a J-shaped manner to form the *inguinal ligament* in the groin. From the pubic tubercle the aponeurosis extends to the iliopectineal line forming the *pectineal part of the inguinal ligament*. From the pubic crest the aponeurosis extends upwards to the xiphoid cartilage, blending with the aponeuroses of the internal oblique and transversus abdominis to form the *linea alba*. From here it extends over the front of the abdominal wall forming the anterior boundary of the rectus sheath.

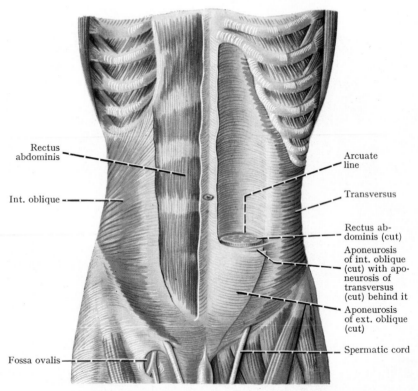

Rectus abdominis

Int. oblique

Fossa ovalis

Arcuate line

Transversus

Rectus abdominis (cut)

Aponeurosis of int. oblique (cut) with aponeurosis of transversus (cut) behind it

Aponeurosis of ext. oblique (cut)

Spermatic cord

FIG. 127.—The deeper muscles of the abdominal wall.

Above and medial to the pubic tubercle the aponeurosis of the external oblique is evaginated at the *external abdominal ring* by the spermatic cord or round ligament of the uterus (figs. 126 and 127). Some fibres of the aponeurosis are prolonged on to those structures in the form of a sheath called the external spermatic fascia.

Obliquus Internus Abdominis (figs. 127 and 128)

Origin. From the lateral two-thirds of the inguinal ligament, from the anterior two-thirds of the middle lip of the iliac crest and from the posterior lamella of the lumbar fascia.

Insertion. The innermost fibres from the inguinal ligament arch over the spermatic cord (or round ligament) and becoming aponeurotic join with the distal and medial fibres of the transversus abdominis muscle to form the *conjoined tendon* which lies behind the inner end of the spermatic cord (or round ligament) and is attached to the pubic crest and iliopectineal line. The outermost fibres from the inguinal ligament end in an aponeurosis which runs in front of the rectus muscle to join the linea alba. The fibres arising from the iliac crest pass upwards and medially and becoming aponeurotic at the lateral border of the rectus (linea semilunaris) split into two lamellae which ensheathe the rectus before passing to the linea alba. These fibres are attached above to the 7th, 8th and 9th costal cartilages. The fibres arising from the lumbar fascia pass almost vertically upwards to be inserted into the 10th, 11th and 12th ribs (fig. 128).

Transversus abdominis (fig. 127)

Origin. From the lateral third of the inguinal ligament, from the anterior two-thirds of the medial lip of the iliac crest, from the lumbar fascia and from the medial surfaces of the cartilages of the lower six ribs interdigitating with the diaphragm.

Insertion. The fibres arising from the inguinal ligament arch over the spermatic cord (or round ligament) and fusing with the internal oblique form the conjoined tendon. The remaining fibres run transversely and becoming aponeurotic at the lateral border of

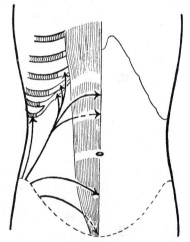

Fig. 128.—A diagrammatic representation of the direction taken by the fibres of the internal oblique muscle.

the rectus abdominis (linea semilunaris) help to form the sheath of that muscle before passing to the linea alba. From the xiphoid process to a point midway between the umbilicus and the pubis the aponeurosis passes behind the rectus, below this point it passes in front of the rectus.

Nerve supply to the muscles on the abdominal wall is from the lower six or seven intercostal nerves. The first lumbar nerve via the iliohypogastric and ilio-inguinal nerves also supplies the oblique muscles and the transversus abdominis.

Action of the muscles of the abdominal wall. The abdominal muscles and more especially the transversus abdominis are concerned with the control of intra-abdominal pressure. Thus they help to keep the viscera in position and materially assist the flow of venous blood and lymph against gravity. By their contraction they increase intra-abdominal pressure and so force the diaphragm upwards into the chest thus emptying the lungs. They assist in all expulsive efforts, e.g., defaecation and parturition. On contraction they form a rigid wall which can protect the abdominal viscera from injury.

The rectus abdominis with iliopsoas initiates flexion of the trunk on the hips which is afterwards continued by gravity. The oblique muscles act as rotators of the trunk (p. 328), the external oblique muscle of one side acting with the internal oblique muscle of the opposite side, i.e., the more mobile thorax rotates around the more fixed pelvis.

The rectus acts powerfully in drawing up the pelvis and lower limbs towards the trunk, e.g., when climbing with the hands.

The abdominal muscles in women who have borne children are often weak and flabby, and thus it may be much easier to palpate the abdominal viscera in women than men.

Cessation of abdominal breathing may be an indication of serious abdominal disease (general peritonitis) and is one of the signs commonly looked for when this condition is suspected.

The Rectus Sheath

The rectus muscle is enveloped in an aponeurotic sheath which is, however, deficient in certain regions.

In the thorax the muscle is covered only by the aponeurosis of the external oblique and lies directly on the 5th, 6th and 7th costal cartilages.

From the xiphoid process to a point midway between the umbilicus and the pubis the muscle is completely enveloped in a sheath which is formed by the

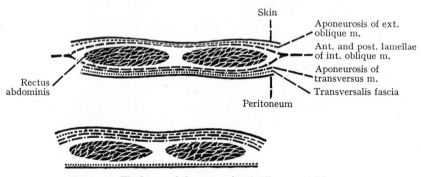

FIG. 129.—The layers of the rectus sheath (diagrammatic).
The upper figure represents the arrangement in the upper two-thirds and the lower figure in the lower one-third of the abdominal wall.

splitting of the aponeurosis of the internal oblique. In this region, therefore, the muscle is covered in front by the aponeurosis of the external oblique and the anterior lamella of the aponeurosis of the internal oblique and behind by the posterior lamella of the aponeurosis of the internal oblique and the aponeurosis of the transversus abdominis muscle, the transversalis fascia, the extra-peritoneal fat and the peritoneum.

Below a point midway between the umbilicus and the pubis the posterior wall is deficient and the muscle lies on the transversalis fascia, the extra-peritoneal fat and the peritoneum. The sheath is here represented in front by the aponeuroses of the external oblique, internal oblique and transversus abdominis muscles.

The point midway between the umbilicus and the pubis marks the distal extremity of the posterior wall of the sheath which ends in a free crescentic border known as the *arcuate line* (fig. 127).

The *sheath contains* the rectus abdominis and pyramidalis muscles, the lower five intercostal nerves and the last thoracic nerve and also the superior and inferior epigastric vessels which anastomose within the sheath.

The Inguinal Canal

The inguinal canal lies obliquely in the abdominal wall immediately above the medial half of the inguinal ligament. It is about 4 cm. long and presents an inlet called the *deep inguinal ring* and an outlet called the *superficial inguinal ring* (q.v.).

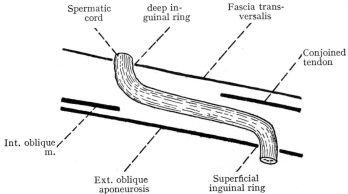

FIG. 130.—Transverse section through the inguinal canal showing the position of the spermatic cord (diagrammatic).

Its *anterior wall* is formed by the aponeurosis of the external oblique reinforced laterally by muscle fibres from the internal oblique.

Its *posterior wall* is formed by the fascia transversalis and is reinforced medially by the conjoined tendon.

Its *roof* is formed by the arching fibres of internal oblique and transversus abdominis muscles as they pass to form the conjoined tendon.

Its floor is formed by the gutter-shaped inguinal ligament and its pectineal reflection.

The canal transmits the spermatic cord in the male and the round ligament of the uterus in the female and also the terminal part of the ilio-inguinal nerve.

When intra-abdominal pressure is raised the anterior and posterior walls come into apposition and close the canal, thus strengthening a potential weakness.

Hernia (rupture) of the inguinal type is due to a muscular weakness in this region which allows an organ or part of an organ (most commonly small intestines or omentum) to enter the canal, whence it usually passes through the external ring and may descend into the scrotum (scrotal hernia).

The muscles of the posterior abdominal wall (fig. 124). The posterior abdominal wall is formed by the transversus abdominis, quadratus lumborum, psoas major, iliacus and, when present, the psoas minor muscles. Of these only the quadratus lumborum will be considered here.

Quadratus Lumborum (fig. 119)

Origin. From the iliac crest, iliolumbar ligament and transverse processes of the lower lumbar vertebrae.

Insertion. Into the transverse processes of the upper four lumbar vertebrae and into the last rib.

Nerve supply. From the twelfth thoracic and upper four lumbar nerves.

Action. Flexes the vertebral column laterally. This muscle also plays an important part in respiration, since by fixing the last rib it greatly increases the power of the diaphragm in inspiration.

The Pelvic Floor (fig. 131)

The pelvic floor is a muscular diaphragm, concave upwards, perforated by the urethra and rectum in the male and by the urethra, vagina and rectum in

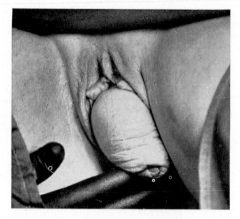

FIG. 133.—A case of prolapse.

the female. It acts in conjunction with the musculature of the abdominal walls and with the diaphragm in helping to regulate intra-abdominal pressure and in addition it has certain specialised functions in the female in whom it is sometimes stretched or torn at parturition (child-birth), and since it is designed to support the pelvic viscera and to act as an auxiliary sphincter for the anal orifice, it follows that such injuries are liable to cause a prolapse of the vagina, followed by the uterus and its appendages (fig. 133) and also some degree of faecal incontinence.

The muscles forming the pelvic floor are the levatores ani and coccygei which blend with their fellows of the opposite side in the mid-line of the body. For all practical purposes these two muscles can be considered as one.

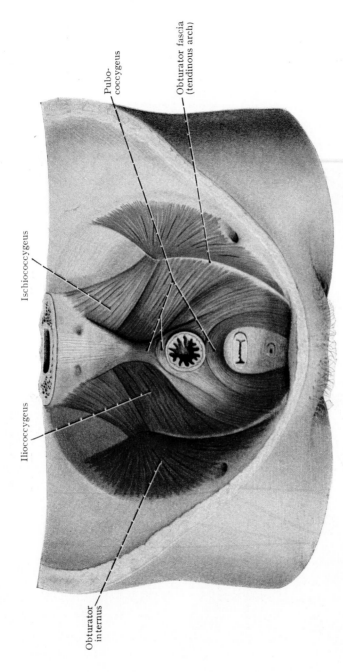

Pubo-
coccygeus

Obturator fascia
(tendinous arch)

Ischiococcygeus

Iliococcygeus

Obturator
internus

Fig. 131.—The pelvic floor in the female as seen from above.

The urethra and vagina are seen piercing the pelvic fascia (yellow). The rectum is seen behind the vagina. Note the three divisions of the pubococcygeus, viz., the pubovaginalis forming a U-loop around the vagina, the puborectalis surrounding the rectum and the pubococcygeus proper, which has a Y-shaped attachment to the sacrum and coccyx.

[facing page 140]

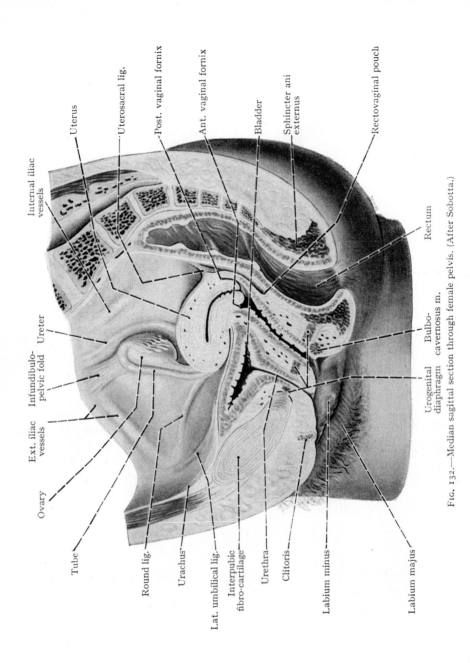

Internal iliac vessels

Uterus

Uterosacral lig.

Post. vaginal fornix

Ant. vaginal fornix

Bladder

Sphincter ani externus

Rectovaginal pouch

Rectum

Ureter

Infundibulo-pelvic fold

Ext. iliac vessels

Ovary

Tube

Round lig.

Urachus

Lat. umbilical lig.

Interpubic fibro-cartilage

Urethra

Clitoris

Labium minus

Labium majus

Urogenital diaphragm

Bulbo-cavernosus m.

FIG. 132.—Median sagittal section through female pelvis. (After Sobotta.)

[facing page 141]

Levator Ani and Coccygeus (fig. 131)

Origin. From the pelvic aspect of the body of the pubis and from the ischial spine. Between these two bony points the muscle takes an extensive origin from the obturator fascia.

Insertion into the lateral and posterior vaginal walls, into the central point of the perineum, into the anal canal between the internal and external sphincters, into the anococcygeal body and into the lateral border of the lower end of the sacrum and the coccyx.

Nerve supply. Inferior haemorrhoidal nerve, the perineal branch of S4 and branches from S3, 4 and 5, direct from the sacral plexus.

Action. It helps to regulate intra-abdominal pressure and its specialised functions in the female are as follows:—The portion of the pelvic floor arising from the pubis and forming a U-loop around the vagina is known as the *pubovaginalis* (fig. 131). Its function is to support the vagina and so it is an important indirect support for the uterus and its appendages. The portion of the pelvic floor which surrounds the anal canal is known as the *pubo-rectalis* (fig. 131). It blends with the anal sphincters and powerfully augments their action. The portion of the pelvic floor arising from the pubis and inserted into the coccyx is known as the *pubococcygeus* (fig. 131). This muscle flexes the coccyx forwards, and by increasing the anorectal kink controls the descent of the faeces as they pass into the lowest part of the bowel.

The terms central point of the perineum and anococcygeal body need further elaboration.

The *central point of the perineum* refers to a region between the vulva and anal orifice in the female or the bladder and rectum in the male where several muscles, the levatores ani chiefly, meet and fuse. It is particularly important in the female because it lies in a vulnerable position at parturition and is not infrequently torn. The *anococcygeal body* is the name given to that part of the perineum which lies between the anal orifice and the coccyx.

THE FASCIA AND MUSCLES OF THE UPPER EXTREMITY

The deep fascia in the region of the Shoulder and Arm

The deep fascia lines the walls of the axilla and with the integument is solely responsible for the formation of its floor. The deep fascia is perforated by that portion of the breast known as the axillary tail (fig. 236). The axillary lymph nodes lie beneath the deep fascia.

The axillary vessels and the cords of the brachial plexus are enveloped in a sheath of deep fascia.

A specialised band of deep fascia known as the *clavipectoral fascia* forms the floor of the deltopectoral triangle (fig. 134). It is continuous above with the fascia enclosing the subclavius muscle and below with that enclosing the pectoralis minor. Medially the clavipectoral fascia is attached to the first rib and blends with the fascia over the intercostal muscles, while laterally it is attached to the coracoid process and blends with the axillary fascia. It is pierced by the lateral pectoral nerve, branches of the axillary artery passing to the pectoral muscles and the cephalic vein as it passes deeply to enter the subclavian vein.

The deep fascia of the arm gives off septa which separate the muscles, two of which are especially strong and are known as the *lateral and medial intermuscular septa.* These septa divide the arm into anterior and posterior compartments and are attached respectively to the lateral and medial supracondylar ridges on the humerus.

The Shoulder and Arm muscles

The muscles connecting the upper limb to the trunk comprise the trapezius, latissimus dorsi, levator scapulae, rhomboids, pectorales, subclavius and serratus anterior.

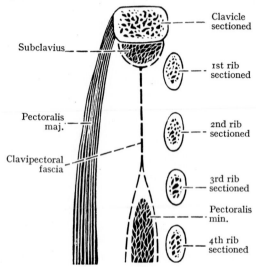

FIG. 134.—Sagittal section through the upper part of the thorax to show the arrangement of the clavipectoral fascia (diagrammatic).

Trapezius (fig. 135)

Origin. From the medial third of the superior nuchal line on the occipital bone and the external occipital protuberance, from the ligamentum nuchae, from the spines of the 7th cervical and all the thoracic vertebrae and the supraspinous ligaments.

Insertion. Into the superior border of the crest of the spine of the scapula, the adjacent acromion process and into the posterior border of the lateral third of the clavicle.

The upper fibres are directed downwards and laterally before sweeping forwards to be inserted into the clavicle. The middle fibres are directed horizontally and the lower fibres upwards and laterally as they pass to their insertion into the spine of the scapula (fig. 135).

Nerve supply. From the spinal accessory and 3rd and 4th cervical nerves.

Action. The upper fibres of trapezius elevate the scapula, the lower fibres depress it while the middle and lower fibres assist the serratus anterior to rotate the scapula outwards when the arm is raised above the head. The middle fibres of trapezius adduct the scapula. By its inherent tonus it braces the shoulder and when the muscle is paralysed the shoulder droops and its contour is altered considerably, giving to it a characteristically flattened appearance. Drooping shoulders especially in children indicate poor muscle tone throughout the body. Acting in reverse the trapezius may extend or laterally flex the head.

Latissimus Dorsi (fig. 135)

Origin. From the posterior part of the lateral lip of the iliac crest, the lumbar fascia, the spines of the lower six thoracic vertebrae (deep to trapezius), from the lower three or four ribs, and sometimes by a few fibres from the inferior angle of the scapula.

Insertion. Its flattened tendon turns on itself and crosses in front of teres major to be inserted into the floor of the bicipital groove on the humerus. The general direction of the fibres of this muscle is obliquely upwards and laterally. Note how its upper fibres strap the scapula to the chest wall (fig. 135).

Nerve supply. Nerve to latissimus dorsi from the posterior cord.

Action. Extends, adducts and medially rotates the arm.

It sometimes acts in reverse, when with the upper limbs fixed, it draws the trunk upwards (e.g., in climbing with the hands).

Note the derivation of its name, it is the broadest muscle of the back.

Levator Scapulae (fig. 135)

Origin. From the transverse processes of the upper four cervical vertebrae.

Insertion. Into the vertebral margin of the scapula from the superior angle to the root of the spine.

Nerve supply. By branches from the 3rd and 4th cervical nerves and also by the 5th cervical nerve via the nerve to the rhomboids.

Action. Raises the shoulder by elevating the scapula.

It acts in conjunction with the rhomboids when the scapula is rotated and with the trapezius when the scapula is elevated.

Rhomboideus Major (fig. 135)

Origin. From the 2nd, 3rd, 4th and 5th thoracic spines and the supraspinous ligaments.

Insertion. Into the vertebral border of the scapula from the root of the spine to the inferior angle.

Nerve supply. Nerve to rhomboids (C.5).

Rhomboideus Minor (fig. 135)

Origin. From the ligamentum nuchae, the spines of the 7th cervical and 1st thoracic vertebrae and the supraspinous ligaments.

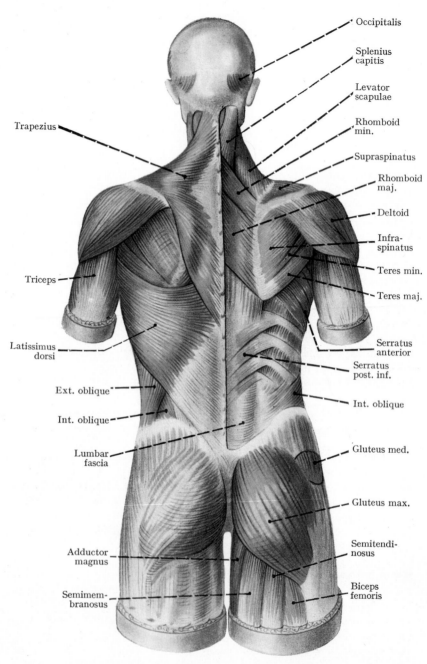

Occipitalis

Splenius
capitis

Levator
scapulae

Rhomboid
min.

Supraspinatus

Rhomboid
maj.

Deltoid

Infra-
spinatus

Teres min.

Teres maj.

Serratus
anterior

Serratus
post. inf.

Int. oblique

Gluteus med.

Gluteus max.

Semitendi-
nosus

Biceps
femoris

Trapezius

Triceps

Latissimus
dorsi

Ext. oblique

Int. oblique

Lumbar
fascia

Adductor
magnus

Semimem-
branosus

FIG. 135.—The superficial muscles of the back; trapezius, latissimus dorsi and external
oblique have been removed on the right side to show the deeper structures.

144

Insertion. Into the vertebral border of the scapula at the root of the spine.

Nerve supply. Nerve to rhomboids (C.5).

Action of Rhomboids. They act with levator scapulae in elevating the scapula and drawing it backwards and are thus the antagonists of serratus anterior.

Subclavius (fig. 137)

Origin. From the first costal cartilage and adjacent first rib.

Insertion. Its fibres pass upwards and laterally to be inserted into the subclavian groove on the under surface of the clavicle.

Nerve supply. Nerve to subclavius (C.5 and 6).

Action. Is a depressor of the clavicle and steadies this bone during movements of the shoulder girdle.

Pectoralis Major (fig. 126)

Origin. From the medial half of the anterior surface of the clavicle, from the anterior aspect of the sternum and the upper six costal cartilages, and a small but important head from the aponeurosis of the external oblique muscle.

Insertion. Its upper fibres curl round its lower fibres and pass to a tendinous bilaminar insertion into the lateral lip of the bicipital groove on the humerus. It gives a fibrous expansion into the capsule of the shoulder joint. The muscle forms the anterior wall of the axilla.

Its upper fibres pass downwards and laterally and its lower fibres upwards and laterally.

Nerve supply. Medial and lateral pectoral nerves.

Action. Is a powerful adductor and medial rotator of the arm. Its clavicular head also assists in flexion.

Pectoralis Minor (fig. 137)

Origin. From the third, fourth and fifth ribs (or second, third and fourth) near the costal cartilages.

Insertion. The muscle lies under cover of the pectoralis major and is inserted into the medial border of the coracoid process of the scapula.

Nerve supply. Medial and lateral pectoral nerves.

Action. This muscle is the antagonist of the levator scapulae. Its fibres pass upwards and laterally and pull the scapula downwards and forwards.

Serratus Anterior (figs. 126 and 135)

Origin. By digitations from the lateral surfaces of the upper eight ribs and the fascia covering the intercostal muscles, the lower four interdigitating with the external oblique muscle of the abdomen. The first digitation arises from the second as well as the first rib.

Insertion. The muscle is inserted into the costal surface of the vertebral border of the scapula as follows—the first digitation is thick and quadrate and is attached to the superior angle; the next three digitations form a thin sheet which is attached to the vertebral border and the last four digitations converge on to the inferior angle of the scapula.

Nerve supply. Nerve to serratus anterior from C.5, 6 and 7.

Action. Draws the scapula towards the chest wall and thus steadies it in the initial movements of elevation of the upper limb. When the limb has been raised to the horizontal by the deltoid, a movement which takes place principally at the shoulder joint; the serratus anterior assisted by the lower fibres of the trapezius rotates the scapula in elevating the limb to the vertical, a movement which takes place at the joints of the shoulder girdle (*vide* p. 327). The serratus anterior has been described as the muscle of "forward punch" since it comes into action when the upper limb is pushed forward in the horizontal position.

Paralysis of this muscle gives rise to a characteristic deformity known as *winged scapula* when the vertebral border of the scapula protrudes from the chest wall.

Muscles of the Shoulder Girdle

The Muscles of the Shoulder Girdle comprise deltoid, supraspinatus, infraspinatus, teres major and minor, subscapularis and coracobrachialis.

Deltoid (figs. 135 and 143)

Origin. From the inferior border of the crest of the spine of the scapula, the lateral border of the acromion, and the anterior border of the lateral third of the clavicle.

Insertion. Into the deltoid tuberosity, on the middle of the lateral surface of the shaft of the humerus.

The deltoid is a powerful multipennate muscle. It is triangular in shape and its fibres converge from a broad origin to a narrow insertion, thereby increasing its power.

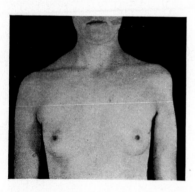

Nerve supply. Circumflex nerve.

Action. With the aid of the supraspinatus the deltoid is *the* abductor of the upper limb, its direct antagonist in this circumstance being the pectoralis major. Its anterior fibres help to flex and medially rotate, and its posterior fibres to extend and laterally rotate the arm.

This muscle gives the rounded contour to the shoulder and when paralysed the shoulder is flat (fig. 136). Elevation of the upper limb is then seriously hampered.

Fig. 136.—Wasting of the left deltoid muscle following paralysis of the circumflex nerve.

Supraspinatus (fig. 135)

Origin. From the supraspinous fossa on the scapula.

Insertion. Into the uppermost facet on the greater tuberosity of the humerus and into the capsule of the shoulder joint.

Nerve supply. Suprascapular nerve.

Action. This muscle initiates abduction by fixing the head of the humerus as the deltoid elevates the limb. Watson-Jones likens it to the workman's mate who places his foot at the bottom of a ladder to prevent the ladder sliding while it is being elevated. When the supraspinatus is ruptured, "weak abduction to 60° by scapular movement is all that is possible."

Infraspinatus (figs. 143 and 145)
Origin. From the infraspinous fossa on the scapula.
Insertion. Into the middle facet on the greater tuberosity of the humerus and into the capsule of the shoulder joint.
Nerve supply. Suprascapular nerve.
Action. Laterally rotates the arm in conjunction with teres minor, their antagonists in this action being latissimus dorsi, subscapularis, teres major and pectoralis major.

Teres Major (figs. 143 and 145)
Origin. From the posterior surface of the lateral border and inferior angle of the scapula.
Insertion. Into the medial border of the bicipital groove on the humerus.
Nerve supply. Lower subscapular nerve.
Action. Medially rotates, adducts and extends the upper limb.

Teres Minor (figs. 143 and 145)
Origin. From the posterior surface of the lateral border of the scapula above teres major.
Insertion. Into the lowest facet on the greater tuberosity of the humerus and into the capsule of the shoulder joint.
Nerve supply. Circumflex nerve.
Action. Acts with infraspinatus in laterally rotating the arm.
Note the teres minor passes to its insertion behind the humerus and the teres major in front of it, hence the minor is a lateral rotator and the major a medial rotator.

Subscapularis (fig. 137)
Origin. By fleshy fibres and tendinous intersections from the subscapular fossa on the anterior aspect of the scapula.
Insertion. Into the lesser tuberosity of the humerus and into the capsule of the shoulder joint.
Nerve supply. Upper and lower subscapular nerves.
Action. Acts with latissimus dorsi in medially rotating the arm.

One of the main functions of the short muscles of the shoulder joint, viz., supraspinatus, infraspinatus, subscapularis and teres minor is to retain the head of the humerus in contact with the glenoid cavity while the larger muscles, viz., teres major, latissimus dorsi, pectoralis major, deltoid and coracobrachialis perform the movements. The long head of biceps is also an important factor in maintaining the integrity of the shoulder joint. It should be noted that the short muscles are also inserted into the capsule and thus they keep this structure tense during movements of the shoulder joint.

Coracobrachialis (fig. 126)

Origin. From the tip of the coracoid process by a tendon common to it and the short head of biceps.

Insertion. Into the middle of the medial surface of the shaft of the humerus, opposite the deltoid insertion.

Nerve supply. Musculocutaneous nerve.

Action. Flexes the arm, its direct antagonists being the teres major and latissimus dorsi. It is also a weak adductor of the upper limb.

Two spaces called the quadrilateral and triangular spaces are described n the shoulder region. They are potential spaces seen only when the limb ; dissected.

The quadrangular space (fig. 145) is bounded above by the subscapularis front and the teres minor behind, while between these two muscles is the psule of the shoulder joint. The space is bounded laterally by the humerus d lateral head of triceps, medially by the long head of triceps and in-iorly by the teres major. The circumflex nerve enters the space in close ›ximity to the capsule of the shoulder joint and passes backwards to ›ply the deltoid and teres minor muscles. A small branch of the axillary ery (the posterior humeral circumflex) accompanies the nerve.

The triangular space is bounded above by the subscapularis in front l the teres minor behind, while between these two muscles is the axillary der of the scapula. The space is bounded laterally by the long head of eps and inferiorly by the teres major. A branch of the subscapular ery—the circumflex scapular—is seen in the space as it passes beneath the s minor muscle to enter the infraspinous fossa.

The Muscles of the Arm

he Muscles of the Arm comprise the biceps brachii, brachialis and t eps brachii.

iceps (fig. 137)

rigin. *Long head* from the supraglenoid tubercle, *short head* in common w ι coracobrachialis, from the tip of the coracoid process of the scapula. T tendon of the long head lies in the bicipital groove on the humerus h‹ ing traversed the shoulder joint where it is ensheathed by synovial m nbrane. The two heads unite at the junction of the middle and lower th ds of the arm and the muscle becomes tendinous at the level of the hu ιeral epicondyles.

nsertion. Into the posterior part of the bicipital tuberosity on the radius an by a fascial slip called the bicipital aponeurosis into the deep fascia on th medial aspect of the forearm.

erve supply. Musculocutaneous nerve.

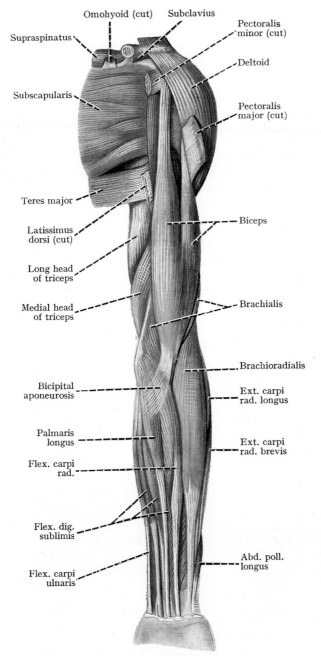

Supraspinatus

Omohyoid (cut) Subclavius

Pectoralis
minor (cut)

Subscapularis

Deltoid

Pectoralis
major (cut)

Teres major

Latissimus
dorsi (cut)

Biceps

Long head
of triceps

Medial head
of triceps

Brachialis

Brachioradialis

Bicipital
aponeurosis

Ext. carpi
rad. longus

Palmaris
longus

Ext. carpi
rad. brevis

Flex. carpi
rad.

Flex. dig.
sublimis

Abd. poll.
longus

Flex. carpi
ulnaris

FIG. 137.—The superficial muscles on the anterior aspect of the arm and forearm.
(After Sobotta.)

Action.   The biceps acts more powerfully as a supinator than as a flexor of the forearm for if the forearm be flexed in the pronated position the muscle is only feebly contracted, but contracts forcibly on supination.   The muscle is an important flexor when the forearm is supinated.

The long head of biceps also helps to retain the head of the humerus in contact with the glenoid cavity of the scapula during movements of the shoulder joint and it is also a flexor of that joint.

The bicipital aponeurosis holds down its tendon of insertion and protects the brachial artery and median nerve which lie immediately beneath it.

Brachialis (figs. 137 and 145)

Origin.   From the lower half of the anterior surface of the shaft of the humerus and the intermuscular septa.

Insertion.   Into the lower part of the anterior aspect of the coronoid process of the ulna.

Nerve supply.   Musculocutaneous and radial nerves.

Action.   This muscle is *the* great flexor of the forearm.   The triceps is its antagonist.

Triceps (figs. 137 and 145)

Origin.   *Long head* from the infraglenoid tubercle on the scapula and the capsule of the shoulder joint, *lateral head* by a linear origin from the upper half of the posterior surface of the shaft of the humerus, *medial head* by a broad origin from the posterior surface of the lower half of the shaft of the humerus and from the lateral and medial intermuscular septa.

Insertion.   The long and lateral heads form the superficial part of the muscle.   They fuse into a broad tendon which receives the medial head before the muscle passes to its insertion into the olecranon process of the ulna and into the fascia of the forearm.   This fascial insertion of the triceps is important for in fractures of the olecranon process it prevents the upward displacement of the upper fragment.

Nerve supply.   Radial nerve.

Action.   This muscle is *the* extensor of the forearm in which action it is assisted by the anconeus.   The brachialis is the natural antagonist of these muscles.

The Fascia of the Forearm and Hand

Certain specialised bands of deep fascia are seen in the vicinity of the wrist and hand, viz., the flexor and extensor retinacula, the palmar aponeurosis, the superficial transverse ligament of the palm and the osseo-aponeurotic sheaths of the digits.

The *flexor retinaculum* lies on the front of the wrist and converts the concave carpal arch into a tunnel.   It is attached medially to the pisiform and the hook of the hamate, laterally to the scaphoid and trapezium.   The attachment to the trapezium consists of a superficial and a deeper part.   The tunnel so formed is lined by synovial membrane through which passes the tendon of flexor carpi radialis (fig. 138).   Proximally the flexor retinaculum blends with the deep fascia of the forearm and distally with the palmar aponeurosis.   It receives part of the insertions of palmaris longus and flexor carpi ulnaris, whilst it is pierced by the flexor carpi radialis.   It gives origin

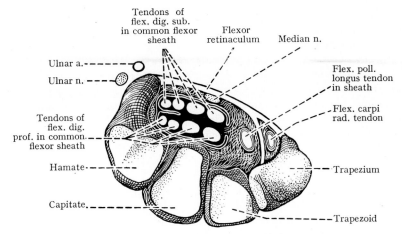

Fig. 138.—The flexor retinaculum (diagrammatic).

to all the short muscles of the thumb and little finger, except the abductor digiti minimi, and also to the palmaris brevis. On it lie the ulnar artery and nerve covered by a further band of deep fascia, whilst lying in the carpal tunnel beneath the ligament are the tendons of flexores sublimis, profundus and pollicis longus, and also the median nerve.

The *extensor retinaculum* lies on the dorsum of the wrist and is attached medially to the styloid process of the ulna and to the triquetral and pisiform bones and laterally to the distal end of the radius.   It converts the grooves on the distal ends of the radius and ulna into six separate tunnels by sending down septa which are attached to the adjacent ridges.   Details of these tunnels have already been described (see p. 47).

The Palmar Aponeurosis (fig. 146) is triangular in shape, with an apex which receives part of the insertion of palmaris longus and a base which divides at the bases of the fingers into four slips.   Each slip divides into two bands, one passing superficially to the skin and the other deeply into the palm where it diverges around the flexor tendons, before merging with the deep transverse ligament of the palm and the osseo-aponeurotic sheath of the digits.   These fascial slips are attached to the whole length of the margins of the proximal phalanx and to the margins of the proximal end of the middle phalanx of each finger.   This is a point of some practical importance for chronic inflammation of the palmar fascia (due to irritation) may give rise to a Dupuytren's contraction in which the metacarpophalangeal and proximal interphalangeal joints are flexed and the distal interphalangeal joint extended.   This condition usually affects the ring finger.

The palmar aponeurosis blends with the deep fascia covering the thenar and hypothenar eminences and from the union of these fascial bands septa pass deeply into the palm dividing it into three palmar spaces.

The *superficial transverse metacarpal ligaments* (fig. 146) pass transversely in the superficial fascia across the palm on a level with the heads of the metacarpal bones.

The *osseo-aponeurotic sheaths of the digits* will be discussed with the synovial sheaths of the flexor tendons (*q.v.*).

The Muscles on the anterior aspect of the Forearm comprise a superficial group consisting of *flexor carpi radialis, palmaris longus, flexor carpi ulnaris* and *pronator teres*; an intermediate group consisting of *flexor digitorum, sublimis* and a deep group consisting of *flexor digitorum profundus, flexor pollicis longus* and *pronator quadratus*.

Flexor Carpi Radialis (fig. 137)

Origin.   From the common flexor tendon.

Insertion.   Its long tendon pierces the flexor retinaculum and runs in a groove on the trapezium bone to reach its insertion into the bases of the second and third metacarpal bones.

Nerve supply.   Median nerve.

Action.   Flexes and abducts the hand.

Palmaris Longus (fig. 137)

This is a vestigial muscle, often absent.

Origin.   From the common flexor tendon.

Insertion.   Into the palmar fascia and flexor retinaculum.

Nerve supply.   Median nerve.

Action.   Makes tense the palmar fascia and flexes the hand.

Flexor Carpi Ulnaris (figs. 137 and 139)

Origin.   The muscle arises by two heads—*humeral head* from the common flexor tendon and an *ulnar head* from the medial aspect of the olecranon process, the capsule of the elbow joint and from the aponeurosis on the posterior border of the ulna.

Insertion.   The two heads merge into a long tendon which passes to be inserted into the pisiform bone, the hook of the hamate and the base of the fifth metacarpal bone.

Nerve supply.   Ulnar nerve.

Action.   Flexes and adducts the hand.

Pronator Teres (fig. 139)

Origin.   The muscle arises by two heads—a large *humeral head* from the common flexor tendon, and from the medial epicondyle of the humerus; and a small *ulnar head* from the middle facet on the medial border of the coronoid process of the ulna.   A tearing of the ulnar head of pronator teres is the cause of tennis elbow.

Insertion. Into the pronator tuberosity on the lateral aspect of the shaft of the radius.

Nerve supply. Median nerve.

Action. Flexes and pronates the forearm.

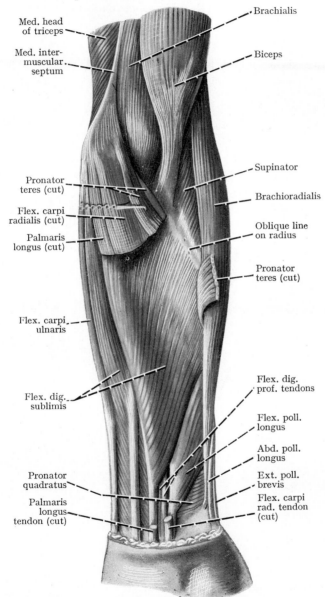

Med. head of triceps

Med. inter-muscular septum

Brachialis

Biceps

Pronator teres (cut)

Flex. carpi radialis (cut)

Palmaris longus (cut)

Flex. carpi ulnaris

Flex. dig. sublimis

Pronator quadratus

Palmaris longus tendon (cut)

Supinator

Brachioradialis

Oblique line on radius

Pronator teres (cut)

Flex. dig. prof. tendons

Flex. poll. longus

Abd. poll. longus

Ext. poll. brevis

Flex. carpi rad. tendon (cut)

Fig. 139.—The muscles of the anterior aspect of the forearm (deeper layer). (After Sobotta.)

Flexor Digitorum Sublimis (fig. 139)

Origin. The muscle arises by two heads—a *humero-ulnar head* from the common flexor tendon, from the upper facet on the medial margin of the coronoid process of the ulna and from the medial ligament of the elbow joint; and a *radial head* from the oblique line on the shaft of the radius.

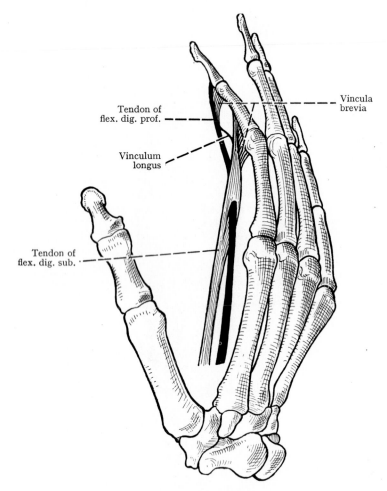

Tendon of flex. dig. prof.

Vinculum longus

Tendon of flex. dig. sub.

Vincula brevia

FIG. 140.—Showing the relationship of a tendon of flexor sublim is with that of profundus as they pass to their insertions.

Insertion. The muscle divides into four tendons which pass beneath the flexor retinaculum to be inserted into the fingers. On reaching the proximal phalanges, each tendon divides, then reunites and finally divides again to be inserted into the sides of the middle phalanx. The corresponding tendon of the flexor digitorum profundus passes through the division to be inserted into the distal phalanx. In this way the tendons of sublimis form levers for the tendons of profundus which considerably enhance their pulling power (fig. 140).

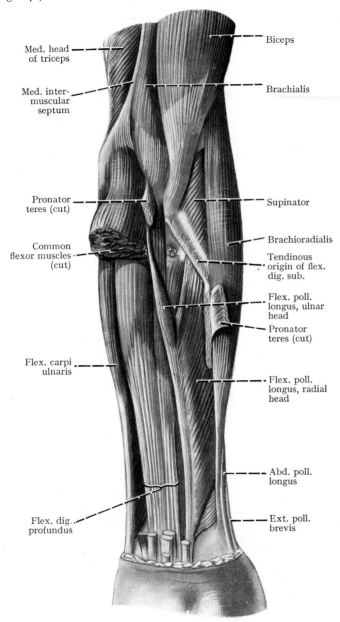

Med. head of triceps

Med. intermuscular septum

Pronator teres (cut)

Common flexor muscles (cut)

Flex. carpi ulnaris

Flex. dig. profundus

Biceps

Brachialis

Supinator

Brachioradialis

Tendinous origin of flex. dig. sub.

Flex. poll. longus, ulnar head

Pronator teres (cut)

Flex. poll. longus, radial head

Abd. poll. longus

Ext. poll. brevis

FIG. 141.—The muscles of the anterior aspect of the forearm (deepest layer). (After Sobotta.)

These tendons are bound to the digits by bands of fibrous tissue called vincula which carry blood vessels to the tendons (fig. 140).

Nerve supply. Median nerve.

Action. Flexes the middle and proximal phalanges of the fingers and also assists in flexing the wrist.

Flexor Digitorum Profundus (fig. 141)

Origin. From the upper two-thirds of the anterior and medial surfaces of the shaft of the ulna, from the aponeurosis on the dorsal border of that bone and from the interosseous membrane.

Insertion. The muscle divides into four tendons which pass beneath the flexor retinaculum. Each tendon passes through a division in the corresponding tendon of sublimis to be inserted into the base of the distal phalanx. These tendons are bound to the digits by vincula (fig. 140).

Nerve supply. Anterior interosseous branch of the median nerve supplies the lateral half of the muscle and the ulnar nerve the medial half.

Action. Flexes the phalanges and assists in flexing the wrist.

Flexor Pollicis Longus (fig. 141)

Origin. From the middle of the anterior surface of the shaft of the radius, from the interosseous membrane and sometimes from the lowest facet on the medial border of the coronoid process of the ulna.

Insertion. This is a typical unipennate muscle the tendon of which passes beneath the flexor retinaculum to be inserted into the base of the distal phalanx of the thumb.

Nerve supply. Anterior interosseous branch of the median nerve.

Action. Flexes the distal phalanx of the thumb.

The Synovial Sheaths of the Flexor Tendons (figs. 142 and 146)

The tendons of flexores digitorum sublimis et profundus are enclosed in the *common flexor sheath*, the tendon of flexor pollicis longus is enclosed in a smaller tubular mucous sheath of its own. Sometimes these sheaths are separate but in most cases they communicate beneath the flexor retinaculum. They commence about 2·5 cm. proximal to the flexor retinaculum and the sheath surrounding the flexor pollicis longus tendon extends as far as the insertion of that tendon into the base of the distal phalanx of the thumb. That part of the common flexor sheath which surrounds the tendons of sublimis and profundus passing to the 2nd, 3rd and 4th digits, ends at the middle of the palm, but the portion which surrounds the tendons to the 5th digit is carried with the tendon of profundus to the base of the distal phalanx of that digit. The tendons to the 2nd, 3rd and 4th digits on reaching the fingers are enclosed in *synovial sheaths* (figs. 142 and 146) which are entirely separate from the common flexor sheath. The tendons in the fingers and their covering synovial sheaths run in *osseo-aponeurotic canals*. These are formed behind by the phalanges and in front by fibrous sheaths arching over the tendons and attached to the margins of the bone.

An infected synovial sheath of the little finger or thumb is likely to be much more serious than an infection of the other digits since the infection may extend rapidly into the hand and forearm.

An adhesion between a tendon and its sheath is the cause of trigger finger.

Pronator Quadratus (fig. 139)

Origin. From the lowest quarter of the anterior surface of the shaft of the ulna.

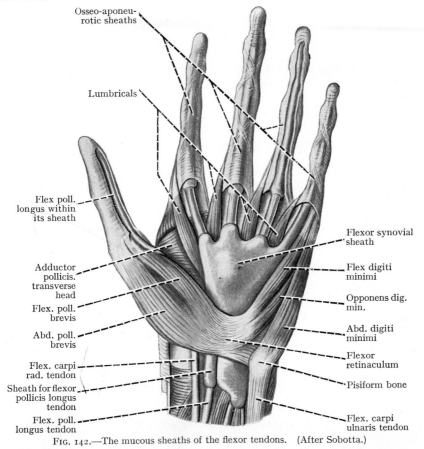

Osseo-aponeu-
rotic sheaths

Lumbricals

Flex poll.
longus within
its sheath

Flexor synovial
sheath

Adductor
pollicis.
transverse
head

Flex digiti
minimi

Flex. poll.
brevis

Opponens dig.
min.

Abd. poll.
brevis

Abd. digiti
minimi

Flex. carpi
rad. tendon

Flexor
retinaculum

Sheath for flexor
pollicis longus
tendon

Pisiform bone

Flex. poll.
longus tendon

Flex. carpi
ulnaris tendon

FIG. 142.—The mucous sheaths of the flexor tendons. (After Sobotta.)

Insertion. Into the distal quarter of the anterior surface of the shaft of the radius.

Nerve supply. Anterior interosseous branch of the median nerve.

Action. Pronates the forearm.

Muscles on the posterior aspect of the Forearm comprise a superficial group consisting of *brachioradialis, extensores carpi radialis longus et brevis, extensor digitorum, extensor digiti minimi, extensor carpi ulnaris* and *anconeus*—a deep group consisting of *supinator, abductor pollicis longus, extensor pollicis longus, extensor pollicis brevis* and *extensor indicis.*

Brachioradialis (figs. 137, 139 and 141)

Origin. From the lateral supracondylar ridge on the humerus and the lateral intermuscular septum.

Insertion. Into the base of the radial styloid process.

Nerve supply. Radial nerve.

Action. This muscle is a pure flexor of the forearm. It can, however, assist in restoring the forearm to the mid-position from either full pronation or full supination.

Extensor Carpi Radialis Longus (figs. 137 and 143)

Origin. From the lateral supracondylar ridge on the humerus and the lateral intermuscular septum (below brachioradialis).

Insertion. Into the posterior aspect of the base of the second metacarpal bone.

Nerve supply. Radial nerve.

Action. Extends and abducts the hand. This muscle with the brevis is frequently called upon to act synergically as an extensor of the wrist when the fist is clenched.

Extensor Carpi Radialis Brevis (figs. 137 and 143)

Origin. From the common extensor tendon and the lateral ligament of the elbow joint.

Insertion. Into the posterior aspect of the base of the third metacarpal bone chiefly, but it also gives a slip to the second metacarpal bone.

Nerve supply. Posterior interosseous branch of the radial nerve.

Action. Extends and abducts the hand.

Extensor Digitorum (figs. 143 and 144)

Origin. From the common extensor tendon.

Insertion. The muscle divides into four tendons, which pass to the dorsum of the fingers, mainly into the bases of the middle and distal phalanges but may give small slips into the bases of the proximal phalanges. On the proximal phalanx each tendon is incorporated in a fascial expansion called the *extensor expansion* which is common to the lumbricals and interossei.

Nerve supply. Posterior interosseous branch of the radial nerve.

Action. The main action of the muscle is to extend the phalanges but it also assists in extending the hand.

Fibrous slips connect the tendons to the 3rd, 4th and 5th digits so that it is impossible to fully extend these digits independently. The tendon to the index finger is independent of the other tendons and this allows greater freedom of movement of this digit.

Extensor Digiti Minimi (fig. 143)

Origin. From the common extensor tendon.

Insertion. Into the extensor expansion to the little finger.

Nerve supply. Posterior interosseous branch of the radial nerve.

Action. It has a feeble action in assisting to extend the little finger.

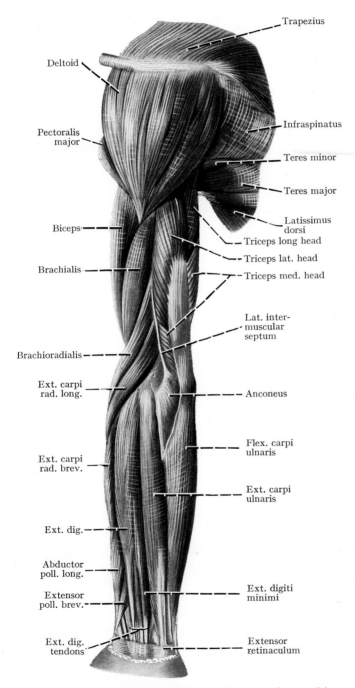

Deltoid

Pectoralis
major

Biceps

Brachialis

Brachioradialis

Ext. carpi
rad. long.

Ext. carpi
rad. brev.

Ext. dig.

Abductor
poll. long.

Extensor
poll. brev.

Ext. dig.
tendons

Trapezius

Infraspinatus

Teres minor

Teres major

Latissimus
dorsi

Triceps long head

Triceps lat. head

Triceps med. head

Lat. inter-
muscular
septum

Anconeus

Flex. carpi
ulnaris

Ext. carpi
ulnaris

Ext. digiti
minimi

Extensor
retinaculum

FIG. 143.—The superficial muscles of the posterior aspect of arm and forearm.
(After Sobotta.)

159

Extensor Carpi Ulnaris (fig. 143)

Origin. From the common extensor tendon and from the fibrous expansion on the posterior border of the ulna.

Insertion. Into the dorsal aspect of the base of the fifth metacarpal bone.

Nerve supply. Posterior interosseous branch of the radial nerve.

Action. Extends and adducts the hand.

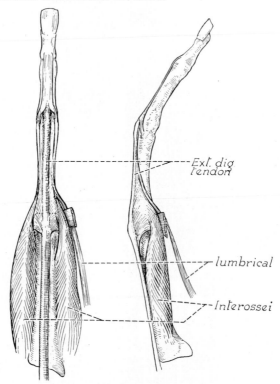

Ext. dig tendon

lumbrical

Interossei

FIG. 144.—The insertion of extensor digitorum.

Anconeus (figs. 143 and 145)

Origin. From the posterior aspect of the lateral epicondyle of humerus.

Insertion. Into the lateral surface of the olecranon process of the ulna.

Nerve supply. Radial nerve.

Action. Assists the triceps to extend the forearm.

Supinator (figs. 139, 141 and 145)

Origin. The muscle has an extensive origin—from the lateral condyle of the humerus, from the lateral ligament of the elbow joint, from the annular ligament and from the supinator crest and fossa on the ulna.

Insertion. The muscle winds round the lateral aspect of the upper part of the radius to be inserted into the neck and shaft as far down as the oblique line.

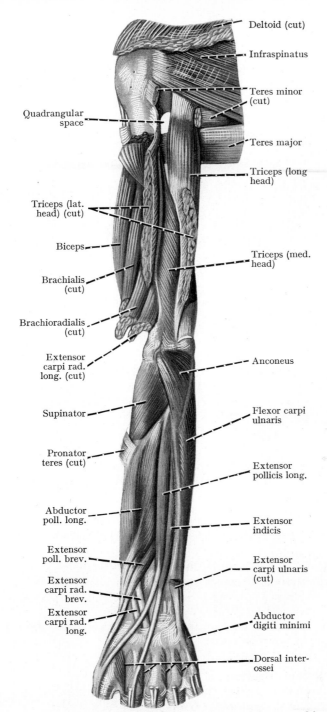

Deltoid (cut)

Infraspinatus

Teres minor (cut)

Quadrangular space

Teres major

Triceps (long head)

Triceps (lat. head) (cut)

Biceps

Brachialis (cut)

Triceps (med. head)

Brachioradialis (cut)

Extensor carpi rad. long. (cut)

Anconeus

Supinator

Flexor carpi ulnaris

Pronator teres (cut)

Extensor pollicis long.

Abductor poll. long.

Extensor indicis

Extensor poll. brev.

Extensor carpi ulnaris (cut)

Extensor carpi rad. brev.

Extensor carpi rad. long.

Abductor digiti minimi

Dorsal inter-ossei

FIG. 145.—The deep layer of the muscles on the dorsum of the arm and forearm. (After Sobotta.)

161

Nerve supply. Posterior interosseous branch of the radial nerve.
Action. Supinates the forearm.

Abductor Pollicis Longus (fig. 145).
Origin. From the middle of the posterior surface of the shaft of the ulna and radius and the intervening interosseous membrane.
Insertion. Into the dorsal aspect of the base of the first metacarpal bone.
Nerve supply. Posterior interosseous branch of the radial nerve.
Action. Abducts and extends the thumb at the carpometacarpal joint.

Extensor Pollicis Brevis (fig. 145)
Origin. From the posterior surface of the radius and adjacent interosseous membrane.
Insertion. Into the dorsal surface of the base of proximal phalanx of thumb.
Nerve supply. Posterior interosseous branch of the radial nerve.
Action. Extends the proximal phalanx of the thumb.
Note how the tendons of the abductor and the short extensor of the thumb run together (fig. 145) crossing first the insertion of brachioradialis and then the tendons of extensor carpi radialis longus and brevis.

Extensor Pollicis Longus (fig. 145)
Origin. From the posterior surface of the ulna and adjacent interosseous membrane.
Insertion. Into the dorsal surface of the base of distal phalanx of thumb.
Nerve supply. Posterior interosseous branch of the radial nerve.
Action. Extends the distal phalanx of the thumb.

Extensor Indicis
Origin. From the posterior surface of the ulna, below extensor pollicis longus.
Insertion. Into the extensor digitorum tendon to index finger.
Nerve Supply. Posterior interosseous branch of radial nerve.
Action. Assists in extending the index finger and wrist.

Short Muscles of the Hand include the muscles of the thenar and hypothenar eminences, the palmaris brevis, the interossei and the lumbricals.

Muscles of the Thenar Eminence

Abductor Pollicis Brevis (figs. 142 and 146)
Origin. From the scaphoid bone, the crest on the trapezium bone and the flexor retinaculum.
Insertion. Into the lateral aspect of the base of proximal phalanx of thumb.
Nerve supply. Median nerve.
Action. Abducts the thumb.

Flexor Pollicis Brevis (figs. 142 and 146)
Origin. The muscle arises from the crest on the trapezium bone and the flexor retinaculum.
Insertion. Into the lateral side of the base of proximal phalanx of thumb.

Nerve supply.   Median nerve.

Action.   Flexes the proximal phalanx of the thumb.

Opponens Pollicis (fig. 147)

Origin.   From the trapezium bone and the flexor retinaculum.

Insertion.   Into the lateral border of the shaft of the first metacarpal bone.

Nerve supply.   Median nerve.

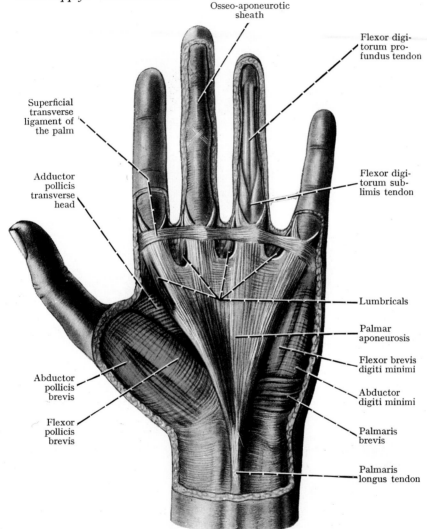

Osseo-aponeurotic
sheath

Flexor digi-
torum pro-
fundus tendon

Superficial
transverse
ligament of
the palm

Adductor
pollicis
transverse
head

Flexor digi-
torum sub-
limis tendon

Lumbricals

Palmar
aponeurosis

Flexor brevis
digiti minimi

Abductor
pollicis
brevis

Abductor
digiti minimi

Flexor
pollicis
brevis

Palmaris
brevis

Palmaris
longus tendon

FIG. 146.—The superficial dissection of the palm.   (After Sobotta.)

Action.   Draws the thumb medially and forwards across the hand and enables it to come into apposition with the bases of the other digits.   It enables the thumb to form one claw in "the pincer action" so essential in picking up objects.　This is one of the most important muscles in the body and when paralysed the usefulness of the upper limb is seriously impaired.

Adductor Pollicis (fig. 147)

Origin.　The muscle arises by two heads—an *oblique head* from the trapezoid and capitate bones and from the bases of the second and third metacarpal bones and from the tendon of flexor carpi radialis, and a *transverse head* from the palmar surface of the shaft of the third metacarpal bone.

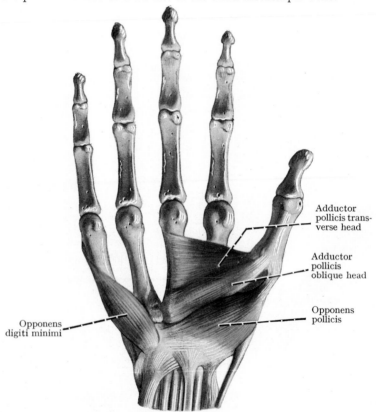

Adductor
pollicis trans-
verse head

Adductor
pollicis
oblique head

Opponens
pollicis

Opponens
digiti minimi

Fɪɢ. 147.—Dissection of the hand to show the deeper muscles of the thenar and hypothenar eminences.

Insertion.　Into the medial and lateral sides of the base of the proximal phalanx of the thumb.

Nerve supply.　Ulnar nerve.

Action.　Draws the thumb medially, flush with the palm of the hand.

Short Muscles of Little Finger

Abductor Digiti Minimi (fig. 146)

Origin.　From the pisiform bone, the tendon of flexor carpi ulnaris and the pisohamate ligament.

Insertion.   Into the medial aspect of the base of the proximal phalanx of the little finger.
Nerve supply.   Ulnar nerve.
Action.   Abducts the little finger.

Flexor Brevis Digiti Minimi (fig. 146)

Origin.   From the hook of the hamate and the flexor retinaculum.
Insertion.   Into the medial side of the base of the proximal phalanx of the little finger.
Nerve supply.   Ulnar nerve.
Action.   Helps to flex the little finger.

Opponens Digiti Minimi (fig. 147)

Origin.   From the hook of the hamate and the flexor retinaculum.
Insertion.   Into the medial side of the shaft of the fifth metacarpal bone.
Nerve supply.   Ulnar nerve.
Action.   Opposes the little finger to the thumb, thereby deepening the palm of the hand.

Short Muscle of Palm

Palmaris Brevis (fig. 146)

Origin.   This small muscle is not always present.   It arises from the flexor retinaculum and the palmar aponeurosis.
Insertion.   Into the skin of the palm.
Nerve supply.   Ulnar nerve.
Action.   Corrugates the skin at the base of the hypothenar eminence.

The Lumbrical Muscles (fig. 146)

Origin.   The lumbricals are four small worm-like muscles which arise in the middle of the palm from the tendons of flexor digitorum profundus.

The first and second lumbricals arise from the lateral aspect of the tendons to the index and middle fingers, the third and fourth lumbricals from the contiguous sides of the tendons to the middle, ring and little fingers.

Insertion.   Each muscle is inserted by a tendon into the lateral side of the corresponding extensor expansion and by a small slip into the base of the proximal phalanx.
Nerve supply.   The first and second lumbrical muscles are supplied by the median nerve, the third and fourth muscles by the ulnar nerve.
Action.   Assisted by the interossei, they flex the proximal phalanges of the fingers.

The Interossei (fig. 148)

Origin.   The interossei comprise four palmar and four dorsal muscles. They fill the spaces between the metacarpal bones.   The dorsal muscles arise by two heads and are much larger than the palmar which have one head only.   When it is remembered that the palmar muscles adduct the fingers towards the mid-line (i.e., towards the centre of the 3rd digit) and that the dorsal muscles abduct the fingers, including the middle finger from the midline, their precise attachments are not difficult to visualise.

The first palmar interosseous muscle arises from the medial side of the base of the first metacarpal bone, the second from the medial side of the shaft of the second metacarpal bone, the third and fourth from the lateral sides of the shafts of the fourth and fifth metacarpal bones.

The four dorsal interossei arise from the contiguous side of the first and second, second and third, third and fourth, and fourth and fifth metacarpal bones respectively.

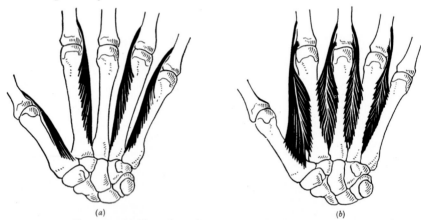

(a)   (b)

FIG. 148.—(a) The palmar interossei. (b) The dorsal interossei

Insertion. One muscle is inserted into the thumb—the first palmar interosseous and is attached to the medial side of the base of the proximal phalanx and to the capsule of the metacarpophalangeal joint. The second palmar interosseous is inserted into the medial side and the first dorsal interosseous into the lateral side of the base of the proximal phalanx of the index finger. The second and third dorsal interossei are inserted into the lateral and medial sides respectively of the base of the proximal phalanx of the middle finger. The third palmar interosseous is inserted into the lateral side and the fourth dorsal interosseous into the medial side of the base of the proximal phalanx of the ring finger. The fourth palmar interosseous is inserted into the lateral side of the base of the proximal phalanx of the little finger. All are inserted into the capsule of the metacarpophalangeal joint and the extensor expansion of the digit on which they act. These attachments will be more easily understood by consulting fig. 148.

Nerve supply. All the interossei are supplied by the ulnar nerve.

Action. While these muscles acting with the lumbricals flex the metacarpophalangeal joints the main action of the palmar interossei is to adduct the digits and that of the dorsal interossei to abduct the digits. It should be noted that they act to and from the middle finger which is in the neutral position.

The thumb and little finger have special abductors and the thumb a special adductor.

THE FASCIA OF THE BUTTOCK AND THIGH

The superficial fascia in the buttock is unusually thick and is impregnated with large quantities of fat. This feature is more pronounced in women than men.

The deep fascia of the buttock and thigh is known as the *fascia lata*. As in other parts of the body, it dips down between the muscles to form septa which blend with the periosteum. Two of these septa, larger than the rest, are attached to the supracondylar ridges on the femur and form the *lateral and medial intermuscular septa* which divide the thigh into anterior and posterior compartments.

Another specialised band of deep fascia, known as the *iliotibial tract*, lies on the lateral aspect of the thigh and is attached above to the iliac crest and below to the lateral condyle of the tibia. It ensheathes the tensor fasciae latae muscle and receives the major insertion of gluteus maximus.

The fascia lata is perforated by the long saphenous vein at a point 3·5 cm. below and lateral to the pubic tubercle. This oval opening in the fascia lata is called the *saphenous opening* (fig. 200). It is important because it overlies the femoral sheath, and through it a femoral hernia, when present, emerges.

THE MUSCLES OF THE LOWER EXTREMITY

Muscles on the front of the thigh comprise *sartorius, iliacus, psoas, pectineus* and the *quadriceps femoris* muscles.

Sartorius (fig. 149)

Origin. The sartorius is a thin strap-like muscle—the longest in the body. It arises from the anterior superior spine on the innominate bone and the notch below.

Insertion. The muscle fibres are directed downwards and medially and pass to a semilunar insertion on the medial aspect of the upper part of the shaft of the tibia which overhangs the tendons of gracilis and semitendinosus.

Nerve supply. Femoral nerve.

Action. Flexes, abducts and laterally rotates the thigh. Flexes and medially rotates the leg. It helps to perform a wide range of movements but its power is limited.

Iliacus and Psoas (figs. 124 and 149)

Origin of Iliacus. From the iliac fossa, the ala of the sacrum, the iliolumbar ligament and the anterior ligaments of the sacro-iliac joint.

Origin of Psoas. From the bodies and transverse processes of all the lumbar vertebrae and from the intervertebral discs, including that between the twelfth thoracic and first lumbar vertebrae, from the aponeurotic arches covering the lumbar vessels.

Insertion. The tendon of iliacus fuses with that of psoas to form the iliopsoas muscle which runs beneath the inguinal ligament and immediately in front of the hip joint to reach its insertion into the lesser trochanter and adjacent shaft of the femur. A bursa intervenes between the psoas and the hip joint (fig. 149).

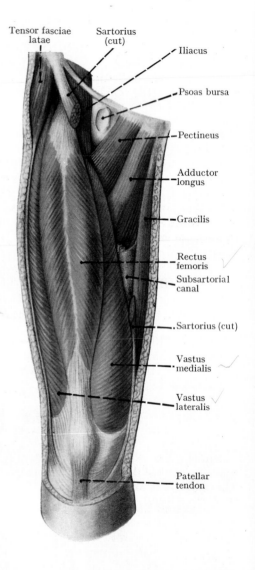

FIG. 149.— The superficial muscles on the front of the thigh: psoas has been removed to show the bursa.
(After Spalteholz.)

Tensor fasciae latae

Sartorius (cut)

Iliacus

Psoas bursa

Pectineus

Adductor longus

Gracilis

Rectus femoris

Subsartorial canal

Sartorius (cut)

Vastus medialis

Vastus lateralis

Patellar tendon

Nerve supply. Femoral nerve (to iliacus) and the second, third and fourth lumbar nerves directly (to psoas).

Action. The combined muscle is by far the most powerful flexor of the thigh when the lower limb is free from the ground. It also assists in medial rotation. When rising from the supine position the muscle flexes the trunk on the thigh.

Certain pathological conditions in the abdomen, e.g., an acutely inflamed appendix, or a tubercular infection of the lower thoracic or lumbar vertebrae occasionally cause the muscle to go into spasm, when the lower limb is characteristically flexed. Extension of the lower limb under such circumstances causes the contracted psoas to arch the lumbar vertebrae (lordosis).

The fascia ensheathing the muscle, known as the *psoas sheath*, commences in the upper abdomen as the medial arcuate ligament (fig. 124) and is carried down with the muscle to its insertion into the lesser trochanter. A tubercular infection (caries) of the lower thoracic or lumbar vertebrae may give rise to an abscess (cold abscess) which has a tendency to point anywhere along the psoas sheath.   Not infrequently it points below the inner end of the inguinal ligament opposite the lesser trochanter.

Psoas Minor
Origin.   From the bodies of the twelfth thoracic and first lumbar vertebrae and the intervening disc.
Insertion.   Into the pelvic brim and into the fascia covering iliopsoas muscle.
Nerve supply.   First lumbar nerve.
Action.   It is a vestigial muscle, absent in 50 per cent of persons.   It has a feeble action in flexing the vertebral column.

Pectineus (fig. 149)
Origin.   From the pectineal line and superior ramus of the pubis.
Insertion.   Into the upper part of the linea aspera just below the lesser trochanter.
Nerve supply.   Femoral and sometimes obturator nerves.
Action.   The muscle is chiefly a flexor of the thigh but assists in adduction and lateral rotation.

The Quadriceps Femoris Muscles comprise *rectus femoris, vastus lateralis, vastus medialis* and *vastus intermedius.*   They have a common insertion, nerve supply and action.

Rectus Femoris (fig. 149)
Origin.   This large bipennate muscle whose fibres diverge from a central tendon, arises from the innominate bone by two heads—a *straight head* from the anterior inferior spine and a *reflected head* from a rough area above the acetabulum.   The muscle also arises from the iliofemoral ligament of the hip joint which lies immediately between the two heads of the muscle.

Vastus Lateralis (fig. 149)
Origin.   From the lateral lip of the linea aspera extending to the front of the bone as far as the intertrochanteric line and from the lateral intermuscular septum.   Its fibres pass downwards and medially to their insertion.

Vastus Medialis (fig. 149)
Origin.   From the medial lip of the linea aspera extending to the front of the bone as far as the lower part of the intertrochanteric line and from the medial intermuscular septum.   Its fibres pass downwards and laterally to their insertion, but its lower fibres are almost horizontal in direction.   These lower fibres arise from the lower part of the tendon of adductor magnus and prevent the patella from being pulled laterally during contraction of quadriceps.   They atrophy rapidly in affections of the knee joint.

Vastus Intermedius
Origin.   From the upper two-thirds of the anterior and lateral surfaces of the shaft of the femur and from the lateral intermuscular septum.
Insertion of Quadriceps Femoris.   The quadriceps converge into a tendon called the ligamentum patellae which is inserted into the upper part of the

tuberosity of the tibia and from here expansions of the tendon called the *patellar retinacula* reinforce the capsule of the knee joint.

Nerve supply. All the quadriceps are supplied by the femoral nerve.

Action. These muscles are powerful extensors of the leg and are the main factors in the maintenance of the erect posture. The rectus femoris is also a powerful flexor of the thigh.

The patella is a sesamoid bone developed in the quadriceps tendon. It causes the quadriceps to pull on the tibia at an angle and thus considerably increases its power. Should the quadriceps contract forcibly at a time when the hamstrings fail to relax fully, the power of the quadriceps may fracture the patella.

Articularis genu (fig. 107)

This muscle is composed of a few detached fibres from vastus intermedius although it is not part of the quadriceps. It is a small muscle with an important function.

Origin. From the lower part of the anterior aspect of the shaft of the femur.

Insertion. Into that part of the synovial membrane of the knee joint which forms the suprapatellar bursa.

Nerve supply. Femoral nerve.

Action. It supports the suprapatellar bursa.

Muscles on the medial aspect of the thigh

This group comprises the *gracilis, adductor longus, adductor brevis* and *adductor magnus.*

Gracilis (figs. 149 and 151) is the most medial muscle of the thigh.

Origin. From the lateral surface of the inferior ramus of the pubis and ischium.

Insertion. Into the upper part of the medial aspect of the shaft of the tibia.

Nerve supply. Obturator nerve.

Action. The muscle acts primarily on the knee joint, flexing the leg. It is also a feeble flexor and adductor of the thigh.

Adductor Longus (fig. 150)

Origin. From the angle between the superior and inferior rami of the pubis. Its rounded tendon of origin is a well-defined landmark on the medial aspect of the upper part of the thigh.

Insertion. Its fibres are directed downwards, laterally and posteriorly into the medial lip of the linea aspera.

Nerve supply. Obturator nerve.

Action. Adducts the thigh.

Adductor Brevis (fig. 150)

Origin. From the inferior ramus of the pubis.

Insertion. Into the linea aspera.

Nerve supply. Obturator nerve.

Action. Adducts the thigh.

Adductor Magnus (fig. 150)

Origin. From the inferior rami of the pubis and ischium extending on to the ischial tuberosity (hamstring portion).

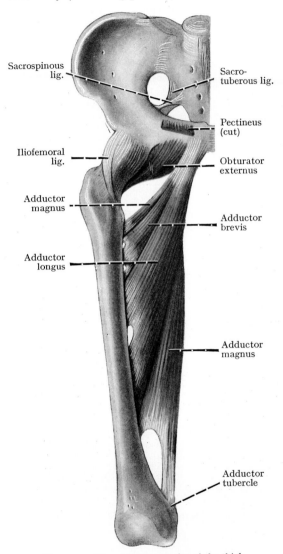

Sacrospinous lig.

Sacro-tuberous lig.

Pectineus (cut)

Iliofemoral lig.

Obturator externus

Adductor magnus

Adductor brevis

Adductor longus

Adductor magnus

Adductor tubercle

FIG. 150.—The adductor muscles of the thigh.

Note the opening in the adductor magnus for the femoral vessels. The smaller openings in adductors longus and brevis are for perforating arteries.

Insertion. The muscle fans out to an insertion which occupies almost the whole length of the femur. The adductor portion is attached to the middle lip of the linea aspera extending from the quadrate tubercle above, to the medial supracondylar ridge below. The hamstring portion passes into the adductor tubercle. There is a gap in its attachment to the supracondylar ridge where the femoral vessels pierce the insertion of the muscles as they pass into the popliteal fossa.

Nerve supply. The obturator nerve supplies the adductor portion and the sciatic nerve, the hamstring portion.

Action. This muscle is the most powerful adductor of the thigh. Its hamstring portion materially assists in extending the thigh.

The Muscles of the Buttock comprise the *gluteus maximus, gluteus medius* and *gluteus minimus*, the *tensor fasciae latae*, the deeply placed lateral rotators of the thigh, viz., the *piriformis, obturator internus et gemelli, quadratus femoris* and *obturator externus*.

Gluteus Maximus (figs. 135 and 151)

Origin. From the dorsal surface of the ilium behind the posterior gluteal line, from the adjacent posterior surface of the sacrum and from the sacrotuberous ligament.

Insertion. Its fibres pass downwards and laterally to be inserted into the iliotibial tract of fascia lata (chiefly) and into the gluteal tuberosity on the femur.

Nerve supply. Inferior gluteal nerve.

Action. The gluteus maximus is the coarsest muscle in the body. It is the main antagonist of the iliopsoas for it is the most powerful extensor of the thigh and it is also an extensor of the trunk, e.g., when raising the trunk from the sitting or stooping positions.

When rising from the sitting position, the thigh is extended on the leg by the action of quadriceps acting in reverse and the trunk on the thigh by the action of the gluteus maximus (*vide* p. 326).

The muscle is also a lateral rotator of the thigh, and since it has an extensive insertion into the fascia lata it helps to maintain the stability of the extended knee joint.

Gluteus Medius (fig. 151)

Origin. From the dorsal surface of the ilium between the middle and posterior gluteal lines.

Insertion. Its fibres pass downwards and slightly backwards into the oblique line on the lateral aspect of the greater trochanter.

Nerve supply. Superior gluteal nerve.

Action. Acting with gluteus minimus and tensor fasciae latae, the muscle abducts the thigh (see also p. 174).

Gluteus Minimus (fig. 151)

Origin. From the dorsal surface of the ilium between the middle and inferior gluteal lines.

Insertion. Its fibres pass downwards and slightly backwards into the anterior surface of the greater trochanter and the capsule of the hip joint.

Nerve supply. Superior gluteal nerve.

Action. Abducts the thigh (see also p. 174).

Tensor Fasciae Latae (fig. 149)

Origin. From the dorsum of the ilium near the anterior superior spine.

Insertion. Into the iliotibial tract of fascia lata.

Nerve supply. Superior gluteal nerve.

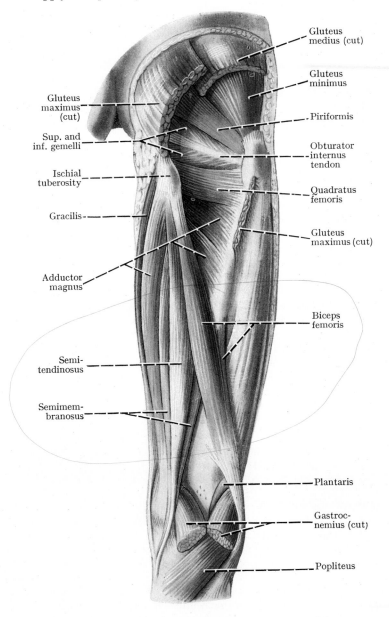

FIG. 151.—The muscles on the posterior aspect of the thigh.

Action. Makes tense the fascia lata and abducts the thigh. It probably modifies the action of gluteus maximus by correcting the obliquity of its pull.

In the normal standing position the gluteal muscles and tensor fasciae latae acting in reverse tend to steady the pelvis on the lower limb. Maintenance of the erect position is due to a co-ordination between these muscles and the flexors of the hip.

The gluteus medius and minimus exercise a most important function in walking. As each limb is successively raised from the ground they pull the pelvis downwards towards the supporting side and the side-flexors of the trunk raise it slightly on the opposite side (*vide* p. 325). This is an essential movement in preserving balance. Paralysis of gluteus medius and minimus is the most serious muscular disability occurring in the region of the hip (Gray).

Piriformis (fig. 151)

Origin. From the pelvic surface of the 2nd, 3rd and 4th sacral vertebrae, from the upper border of the greater sciatic notch and from the sacrotuberous ligament.

Insertion. Its fibres pass downwards and laterally into the superior border of the greater trochanter of the femur behind obturator internus et gemelli.

Nerve supply. S1 and 2.

Action. Laterally rotates the thigh.

Obturator Internus et gemelli (fig. 151)

These three muscles have separate origins but a common insertion.

Origin. *Obturator internus* from the pelvic surface of the obturator membrane and the adjacent bone extending as far back as the greater sciatic notch. *Superior gemellus* from the lateral surface of the ischial spine. *Inferior gemellus*, by a small crescentic origin from the margin of the lesser sciatic notch.

Insertion. The tendon of obturator internus passes out of the pelvis through the lesser sciatic foramen where it is joined by the two gemelli and the three muscles are inserted by a common tendon into the superior border of the greater trochanter of the femur in front of the piriformis.

Nerve supply. L4, 5 and S1 supply inferior gemellus. L5, S1 and 2 supply superior gemellus and obturator internus.

Action. All these muscles laterally rotate the thigh.

Quadratus Femoris (fig. 151)

Origin. From the body of the ischium, lateral to the tuberosity.

Insertion. Into the quadrate tubercle on the intertrochanteric crest.

Nerve supply. L4, 5 and S1.

Action. Laterally rotates the thigh.

Obturator Externus (fig. 150)

Origin. From the obturator membrane and the adjacent margin of the lateral surfaces of the inferior rami of the pubis and ischium.

Insertion. Into the trochanteric fossa on the medial aspect of the greater trochanter.

Nerve supply. Obturator nerve.

Action. Laterally rotates the thigh.

The Hamstring Muscles comprise *biceps femoris, semimembranosus, semitendinosus* and the smaller portion of *adductor magnus.*

Biceps (fig. 151)

Origin. The muscle arises by two heads, a *long head* from the ischial tuberosity in common with the tendon of origin of semitendinosus. The sacrotuberous ligament is believed to be the divorced tendon of long head of biceps and the muscle frequently takes origin from it. The *short head* arises from the linea aspera on the femur, below the gluteal tuberosity and from the lateral intermuscular septum.

Insertion. Into the head of the fibula and adjacent lateral condyle of the tibia. The lateral ligament of the knee joint divides the tendon of insertion into two parts (figs. 104 and 106).

Nerve supply. The medial popliteal portion of the sciatic nerve supplies the long head, and the lateral popliteal portion the short head.

Action. Flexes the leg and rotates it laterally. The long head also extends the thigh.

Semimembranosus (fig. 151)

Origin. From the ischial tuberosity.

Insertion. Into a groove on the posterior surface of the medial condyle of the tibia. From its tendinous insertion it gives off four fascial slips—one passes to the deep fascia of the leg, another to the medial ligament of the knee joint, a third covers the popliteus muscle and passes to its attachment into the soleal line, while a fourth slip runs obliquely upwards and laterally to form the oblique ligament which reinforces the capsule of the knee joint posteriorly.

Nerve supply. The medial popliteal portion of the sciatic nerve.

Action. Flexes and medially rotates the leg and extends the thigh.

Semitendinosus (fig. 151)

Origin. From the ischial tuberosity by a tendon common to it and biceps.

Insertion. Into the upper part of the medial aspect of the shaft of the tibia.

Nerve supply. The medial popliteal portion of the sciatic nerve.

Action. Flexes and medially rotates the leg and extends the thigh.

The hamstring muscles have a rich blood supply from the four perforating arteries, branches of the profunda femoris which reach the posterior compartment of the thigh by perforating the adductors brevis and magnus (fig. 150). They end in the vastus lateralis.

The Fascia of the Leg and Foot

The deep fascia of the leg and foot envelops the limb and forms septa between the muscles. It also forms thickened bands in the region of the ankle joint, viz., the *superior extensor retinaculum* which stretches between the distal ends of the tibia and fibula; the *inferior extensor retinaculum*, a Y-shaped band, the stem of which is attached to the calcaneum and forms a loop for the tendons of extensor digitorum longus and peroneus tertius thus holding them in position when the foot is moved; the upper limb of the Y is attached to the medial malleolus, while the lower limb blends with the plantar fascia on the medial aspect of the foot, both limbs passing over the tendons of the extensor hallucis longus and tibialis anterior (fig. 152). Other thickened bands of deep fascia in this region are the *flexor retinaculum* (fig. 154), which binds the tendons on the inner side of the ankle; the *superior peroneal retinaculum* (fig. 153), which binds the tendons on the outer side of the ankle; and the *inferior peroneal retinaculum* (fig. 153), which binds the tendons of the peroneus longus and peroneus brevis to the peroneal tubercle.

The Plantar aponeurosis (fig. 155) is attached to the tubercles on the calcaneum and passing forward into the sole of the foot divides into five septa. Each septum divides into two slips, a superficial slip which passes to the skin and a deep slip which splits to enclose the flexor tendons before merging with the deep transverse ligament of the sole. The plantar aponeurosis is thick and powerful and helps to preserve the arches of the foot.

Muscles on the front of the Leg comprise the *tibialis anterior, extensor digitorum longus, extensor hallucis longus* and *peroneus tertius*.

Tibialis Anterior (fig. 152)

Origin. From the upper two-thirds of the lateral surface of the tibia and from the interosseous membrane.

Insertion. Into the medial surface of the medial cuneiform bone and the base of the adjacent first metatarsal.

Nerve supply. Anterior tibial nerve.

Action. Dorsiflexes as it inverts the foot and so is the antagonist of peroneus longus.

Extensor Digitorum Longus (fig. 152)

Origin. From the upper two-thirds of the anterior surface of the fibula and adjacent lateral condyle of the tibia and from the interosseous membrane.

Insertion. The muscle divides on the dorsum of the foot into four tendons which are inserted into the middle and distal phalanges of the four outer toes, *c.f.*, the extensor digitorum in the hand.

Nerve supply. Anterior tibial nerve.

Action. Extends the toes. Dorsiflexes the foot.

Extensor Hallucis Longus (fig. 152)

Origin. From the middle of the anterior surface of the shaft of the fibula and the interosseous membrane.

Insertion. Into the base of the distal phalanx of the great toe.

Nerve supply. Anterior tibial nerve.

Action. Extends the great toe, dorsiflexes the foot and assists in inversion.

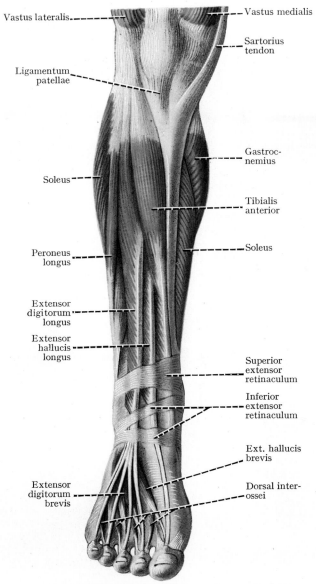

Vastus lateralis

Vastus medialis

Ligamentum patellae

Sartorius tendon

Soleus

Gastroc-nemius

Peroneus longus

Tibialis anterior

Extensor digitorum longus

Soleus

Extensor hallucis longus

Superior extensor retinaculum

Inferior extensor retinaculum

Extensor digitorum brevis

Ext. hallucis brevis

Dorsal inter-ossei

FIG. 152.—The superficial muscles on the front of the leg.

Peroneus Tertius (fig. 153)

This muscle is morphologically part of the extensor digitorum brevis which in some mammals arises in the leg.

Origin. From the lower third of the anterior surface of the shaft of the fibula below the extensor digitorum longus.

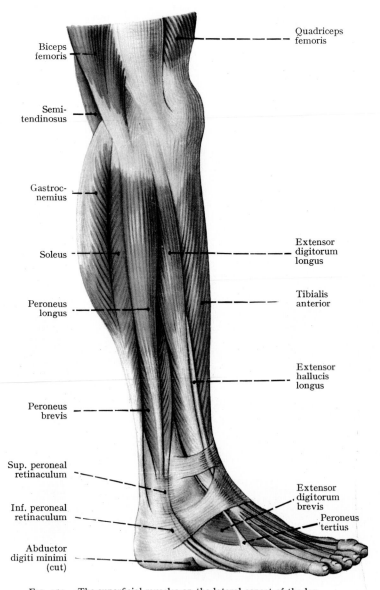

Biceps
femoris

Semi-
tendinosus

Gastroc-
nemius

Soleus

Peroneus
longus

Peroneus
brevis

Sup. peroneal
retinaculum

Inf. peroneal
retinaculum

Abductor
digiti minimi
(cut)

Quadriceps
femoris

Extensor
digitorum
longus

Tibialis
anterior

Extensor
hallucis
longus

Extensor
digitorum
brevis

Peroneus
tertius

FIG. 153.—The superficial muscles on the lateral aspect of the leg.

Insertion. Into the medial side of the dorsal surface of the base of the fifth metatarsal bone.

Nerve supply. Anterior tibial nerve.

Action. Dorsiflexes and assists in everting the foot.

Muscles on the lateral aspect of the Leg comprise *peroneus longus* and *brevis*.

Peroneus Longus (figs. 112 and 153)

Origin. From the upper two-thirds of the lateral surface of the fibula, rarely extending to the lateral condyle of the tibia.

Insertion. Into the lateral aspect of the plantar surface of the medial cuneiform bone and first metatarsal. The tendon of this muscle lies behind the lateral malleolus, posterior to the brevis, it then passes below the peroneal tubercle and runs in a groove on the plantar surface of the cuboid. This groove is converted into a tunnel by the long plantar ligament which spans it. The insertion of peroneus longus is almost continuous with that of the tendon of tibialis anterior and the two tendons are said to contain the foot "within a stirrup."

Nerve supply. Musculocutaneous nerve.

Action. Plantarflexes as it everts the foot and so is the antagonist of tibialis anterior.

Peroneus Brevis (fig. 153)

Origin. From the lower two thirds of the lateral surface of the fibula.

Insertion. The tendon of peroneus brevis is in direct contact with the lateral malleolus whence it passes forwards above the peroneal tubercle to be attached to the base of the fifth metatarsal bone.

Nerve supply. Musculocutaneous nerve.

Action. Plantarflexes as it everts the foot.

Superficial Muscles of the Calf comprise the two heads of *gastrocnemius* and the *soleus* muscles forming the triceps surae and the *plantaris*.

Gastrocnemius (figs. 153 and 154)

Origin. The muscle arises by two heads—medial and lateral—from the posterior aspect of the medial and lateral condyles of the femur respectively and from the capsule of the knee joint.

Soleus (figs. 153 and 154)

Origin. The muscle has a "∩-shaped" origin—from the upper third of the posterior surface of the fibula, from the soleal line and medial border of tibia and from the fibrous arch between the two bones.

Insertion. Gastrocnemius and soleus fuse to form a common tendon in the lower third of the back of the calf called the tendo-calcaneus which is inserted into the posterior surface of the calcaneum. It is an immensely powerful muscle and with one leg off the ground can raise the heel and shift the weight of the body on to the toes.

Nerve supply. The medial popliteal nerve supplies both muscles.

Action. Both muscles plantarflex the foot and gastrocnemius also flexes the knee.

Plantaris (figs. 151 and 154)

The plantaris is a vestigial muscle comparable to the palmaris longus but is rarely absent. It has a small fleshy belly, about the size of a lumbrical

muscle, but its tendon is easily the longest in the body.   It was once connected with the plantar fascia but owing to the growth backwards of the
calcaneum in man, the two parts have become separated.

Origin.   From the posterior aspect of the lateral condyle of the femur

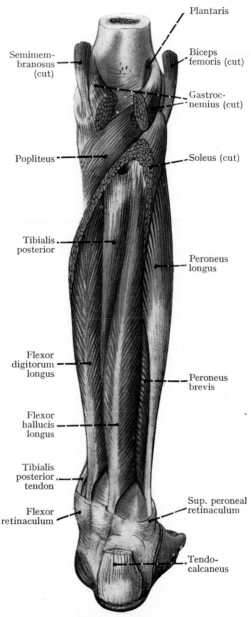

Plantaris

Semimem-
branosus
(cut)

Biceps
femoris (cut)

Gastroc-
nemius (cut)

Popliteus

Soleus (cut)

Tibialis
posterior

Peroneus
longus

Flexor
digitorum
longus

Peroneus
brevis

Flexor
hallucis
longus

Tibialis
posterior
tendon

Sup. peroneal
retinaculum

Flexor
retinaculum

Tendo-
calcaneus

Fig. 154.—The deep muscles of the calf.

above the lateral head of gastrocnemius and from the capsule of the knee joint.

Insertion. Into the posterior surface of the calcaneum, medial to tendo-calcaneus.

Nerve supply. Medial popliteal nerve.

Action. Feebly supplements the action of triceps surae.

The deep Muscles of the Calf comprise *popliteus, tibialis posterior, flexor hallucis longus* and *flexor digitorum longus.*

Popliteus (fig. 154)

Origin. By a tendon from the anterior end of a groove on the lateral condyle of the femur, from the lateral semilunar cartilage and from the arcuate ligament.

The tendon lies within the capsule of the knee joint and separates the lateral ligament of the joint from the lateral semilunar cartilage (fig. 106). When the knee is fully flexed the tendon lies within the groove on the lateral condyle of the femur.

Insertion. Into a triangular area above the soleal line on the tibia.

Nerve supply. Medial popliteal nerve.

Action. While the popliteus can medially rotate the tibia on the femur it more frequently laterally rotates the femur on the tibia. This occurs when the femur is fixed as in the standing position. The movement is known as "unlocking the knee joint" and is an essential precursor to flexing the knee. Before lateral rotation of the femur is effected, the popliteus retracts the lateral semilunar cartilage and draws it out of harm's way. It is because of the mobility of the lateral cartilage that it is less frequently injured than its medial counterpart. The popliteus is in no way a flexor of the knee joint (Last).

Tibialis Posterior (figs. 154 and 157)

Origin. From the upper half of the medial surface of fibula, the inter-osseous membrane and from the middle third of the posterior surface of the tibia, lateral to the origin of flexor digitorum longus.

Insertion. The muscle becomes tendinous at the ankle where it lies immediately behind the medial malleolus. It runs forwards on the sole of the foot, above the sustentaculum tali and beneath the head of the talus to reach the tuberosity of the navicular bone into which it is mainly inserted and the adjacent medial cuneiform bone. From its tendon of insertion small fascial slips pass to the cuboid, the sustentaculum tali, the intermediate and lateral cuneiforms and to the bases of the second, third and fourth meta-tarsals (fig. 157).

Nerve supply. Posterior tibial nerve.

Action. Plantarflexes as it inverts the foot.

Flexor Hallucis Longus (figs. 154 and 156)

Origin. From the middle third of the posterior surface of the shaft of the fibula.

Insertion. The muscle becomes tendinous just above the ankle and, winding around the lower end of the tibia, lies in a deep groove on the posterior surface of the talus. It passes forwards in the foot beneath the

12—A.PH.

sustentaculum tali and reaches the base of the distal phalanx of the great toe by passing between the two heads of flexor hallucis brevis.

Nerve supply. Posterior tibial nerve.

Action. While it is correct to describe this muscle as a flexor of the great toe, it is actually concerned with keeping that digit in apposition with the ground when walking. It has, therefore, been described as the "taking-off" muscle.

Flexor Digitorum Longus (figs. 154 and 156)

Origin. From the middle third of the posterior surface of the shaft of the tibia, medial to the tibial origin of tibialis posterior.

Insertion. The muscle becomes tendinous above the ankle, passes behind the medial malleolus into the foot, where it divides into four tendons which are inserted into the distal phalanges of the four outer toes. Each tendon passes through the corresponding tendon of flexor digitorum brevis, the arrangement being the same as for the corresponding muscle in the hand (fig. 156).

Nerve supply. Posterior tibial nerve.

Action. With the flexor digitorum brevis, the muscle flexes the four outer digits. It also plantarflexes the foot.

The main tendon receives the insertion of the flexor digitorum accessorius in the sole of the foot and on dividing into its four tendons gives origin to the four lumbrical muscles (fig. 156).

Muscle on the Dorsum of the Foot

Extensor Digitorum Brevis (figs. 152 and 153)

Origin. From the anterolateral aspect of the dorsal surface of the calcaneum.

Insertion. The muscle divides into four tendons; the most medial, often called the *extensor hallucis brevis,* is inserted into the base of the proximal phalanx of the great toe (fig. 152). The outer three tendons are inserted into the long extensor tendons passing to the second, third and fourth digits.

Nerve supply. Anterior tibial nerve.

Action. Extends the toes.

Muscles on the Sole of the Foot comprise four layers, numbered one to four, according to the positions they occupy from the superficial to the deep aspect of the sole, viz.,

1st layer: Abductor hallucis.
           Flexor digitorum brevis.
           Abductor digiti minimi.
2nd layer: Flexor digitorum accessorius.
           Lumbricals.
           Flexor digitorum longus tendon.
           Flexor hallucis longus tendon.
3rd layer: Flexor hallucis brevis.
           Adductor hallucis.
           Flexor digiti minimi brevis.

4th layer: Interossei.
　　　　　 Peroneus longus tendon.
　　　　　 Tibialis posterior tendon.

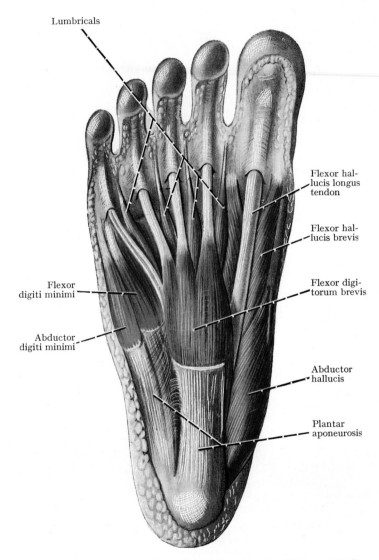

Lumbricals

Flexor hal-
lucis longus
tendon

Flexor hal-
lucis brevis

Flexor
digiti minimi

Flexor digi-
torum brevis

Abductor
digiti minimi

Abductor
hallucis

Plantar
aponeurosis

FIG. 155.—The superficial layer of muscles on the sole. (After Sobotta.)

It should be noted that the origins of the muscles shift forward towards
the toes as the layers get deeper. The action of these muscles is described on
p. 187.

Abductor Hallucis (fig. 155)

Origin. From the medial tubercle on the plantar surface of the calcaneum, from the flexor retinaculum and plantar fascia.

Nerve supply. Medial plantar nerve.

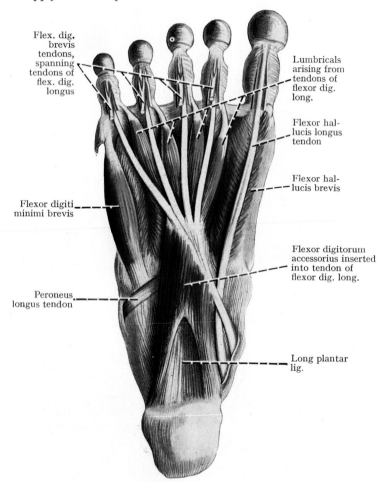

Flex. dig. brevis tendons, spanning tendons of flex. dig. longus

Lumbricals arising from tendons of flexor dig. long.

Flexor hallucis longus tendon

Flexor hallucis brevis

Flexor digiti minimi brevis

Flexor digitorum accessorius inserted into tendon of flexor dig. long.

Peroneus longus tendon

Long plantar lig.

FIG. 156.—The deeper layers of muscles on the sole.

Flexor Digitorum Brevis (fig. 155)

Origin. From the medial tubercle on the plantar surface of the calcaneum and the plantar aponeurosis.

Insertion. The muscle divides into four tendons which are inserted by two slips in the middle phalanx of each of the four outer toes. Each tendon splits to allow the corresponding tendon of flexor digitorum longus to pass through it, *cf.*, flexor digitorum sublimis in the hand.

Nerve supply. Medial plantar nerve.

Abductor Digiti Minimi (fig. 155)

Origin. From the medial and lateral tubercles and the intervening bone on the plantar surface of the calcaneum and from the plantar fascia.

Insertion. Into the lateral side of the base of the proximal phalanx of the little toe.

Nerve supply. Lateral plantar nerve.

Flexor Digitorum Accessorius (fig. 156)

Origin. The muscle arises by two heads, a large medial head from the medial surface of the calcaneum and a much smaller lateral head in front of the lateral tubercle and the long plantar ligament.

Insertion. Into the lateral aspect of the tendon of flexor digitorum longus just before it divides.

Nerve supply. Lateral plantar nerve.

Lumbrical Muscles (figs. 155 and 156)

Origin. The lumbricals are four small muscles which arise from the tendons of flexor digitorum longus; the first from the medial side of the first tendon, the second, third and fourth from the contiguous sides of the first and second, second and third, third and fourth tendons respectively.

Insertion. Each is inserted into the dorsal expansion of the corresponding tendon of extensor digitorum longus.

Nerve supply. The first by the medial plantar nerve and the second, third and fourth by the lateral plantar nerve.

Flexor Hallucis Brevis (fig. 157)

Origin. From the cuboid and lateral cuneiform bones.

Insertion. By two tendons into the medial and lateral aspects of the proximal phalanx of the great toe. A sesamoid bone is developed in each tendon (fig. 157). The medial tendon blends with adductor hallucis and the lateral tendon with abductor hallucis.

Nerve Supply. Medial plantar nerve.

Adductor Hallucis (fig. 157)

Origin. The muscle arises by two heads, an *oblique head* from the bases of the second, third and fourth metatarsal bones and the sheath of peroneus longus, and a *transverse head* from the deep transverse ligaments of the sole and the plantar metatarsophalangeal ligament of the three lateral toes.

Insertion. Into the lateral aspect of the base of the proximal phalanx of the great toe.

Nerve supply. Lateral plantar nerve.

Flexor Digiti Minimi Brevis (fig. 157)

Origin. From the base of the fifth metatarsal bone.

Insertion. Into the base of the proximal phalanx of the fifth digit.

Nerve supply. Lateral plantar nerve.

Interossei (figs. 73, 74 and 157)

Attachments. Consist of seven small muscles—three plantar interossei on the sole and four dorsal interossei on the dorsum of the foot. The plantar muscles are adductors and the dorsal, abductors; but unlike those of the hand they act to and from the second digit instead of the third. The plantar muscles arise from the medial aspect of the third, fourth and fifth metatarsal

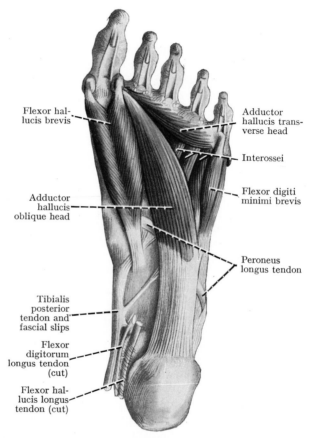

Flexor hallucis brevis

Adductor hallucis transverse head

Interossei

Adductor hallucis oblique head

Flexor digiti minimi brevis

Peroneus longus tendon

Tibialis posterior tendon and fascial slips

Flexor digitorum longus tendon (cut)

Flexor hallucis longus tendon (cut)

FIG. 157.—The deepest layer of muscles on the sole.

bones respectively and are inserted into the corresponding proximal phalanges and extensor expansions.

The dorsal muscles arise from the contiguous sides of the first and second, second and third, third and fourth, and fourth and fifth metatarsal bones respectively. The first and second muscles are inserted into the second digit, the third and fourth muscles into their corresponding digits. In all cases they are attached to the proximal phalanges and the extensor expansions.

Nerve supply. The lateral plantar nerve supplies all the interossei, but the first and second dorsal interosseous muscles are also innervated by the anterior tibial nerve with fibres which are said to be afferent.

Action of the Muscles on the sole of the Foot

The functions of the short muscles on the sole of the foot are twofold. They facilitate the movement of walking and they preserve the arches of the foot. Movements such as abduction and adduction of the digits are very limited in man, e.g., few people can abduct the great toe, although the abductor hallucis remains a large and powerful muscle. The muscles of the sole are concerned with holding the toes firmly in apposition with the ground and propelling the body forward in walking. Since they span the pillars of the arch of the foot, they are powerful factors in its maintenance. The lumbricals and interossei in the foot are much less important than their counterparts in the hand.

CHAPTER V

THE NERVOUS SYSTEM

The Nervous System is divided into the *central nervous system* which consists of the brain and spinal cord and the *peripheral nervous system* which consists of the cranial and spinal nerves and their ganglia. An important subdivision of the peripheral nervous system is known as the *autonomic nervous system* which includes the sympathetic and parasympathetic systems.

THE CENTRAL NERVOUS SYSTEM

As we have already seen (p. 11) the central nervous system is made up of nerve cells and nerve fibres which are enmeshed in a specialised supporting tissue called neuroglia.

On section, the brain is seen to consist of dark and light areas called, respectively, grey and white matter. The *grey matter* lies chiefly at the periphery of the brain, although there are islands of grey matter lying deep in the interior, and these, since they lie at the base of the brain, are known as the "*basal nuclei*" (fig. 161). The *white matter* is, however, the chief component of the deeper parts of the brain.

When the spinal cord is sectioned it is seen to consist of white matter peripherally and grey matter centrally and thus the arrangement is exactly the opposite to that seen in the brain.

In the grey matter, nerve cells predominate, although there are nerve fibres present also in the form of axons and dendrites of nerve cells. In the white matter nerve fibres predominate while neuroglia is present in abundance in both grey and white matter.

The *function* of the brain is to receive messages from the various parts of the body as the result of which it is constantly effecting certain adjustments designed to bring about an harmonious co-ordination between the various components of the body and between the body as a whole and its environment. The spinal cord transmits these messages to and from the brain.

Fibres which transmit messages to the central nervous system are said to be *afferent*, fibres which convey messages from the central nervous system are said to be *efferent*. Fibres which are passing from the brain to the spinal cord or vice versa are aggregated into bundles called *tracts*.

THE BRAIN

The brain almost fills the cranial cavity and weighs about 1380 gm. in the adult male and about 1250 gm. in the adult female.

It is divisible into *cerebrum, mid-brain, cerebellum, pons* and *medulla oblongata*.

The Cerebrum is composed of two cerebral hemispheres which are united by a sheet of white matter called the *corpus callosum* (fig. 163).

The surface layer of each cerebral hemisphere is known as the *cortex*. This is characteristically fissured and convoluted, and in this way the surface area of the brain is increased without a corresponding increase in bulk. Two fissures or sulci are conspicuous, the *lateral sulcus* extending from the forepart of the brain upwards and backwards, and the *central sulcus* extending downwards and forwards on the lateral surface of the cerebrum from a point just behind the centre of the superior border. Also on this border a small part of the *parieto-occipital sulcus* descends on to the lateral surface, while the inferior border presents the rather inconspicuous *pre-occipital notch* (fig. 158).

If an imaginary line be drawn from the parieto-occipital sulcus to the pre-occipital notch the cerebrum can be divided into its various lobes.

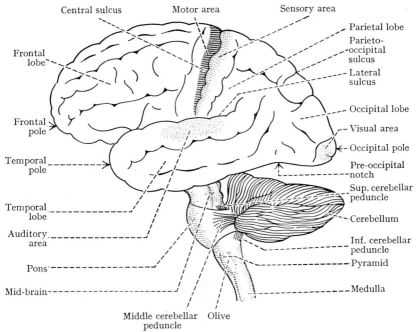

FIG. 158.—The components of the brain, lateral aspect (schematic).

The *frontal lobe* lies in front of the central sulcus and above the lateral sulcus. The *parietal lobe* lies behind the central sulcus and above the lateral sulcus, and is limited by the imaginary line. The portion of brain behind this line is the *occipital lobe* and the portion below the lateral sulcus is the *temporal lobe* (fig. 158).

There is a convolution in front of the central sulcus known as the *pre-central convolution* in which is the *motor area* and a convolution behind the central sulcus known as the *post-central convolution* in which is the *sensory area*. The extremities of the frontal, temporal and occipital lobes are known as the *frontal, temporal* and *occipital poles* respectively (fig. 158).

The precentral convolution controls voluntary movements; the post central convolution is concerned with sensation; the middle of the superior temporal convolution is concerned with hearing (*auditory area*); the occipital pole and adjacent area of brain, on the medial aspect of the hemisphere, are concerned with sight (*visual area*). An area on the frontal lobe near the stem of the lateral sulcus controls the motor element of speech. This is called *Broca's area* and is represented on one side of the brain only, usually the left.

The Mid-brain consists of the two *cerebral peduncles* or crura and the four *corpora quadrigemina.*

The cerebral peduncles are almost hidden on the dorsum of the brain by the cerebral hemispheres but can be seen clearly on the ventral surface or

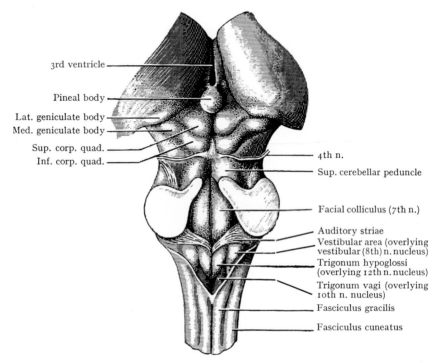

3rd ventricle
Pineal body
Lat. geniculate body
Med. geniculate body
Sup. corp. quad.
Inf. corp. quad.

4th n.
Sup. cerebellar peduncle

Facial colliculus (7th n.)
Auditory striae
Vestibular area (overlying vestibular (8th) n. nucleus)
Trigonum hypoglossi (overlying 12th n. nucleus)
Trigonum vagi (overlying 10th n. nucleus)
Fasciculus gracilis
Fasciculus cuneatus

FIG. 159.—A dissection of the dorsal aspect of the brain stem exposing the fourth ventricle in the floor of which is the deep origin of certain cranial nerves.

base (fig. 158). They contain afferent fibres situated dorsally and efferent fibres situated ventrally as well as the nuclei of the 3rd and 4th cranial nerves and part of the mesencephalic nucleus of the 5th cranial nerve. The mid-brain is tunnelled by the *cerebral aqueduct* (fig. 163).

On the dorsal aspect of the mid-brain are four small rounded bodies, each about the size of a pea, called the *superior* and *inferior corpora quadrigemina* (fig. 159) and adjacent to these, but not in the mid-brain, are the *medial* and *lateral geniculate bodies* (fig. 159). The superior corpora quadrigemina and the lateral geniculate bodies are concerned with sight, the inferior corpora quadrigemina and the medial geniculate bodies are concerned with hearing.

The Pons (fig. 158) appears as a bridge connecting the two halves of the cerebellum. It is composed chiefly of nerve fibres but it also contains the nuclei (nerve cells) of certain important cranial nerves. The fibres which connect the two halves of the cerebellum run transversely through the pons, but the pons also contains vertical fibres which are afferent and efferent tracts passing to and from the cerebrum. The nuclei of the 5th, 6th and 7th cranial nerves arise from that portion of the pons which forms the upper part of the floor of the 4th ventricle (fig. 159).

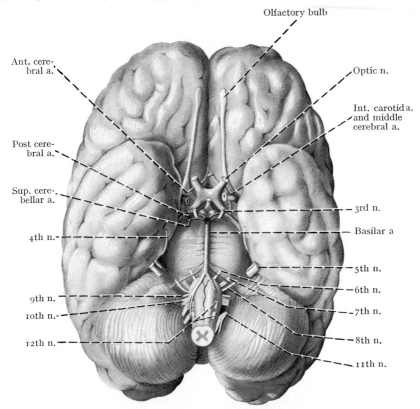

Olfactory bulb

Ant. cerebral a.

Optic n.

Int. carotid a. and middle cerebral a.

Post cerebral a.

Sup. cerebellar a.

3rd n.

4th n.

Basilar a

5th n.

6th n.

9th n.

7th n.

10th n.

12th n.

8th n.

11th n.

FIG. 160.—The base of the brain.

The Medulla Oblongata (fig. 158) lies below the pons and merges imperceptibly into the spinal cord. It contains afferent and efferent fibres, continuous with those of the pons and mid-brain. The *efferent* (*pyramidal*) *tracts* lie on the ventral surface of the medulla where they can be seen as two oval swellings called the *pyramids*. Behind the pyramids are the *olives* formed by the *olivary nuclei* and behind the olives the *inferior cerebellar peduncles* by which the medulla is connected with the cerebellum (fig. 158). The medulla oblongata forms the lower part of the floor of the 4th ventricle and contains the nuclei of the 8th (in part), 9th, 10th, 11th and 12th cranial nerves (fig. 159). Associated with the nuclei of the vagus nerve in the medulla are the three vital centres—the respiratory, vasomotor and cardiac centres. These centres are as vital as their name suggests, if for instance the tracts leading from the respiratory centre to the muscles are damaged as in poliomyelitis, breathing may have to be maintained artificially (iron lung).

The Cerebellum (fig. 158), or small brain, lies behind the pons and medulla. It is connected with the mid-brain by the *superior cerebellar peduncles*, to the pons by the *middle cerebellar peduncles* and to the medulla by the *inferior cerebellar peduncles (restiform bodies)* (fig. 158). It is intricately fissured, consists of two hemispheres and a central connection called the vermis and is concerned with the co-ordination of muscular movement. Proprioceptive impulses from muscles and joints reach the cerebellum by way of the spinocerebellar tracts of the same side. After several relays to bring about the co-ordination of muscles, impulses pass to the cerebrum and via the red nucleus in the mid-brain to the spinal cord. Within the white matter of each cerebellar hemisphere is the *dentate nucleus*. It receives impulses from other parts of the cerebellum and relays them to the red nucleus of the opposite side via the superior cerebellar peduncle.

The points of emergence of the cranial nerves from the base of the brain should be duly noted and particularly those which concern the student of physiotherapy (fig. 160).

The *5th nerve* emerges from the lateral aspect of the pons; the *7th nerve* from the lower border of the pons and between it and the inferior cerebellar peduncle; the *10th and 11th nerves* from the medulla by small thread-like strands which lie between the olive and the inferior cerebellar peduncle.

The Interior of the Brain

When the brain is sectioned horizontally (fig. 161) the following structures come into view. Grey matter is seen lying at the periphery (cortex) of the brain and islands of grey matter called the *basal nuclei* are seen deep in the brain substance. The white matter lies around and between these structures. It will be seen that the interior of the cerebral hemispheres is hollow, for each hemisphere contains a cavity called the *lateral ventricle*. This consists of a central part called the *body*, a part which passes forwards into the frontal lobe called the *anterior horn*, a part which passes backwards into the occipital lobe called the *posterior horn* and a part which passes downwards and forwards into the temporal lobe called the *inferior horn*. This large ventricle communicates with a smaller one which is situated in the mid-line beneath a sheet of white matter called the *fornix* (fig. 163). This is the *3rd ventricle* which is a large central cavity bounded on either side by the thalami (fig. 162). The channel between the lateral and 3rd ventricles is called the *interventricular foramen* (fig. 163). The 3rd ventricle communicates with the *4th ventricle* via the *cerebral aqueduct*, and the 4th ventricle with the *central canal of the spinal cord* (fig. 163).

The Basal Nuclei, which include the *caudate nucleus, lentiform nucleus*, and *claustrum*, can be seen as areas of grey matter in these sections (fig. 161). The caudate and lentiform nuclei together with the intervening fibre tracts constitute the *corpus striatum*, for when cut in coronal section these nuclei and their connections have a striated appearance. The *thalami* bounding the third ventricle have already been referred to.

Between the caudate nucleus and the lentiform nucleus, and between the latter structure and the thalamus, there is an important band of white matter called the *internal capsule* (fig. 161).

The corpus striatum is the motor area in some of the lower animals but in man this function is largely if not entirely taken over by the cerebral

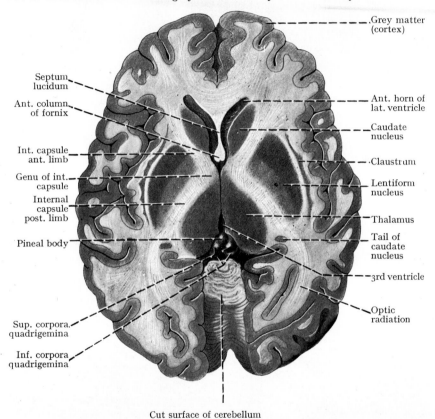

Grey matter (cortex)

Septum lucidum

Ant. column of fornix

Int. capsule ant. limb

Genu of int. capsule

Internal capsule post. limb

Pineal body

Sup. corpora quadrigemina

Inf. corpora quadrigemina

Ant. horn of lat. ventricle

Caudate nucleus

Claustrum

Lentiform nucleus

Thalamus

Tail of caudate nucleus

3rd ventricle

Optic radiation

Cut surface of cerebellum

FIG. 161.—Horizontal section through the brain at the level of the basal nuclei.

cortex. Some authorities believe that the corpus striatum is connected with the extrapyramidal system and is a controlling centre for muscular co-ordination. This is the area of the brain which is affected in encephalitis lethargica (sleeping sickness) and paralysis agitans (Parkinson's disease).

The thalamus is the sensory area in some of the lower animals but in man its function is largely taken over by the cerebral cortex. Only crude sensations especially pain reach consciousness in the thalamus in man but it also functions as an important correlation centre for sensory impulses which

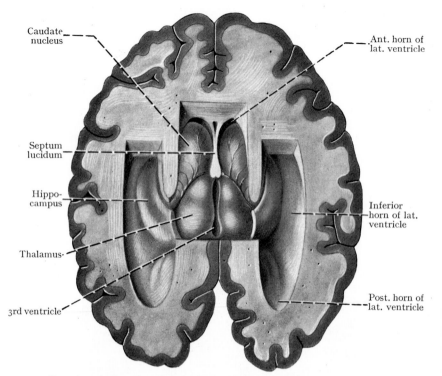

Caudate nucleus

Ant. horn of lat. ventricle

Septum lucidum

Hippo-campus

Inferior horn of lat. ventricle

Thalamus

3rd ventricle

Post. horn of lat. ventricle

FIG. 162.—A dissection of the brain to expose the lateral and 3rd ventricles.

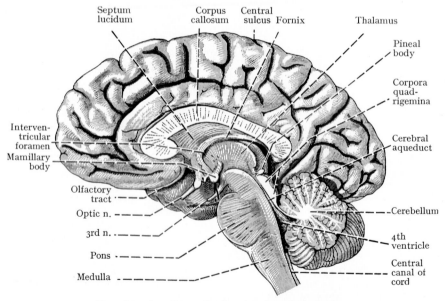

Septum lucidum

Corpus callosum

Central sulcus Fornix

Thalamus

Pineal body

Corpora quad-rigemina

Interventricular foramen

Mamillary body

Cerebral aqueduct

Olfactory tract

Optic n.

3rd n.

Pons

Medulla

Cerebellum

4th ventricle

Central canal of cord

FIG. 163.—A median sagittal section through the brain.

are passing to the postcentral sensory cortex. There is evidence also that it damps down sensory impulses for if its connections with the cortex are cut there is an exaggerated response to trivial stimuli.

The internal capsule is formed by a condensation of nerve fibres passing to and from the cerebral cortex. It consists of an anterior limb, a genu or knee and a posterior limb. The anterior limb contains *frontopontine fibres* which arise in the frontal lobe and pass to the opposite cerebellar hemisphere via the pons and *thalamocortical fibres* passing to the frontal lobe concerned with autonomic activities; behind these occupying the whole of the genu and the anterior two-thirds of the posterior limb are the *cerebrospinal (pyramidal) tracts* which convey motor impulses to the opposite side of the body. The remainder of the internal capsule contains from before back, *thalamocortical fibres* passing to the post-central sensory area, *temporopontine fibres* passing from the temporal lobe to the opposite cerebellar hemisphere via the pons; *auditory fibres* and *visual fibres*. The internal capsule is liable to injury from haemorrhage or thrombosis within the brain substance (stroke) and death or a hemiplegia (paralysis of one side of the body) is the usual sequel.

When the brain is sectioned sagittally (fig. 163) among the structures which come into view are: the *corpus callosum* (sectioned), the *fornix* overlying the *third ventricle*, the *thalamus*, the *corpora quadrigemina*, the *crus, pons, medulla, cerebellum, cerebral aqueduct*, and the *4th ventricle*.

THE SPINAL CORD

The Spinal Cord extends from the foramen magnum to the lower border of the 1st lumbar vertebra and lies within the vertebral canal. In the cervical and lower thoracic regions the cord is thickened to form the cervical and lumbar enlargements, for here the nerves to the upper and lower limbs emerge. The cord ends below in a cone from which a strand of pia mater—the *filum terminale*—passes down to end by blending with the periosteum on the coccyx (fig. 164). The filum terminale is almost hidden by the nerve roots which are emerging from the lumbar enlargement. These nerve roots, together with the filum terminale, are said to resemble a horse's tail and thus are known as the *cauda equina*.

Thirty-one pairs of spinal nerves emerge from the cord; 8 from the cervical region, 12 from the thoracic region, 5 from each of the lumbar and sacral regions and 1 from the coccygeal region.

It should be clearly understood that the terms "lumbar," "sacral" and "coccygeal regions" of the cord do not correspond to similar parts of the vertebral column.

Each nerve has an *anterior* and a *posterior nerve root*, the latter being readily distinguished from the former by the fact that it carries on it a large spindle-shaped ganglion—the *posterior root ganglion* (fig. 165).

When the cord is sectioned it is seen to consist of grey and white matter. The grey matter, composed largely of nerve cells, forms an *anterior horn*

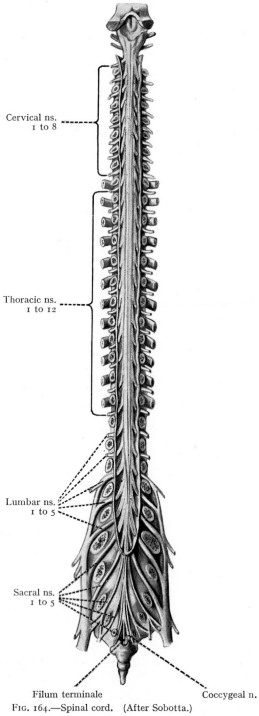

Cervical ns.
1 to 8

Thoracic ns.
1 to 12

Lumbar ns.
1 to 5

Sacral ns.
1 to 5

Filum terminale   Coccygeal n.

FIG. 164.—Spinal cord.   (After Sobotta.)

196

and a *posterior horn* from which the anterior and posterior nerve roots respectively emerge.

The grey matter of one side is united to that of the opposite side by the grey commissure, in the centre of which is the central canal of the spinal cord. In the thoracic and upper lumbar regions there is a lateral enlargement (column) of grey substance and from this area the sympathetic nerves emerge (fig. 167).

A fissure anteriorly and a septum posteriorly separate the white matter into halves, so that the white matter is composed of anterior, lateral and posterior columns.

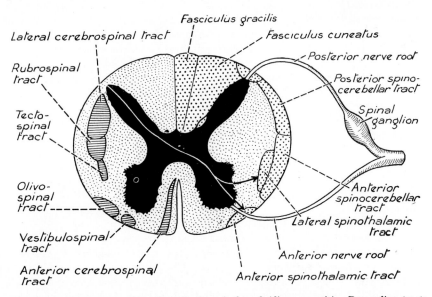

Fig. 165.—A transverse section through the spinal cord (diagrammatic). Descending tracts are represented by dark cross-hatched areas, ascending tracts by stippled areas. The thoracic nucleus or Clarke's column, is seen in the diagram as a light stippled area in the left posterior horn of the cord. It is seen only in the thoracic region of the cord.

Included in the white matter are nerve fibres which pass to and from the brain as the ascending and descending tracts. The ascending tracts carry sensations to the post-central sensory area, the descending tracts convey motor impulses from the pre-central motor area.

The position which these tracts occupy in the cord is indicated in fig. 165.

Ascending Tracts enter the spinal cord via the posterior nerve roots, and convey proprioceptive impulses from muscles, tendons and joints and exteroceptive impulses arising from the surface of the body. These are the fasciculus gracilis and the fasciculus cuneatus, the anterior and posterior spinocerebellar tracts and the spinothalamic tracts. Most of the ascending tracts relay in the spinal cord and those passing to consciousness relay again in the thalamus before passing to the post-central gyrus of the cerebral cortex.

Those carrying proprioceptive impulses do not relay until they get to the medulla and the fasciculus gracilis and cuneatus are the only tracts which degenerate when the posterior nerve roots are cut.   This indeed is how the tracts were discovered.

Awareness of sensation has now been shown to depend on a less discrete tract called *the reticular formation*.   It consists of a series of relays along which impulses pass relatively slowly.   It is paralysed by anaesthetics but the spinocerebral tracts are unaffected.

The fasciculus gracilis and cuneatus (fig. 165) end in nuclei in the upper part of the medulla.   From here the majority of the fibres pass to the post-central sensory cortex in the cerebrum.   These fibres cross in the medulla near the central canal, above and behind the decussation of the pyramids and ascend via the pons, mid-brain (in the medial lemniscus) and thalamus. The remaining fibres pass to the cerebellum.   These tracts convey the finer sensations of touch and proprioceptive impulses to the cortex.

The anterior and posterior spinocerebellar tracts originate in the thoracic nucleus of the same side and in the case of the anterior spinocere-bellar tract of the opposite side also.   The thoracic nucleus lies in the posterior grey column throughout the thoracic region (fig. 165).   The tracts ascend in the lateral column of white matter and then via the superior and inferior cerebellar peduncles respectively, they enter the cerebellar hemispheres. These tracts convey impulses from muscles, tendons and joints to the cere-bellum.   These sensations do not enter consciousness but are entirely con-cerned with the poise of the body and with the co-ordination of muscular movements.

The spinothalamic tract (fig. 165) arises in the posterior horn cells, crosses the cord in the white commissure in close proximity to the central canal and enters the anterior and lateral columns of white matter, forming the *anterior and lateral spinothalamic tracts*.   The *anterior tract* ascends in the anterior white column of the opposite side and from there it ascends through the medulla, pons, and mid-brain to the thalamus via the medial lemniscus. From the thalamus it passes to the post-central sensory cortex.   It is an additional pathway for tactile and pressure sensibility.   The *lateral tract* ascends in the lateral white column of the opposite side, then through the medulla, pons and mid-brain to the thalamus and thence to the post-central sensory cortex.   This tract conveys pain and thermal sensibility to the cortex from the opposite side of the body.

In the condition known as *syringomyelia*, changes take place around the central canal of the spinal cord which cause the canal to enlarge and the nervous tissue around it to be replaced by fibrous tissue.   Invariably the spinothalamic tract is involved and the patient entirely loses the sensations of pain and temperature change, while the sensation of touch will be im-paired.

Descending Tracts commence in the brain, descend in the white matter of the spinal cord and terminate in the anterior horn cells.   From the an-terior horn cells motor nerves convey the impulses to the muscles.

The cerebrospinal (pyramidal) tracts (fig. 165) originate in the cortex of the pre-central motor area as the axons of certain cells found in that region. From the cortex they descend in the internal capsule to the ventral aspect of the mid-brain, pons and medulla. In the medulla about two-thirds of them cross to the opposite side in the decussation of the pyramids forming the *lateral cerebrospinal tract*, which descends in the lateral column of the white matter in the cord. The remainder descend in the anterior column of white matter in the cord as the *anterior cerebrospinal tract* and cross in the cord just prior to their termination. There is evidence that a few of the fibres in the lateral cerebrospinal tract originate from the cortex of the same side. The cerebrospinal tracts finally terminate in the anterior horn cells.

The axons of these anterior horn cells constitute the somatic motor fibres of the peripheral nerves.

Neurones running from the cerebral cortex to the anterior horn cells or to the nuclei of the cranial nerves are known as *upper motor neurones*, while neurones running from the anterior horn cells or the cranial nerve nuclei to the periphery are known as *lower motor neurones*. Paralysis of the upper motor neurones is of the *spastic* type, while paralysis of the lower motor neurones is of the *flaccid* type.

The extra pyramidal tracts (fig. 165) consisting of the *rubrospinal reticulospinal, tectospinal, olivospinal* and *vestibulospinal tracts*, are all concerned with regulating the finer muscle movements, muscular co-ordination and muscle tone. The vestibulospinal tract which originates in the vestibular (Deiters') nucleus in the medulla is especially concerned with antigravity and postural reflexes.

Afferent and efferent impulses to and from the cranial nerves do not, of course, pass down the cord. Motor impulses are conveyed by tracts which, having crossed to the opposite side, end in the cranial nerve nuclei within the brain (upper motor neurone). From here they are conveyed via the cranial nerves to the periphery (lower motor neurone). Sensory impulses are conveyed to the sensory nuclei of the cranial nerves and then crossing to the opposite side proceed via the thalamus and internal capsule to the post-central sensory cortex.

THE MENINGES OF THE BRAIN AND SPINAL CORD

The brain and spinal cord are covered by three fibrous membranes—the dura, arachnoid and pia.

The dura mater consists of two layers of tough fibrous tissue. These two layers are adherent except where they enclose the venous sinuses of the skull. The outer (endosteal) layer lines the interior of the cranial cavity but is not carried into the vertebral column. The inner layer surrounds the brain and spinal cord and within the cranial cavity forms a large, tough partition between the two cerebral hemispheres called the *falx cerebri*, a much smaller partition between the two cerebellar hemispheres called the *falx cerebelli* and a large shelf on which the posterior part of the cerebral hemispheres rest, called the *tentorium*.   The dura also forms a roof for the hypophyseal fossa called the *diaphragma sellae* (fig. 168).

The **arachnoid mater** lies beneath the dura and envelops the brain and spinal cord.   It is a transparent membrane which bridges the fissures on the surface of the cerebral hemispheres.   With the dura, it ends at the level of the 2nd sacral vertebra.

Between the arachnoid and the pia mater is the *subarachnoid space* which is filled with cerebrospinal fluid.

The **pia mater** is a thin vascular membrane of areolar tissue which invests the brain and spinal cord and lies within the arachnoid and dura. It dips into the fissures and is carried into the ventricles of the brain where

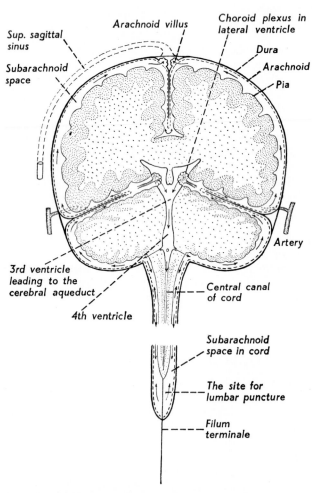

FIG. 166.—This diagram illustrates the formation and circulation of the cerebrospinal fluid over the surface of the brain and spinal cord as indicated by the arrows.

it invests a fringe of blood vessels called the *choroid plexuses*. It is from these plexuses that the cerebrospinal fluid is formed. The pia ends with the cord at the level of the 1st lumbar vertebra but a strand known as the *filum terminale* is carried down within the subarachnoid space. This strand pierces the dura at the level of S2 and fuses with the periosteum on the back of the coccyx (fig. 164).

The Cerebrospinal Fluid arises from the choroid plexuses in the ventricles of the brain and circulates from the lateral ventricle, via the inter-

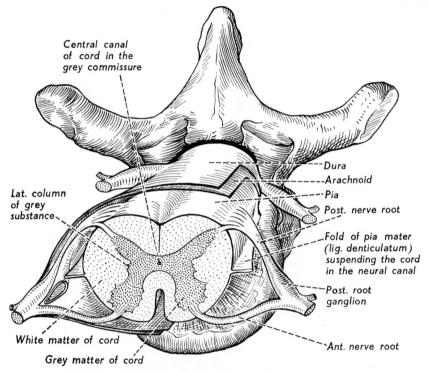

FIG. 167.—The spinal cord and its coverings occupying the vertebral canal.

ventricular foramen to the 3rd ventricle and then via the cerebral aqueduct to the 4th ventricle. From the 4th ventricle a very small part of the fluid passes down the central canal in the spinal cord, but the greater part passes out of this ventricle through a central and two lateral foramina situated in its roof. The cerebrospinal fluid circulates over the surface of the brain and spinal cord in the subarachnoid space. From this space it is absorbed into the venous sinuses in the skull (fig. 168) and so the fluid returns to the venous system.

The cerebrospinal fluid, acting as a fluid buffer, protects the brain from injury, it serves as an exchange for nutrient material and waste products and it helps to regulate the volume of the cranial contents.

If a specimen of cerebrospinal fluid is wanted, a *lumbar puncture* is performed. It is important that this should be done in that part of the subarachnoid space which lies below the level of the spinal cord. The site usually chosen is between L4 and L5, when a hollow needle is pushed between the vertebrae and into the space. Lumbar puncture is performed for diagnostic purposes, to produce spinal anaesthesia, to introduce certain drugs or sera and sometimes to relieve intracranial pressure.

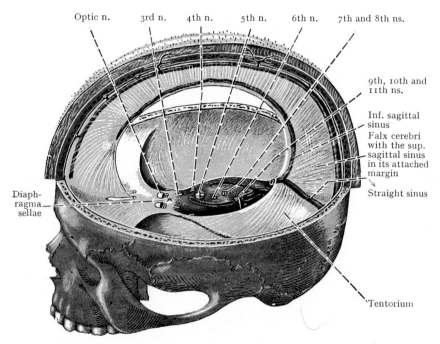

Optic n.   3rd n.   4th n.   5th n.   6th n.   7th and 8th ns.

9th, 10th and 11th ns.

Inf. sagittal sinus

Falx cerebri with the sup. sagittal sinus in its attached margin

Diaphragma sellae

Straight sinus

Tentorium

FIG. 168.—Interior of the skull with the dura mater and its contained sinuses in situ.

THE PERIPHERAL NERVOUS SYSTEM

Under this heading certain cranial and spinal nerves and the autonomic nervous system will be described. The 5th, 7th, 10th and 11th cranial nerves will first be considered.

The Trigeminal or 5th Cranial Nerve (figs. 160 and 169)

This is the largest of the cranial nerves. It arises by elongated sensory and motor roots within the brain stem and emerges on the surface of the base of the brain, lateral to the pons.

The large sensory root enters a semilunar ganglion called the trigeminal ganglion which lies partly in the cavum trigeminale at the apex of the petrous temporal bone and partly on the cartilage which covers the *foramen lacerum* (fig. 36).

The small motor root lies immediately beneath the sensory ganglion and enters the mandibular division of the nerve outside the skull.

From the trigeminal ganglion three large trunks emerge called the ophthalmic, maxillary and mandibular divisions.

The Ophthalmic Division passes forwards in the cavernous sinus to enter the orbit via the superior orbital fissure. Here it breaks up into its three terminal branches, the nasociliary, frontal and lacrimal nerves. The *nasociliary* nerve gives branches to the eye, the ethmoidal air sinus, the

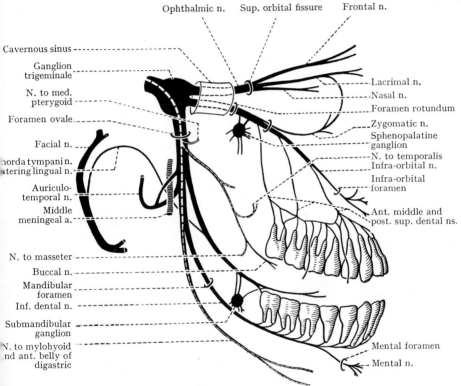

Ophthalmic n.   Sup. orbital fissure   Frontal n.

Cavernous sinus

Ganglion trigeminale

N. to med. pterygoid

Foramen ovale

Facial n.

horda tympani n.
tering lingual n.

Auriculo-temporal n.

Middle meningeal a.

N. to masseter

Buccal n.

Mandibular foramen

Inf. dental n.

Submandibular ganglion

N. to mylohyoid
nd ant. belly of digastric

Lacrimal n.

Nasal n.

Foramen rotundum

Zygomatic n.

Sphenopalatine ganglion

N. to temporalis

Infra-orbital n.

Infra-orbital foramen

Ant. middle and post. sup. dental ns.

Mental foramen

Mental n.

Fig. 169.—The trigeminal nerve (schematic).
The motor portion of the nerve is indicated by white interrupted lines.

interior of the nose and the skin of the lower lid and lateral wall of the nose. The *frontal* nerve divides into the supra-orbital and supratrochlear nerves which supply the skin of the scalp; the former is much the larger and supplies the scalp as far back as the vertex of the skull where its fibres intermingle with the greater occipital nerve. The *lacrimal* nerve supplies the lacrimal gland and the skin of the upper eyelid.

The Maxillary Division passes forwards in the cavernous sinus, leaves the skull via the foramen rotundum and enters the pterygopalatine fossa. It leaves the fossa by passing forwards on the floor of the orbit as the *infra-*

orbital nerve which leaves the orbit by passing through the infra-orbital foramen and at once divides into branches which supply the skin on the front of the face. While in the fossa the nerve gives *branches to the spheno-palatine ganglion,* a *zygomatic* branch which supplies the skin in the temporal region and over the cheek bone and a *posterior superior dental* branch which supplies the molar teeth. While in the orbit the nerve gives off further branches to the teeth.

The Mandibular Division is joined by the motor root of the 5th nerve and leaves the skull through the foramen ovale. It soon divides outside the skull into an *anterior* division and a *posterior* division. The anterior division is chiefly motor but gives off one important sensory branch called

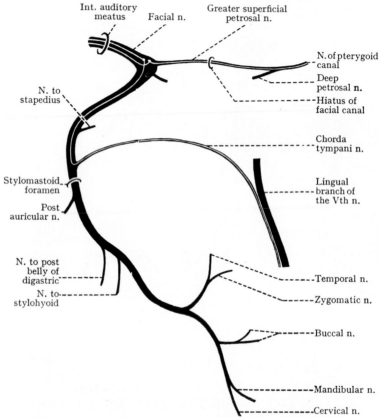

FIG. 170.—The facial nerve (sensory portion is indicated by white lines).

the *buccal* nerve which supplies the skin over the buccinator muscle and the mucous membrane of the mouth on the inner surface of that muscle. The muscle itself is supplied by the facial nerve. The *motor* branches from this anterior division supply the muscles of mastication, viz., the masseter, temporalis and the medial and lateral pterygoids. The *osterior division* of the mandibular nerve gives off three branches, viz., th *auriculo-temporal* nerve which passes back to supply the jaw joint, *. external auditory meatus (ear passage) and the skin over the tempor region; the *lingual* nerve which is the nerve of sensation for the anterior ty thirds of the tongue; and the *inferior dental* nerve which not only supplie ie teeth of the lower jaw but also the skin in this region and gives off a *ylohyoid* branch which supplies the anterior belly of digastric and mylohy l muscles.

The **Facial or 7th Cranial Nerve** (fig. 170) is a m or nerve, although it has a small sensory part. It arises in the pons and erges from the base of the brain between the pons and inferior cerebellar duncle (fig. 160). It passes into the interior of the petrous portion of th temporal bone via the internal auditory m tus. Here it enters the facial canal, cros s the internal ear, turns backwards on t medial wall of the middle ear and then rns downwards behind the posterior wal f the middle ear to leave the skull at th *stylomastoid foramen*. It next crosses the yloid process and enters the substance of ie parotid gland, where it divides into ter *orofacial* and *cervicofacial* divisions. From ese divisions five branches emerge and spre out like the fingers of a hand. These ter nal branches, called from above down th *temporal, zygomatic, buccal, mandibular* d *cervical* branches supply all the muscles of expression.

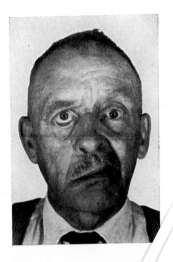

FIG. 171.—A case of paralys of the right facial nerve.

Note the asymmetry of t face, the smoothing out of the c ses on the right side, the droop of the lower eyelid, the slight tw g of the nose to the left and marked obliquity of the mouth. ese manifestations are entirely to a paralysis of the muscle expression (cf. fig. .

While within the petrous portion of the temporal bone, the facial nerve gives off the *greater superficial petrosal* nerve to the spheno-palatine ganglion, the **nerve to the stapedius** muscle (one of the muscles working the ossicles in the ear) and the **chorda tympani** nerve. This nerve supplies the anterior two-thirds of the tongue with taste fibres and innervates the submaxillary and sublingual salivary glands. It is these taste fibres which form the sensory part of the facial nerve.

After the ial nerve leaves the skull and before it enters the parotid gland it giv *nuscular* branches to the muscles of the ear (posterior auricular nerve) an the posterior belly of digastric and stylohyoid muscles.

The *us or 10th Cranial Nerve* (fig. 172) is the longest nerve in the body a has a most extensive distribution.

It es in the medulla and emerges from the base of the brain between the e and the inferior cerebellar peduncle (fig. 160).

asses out of the skull through the jugular foramen and enters the id sheath where it lies behind and between the internal carotid (or common carotid) artery and internal jugular vein. In this way it is carried to the root of the neck where it passes in front of the subclavian artery and enters the thorax lateral to the trachea on the right and over the aortic arch on the left. It then passes behind the lung root to the oesophagus where with its fellow of the opposite side it forms the *oesophageal plexus*. In this way it is carried through the oesophageal opening in the diaphragm into the abdomen, where it lies on the stomach. The left nerve is distributed over the front of that organ and the right nerve behind it, and here the nerves break up into further plexuses which pass with the sympathetic plexuses to the various abdominal viscera.

In the neck it gives branches to the *meninges*, to the *ear passage* and *skin* behind the ear, to the *constrictor muscles of the pharynx*, to the *mucous membrane* and *muscles* of the *larynx* and important *cardiac branches*, some of which arise in the thorax. In the thorax it gives branches to the *trachea, bronchi, lungs* and *oesophagus*.

In the abdomen it gives branches to the *stomach, small intestine, large intestine*, as far as the splenic flexure of the colon, to the *liver* and the *pancreas*.

On emerging from the skull two ganglia placed one above the other called the superior and inferior ganglia are found on the vagus nerve. The cranial root of the accessory nerve blends with the vagus nerve distal to the inferior ganglion and it is probably the 11th nerve and not the 10th which supplies the pharynx and larynx.

The Spinal Accessory or 11th Cranial Nerve (fig. 174) consists of two distinct parts—a *cerebral* portion which arises with the vagus in the medulla and is accessory to that nerve and a *spinal* portion which arises from the upper part of the cervical portion of the spinal cord and supplies the sternomastoid and trapezius muscles. Fibres from the spinal part of the nerve enter the skull through the foramen magnum and there meet the cerebral fibres which have emerged from the medulla between the olive and the inferior cerebellar peduncle and below the vagus (fig. 160). The two parts of the nerve are joined for a short distance only, and on passing out of the skull through the jugular foramen they again divide. The cerebral portion passes into the inferior ganglion of the vagus. The spinal portion runs downwards and backwards deep to the styloid process, crosses the tip of the transverse process of the atlas and enters the deep surface of the sternomastoid muscle and supplies it. Emerging from the posterior border of this muscle, the nerve then enters the posterior triangle of the neck on the levator scapulae. It then runs down on the deep surface of the trapezius and supplies that muscle.

The other cranial nerves are listed with a brief account of their functions for the convenience of students:—

The olfactory or 1st cranial nerve consists of a series of sixteen to twenty fine filaments which arise in the upper part of the nasal cavity and pass through the cribriform plate of the ethmoid at the side of the crista galli to end in the olfactory bulb (fig. 160). It is the nerve of smell.

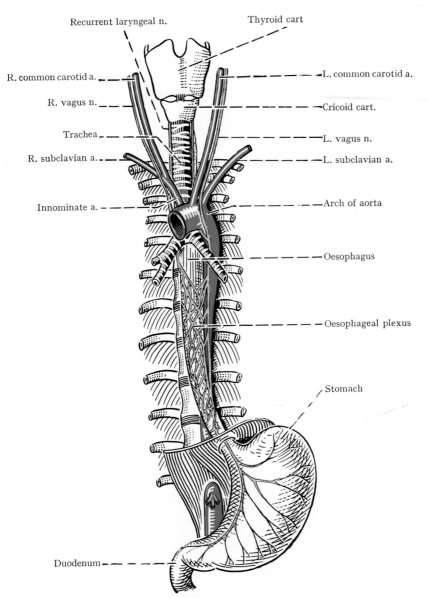

Recurrent laryngeal n.

Thyroid cart

R. common carotid a.

L. common carotid a.

R. vagus n.

Cricoid cart.

Trachea

L. vagus n.

R. subclavian a.

L. subclavian a.

Innominate a.

Arch of aorta

Oesophagus

Oesophageal plexus

Stomach

Duodenum

FIG. 172.—The vagus nerve in the lower part of the neck, the thorax and upper abdomen.

[facing page 206]

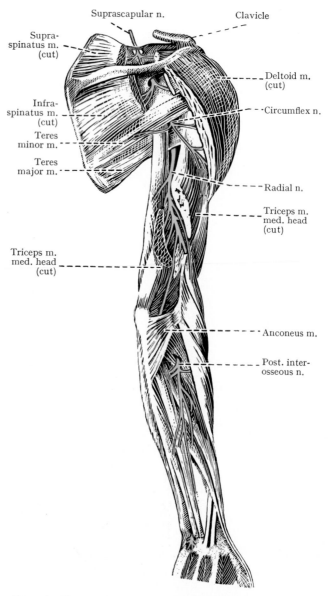

Suprascapular n.

Clavicle

Supra-
spinatus m.
(cut)

Deltoid m.
(cut)

Infra-
spinatus m.
(cut)

Circumflex n.

Teres
minor m.

Teres
major m.

Radial n.

Triceps m.
med. head
(cut)

Triceps m.
med. head
(cut)

Anconeus m.

Post. inter-
osseous n.

FIG. 176.—The nerves on the posterior aspect of the upper limb.
(Redrawn from Gray's "Anatomy.")

[*facing page 207*]

The **optic or 2nd cranial nerve** passes into the orbit through the optic foramen. It is the nerve of sight.

The **oculomotor or 3rd cranial nerve** passes into the orbit via the superior orbital fissure. It supplies the intrinsic and most of the extrinsic muscles of the eyeball including the levator palpebrae superioris, the muscle by which the upper eyelid is raised.

The **trochlear or 4th cranial nerve** passes into the orbit via the superior orbital fissure and supplies the superior oblique muscle of the eyeball.

The **abducent or 6th cranial nerve** passes into the orbit via the superior orbital fissure and supplies the lateral rectus muscle of the eyeball.

The **acoustic or 8th cranial nerve** passes into the internal ear with the seventh nerve through the internal auditory meatus. It divides into a *cochlear portion* which is the nerve of hearing and a *vestibular portion* which passing to the vestibular organs (fig. 298) in the internal ear is concerned with balance.

The **glossopharyngeal or 9th cranial nerve** leaves the skull with the vagus nerve via the jugular foramen. It supplies one of the muscles of the pharynx (stylopharyngeus), is the nerve of taste and common sensation for the posterior third of the tongue and is also responsible for the secretion of saliva from the parotid gland.

The **hypoglossal or 12th cranial nerve** leaves the skull through the anterior condyloid foramen and is a motor nerve to the musculature of the tongue.

THE SPINAL NERVES

Each spinal nerve originates from the spinal cord by two roots, an anterior or motor root and a posterior or sensory root (fig. 167). The latter is easily differentiated from the former because it has a ganglion upon it. These roots unite to form a nerve trunk which almost immediately divides into an anterior and a posterior primary ramus.

The **anterior primary rami** are much larger and more important than the posterior. They unite to form the cervical and brachial plexuses in the neck, and the lumbar, sacral and coccygeal plexuses in their respective regions and are continued as the intercostal nerves in the thorax.

The **posterior primary rami** are for the most part small and relatively unimportant. They supply the skin and muscles of the back but do not form plexuses. A large nerve, the *greater occipital*, emanates from the posterior ramus of C2 and supplies the skin of the back of the scalp extending as far forwards as the vertex of the skull where it meets the terminal fibres of the supra-orbital nerve but, with this exception, the posterior rami are very small.

THE CERVICAL PLEXUS

The cervical plexus (fig. 173) is formed from the anterior rami of the upper four cervical nerves.

A branch from C1 runs in the hypoglossal nerve for a short distance and leaves it as the *descending hypoglossal* nerve. This nerve supplies the genio-hyoid and thyrohyoid muscles and then unites with a branch from C2 and 3 called the *descendens cervicalis* and the two form a loop called the *ansa hypoglossi* which supplies the infrahyoid muscles.

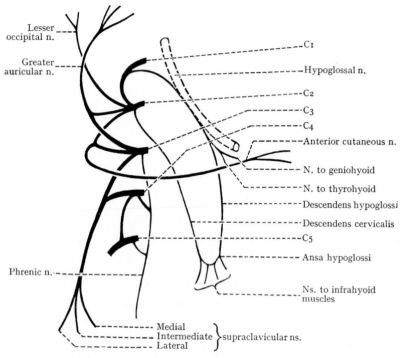

Lesser occipital n.

Greater auricular n.

C1

Hypoglossal n.

C2

C3

C4

Anterior cutaneous n.

N. to geniohyoid

N. to thyrohyoid

Descendens hypoglossi

Descendens cervicalis

C5

Ansa hypoglossi

Phrenic n.

Ns. to infrahyoid muscles

Medial
Intermediate } supraclavicular ns.
Lateral

FIG. 173.—The cervical plexus. (Redrawn from Gray's "Anatomy.")

Four cutaneous branches from the cervical plexus emerge from the posterior border of the sternomastoid. They are the *lesser occipital* nerve from C2 which supplies an area of skin at the back of the scalp; the *greater auricular* nerve from C2 and 3 which supplies the lower part of the pinna of the ear and also an area of skin in front of the ear; the *anterior cutaneous* nerve from C2 and 3 which runs transversely over sternomastoid to supply the skin in the anterior triangle of the neck; the *supraclavicular* nerves from C3 and 4 which descend over the clavicle and divide into medial, intermediate and lateral branches to supply the skin in the upper part of the thorax as far down as the 2nd rib (fig. 174).

The Phrenic Nerve (fig. 173) is the largest motor branch from the cervical plexus. It arises almost directly from C4 but receives small branches from C3 and C5 also. It descends in the neck under cover of the sternomastoid muscle and on the scalenus anterior, enters the thorax between the superior vena cava and mediastinal pleura on the right and be⸜ ⸜n the aortic arch and mediastinal pleura on the left, runs in front of the ⸜ ⸜root and reaches the diaphragm by passing between the pericardium and ʀ⸜ ⸜astinal pleura. It passes through the vena caval opening in the diaphr⸜ ⸜on the right, but pierces the central tendon of the diaphragm indepenɗ⸜ ⸜ly on the left.

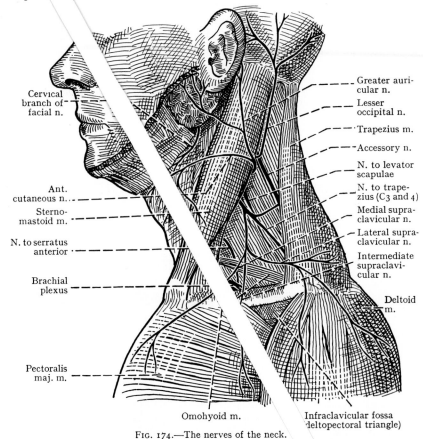

Cervical
branch of
facial n.

Ant.
cutaneous n.

Sterno-
mastoid m.

N. to serratus
anterior

Brachial
plexus

Pectoralis
maj. m.

Greater auri-
cular n.

Lesser
occipital n.

Trapezius m.

Accessory n.

N. to levator
scapulae

N. to trape-
zius (C3 and 4)

Medial supra-
clavicular n.

Lateral supra-
clavicular n.

Intermediate
supraclavi-
cular n.

Deltoid
m.

Omohyoid m.

Infraclavicular fossa
deltopectoral triangle)

FIG. 174.—The nerves of the neck.

Its fibres are two-thirds motor and one-third sensory. ʹts chief function is to supply the diaphragm but it gives branches to all ⸜e serous membranes, viz., the pericardium, pleura and peritoneum (⸜er part only especially in the region of the liver and gall bladder).

THE BRACHIAL PLEXUS

The brachial plexus (fig. 175) commences as roots formed ⸜ the anterior rami of the C5, 6, 7, 8 and T1, augmented by small branchᶜ⸜ ⸜m C4 and T2. The roots of C5 and 6 unite to form the *upper trunk*, the rᶜ⸜ ⸜f

C7 is continued forwards as the *middle trunk*, the roots of C8 and T1 unite to form the *lower trunk*. Each trunk divides into *anterior* and *posterior* divisions. The anterior divisions of the upper and middle trunks unite to form the *lateral cord*, the anterior division of the lower trunk is continued as the *medial cord*, the posterior division of all three trunks unite to form the *posterior cord*. Nerves emerge from all these various parts of the plexus.

The *roots* emerge in the posterior triangle of the neck between the scalenus anterior and scalenus medius muscles and behind the sternomastoid, the *trunks* descend behind the clavicle and the *cords* are arranged around the axillary artery in the axillary space (fig. 195, facing p. 223).

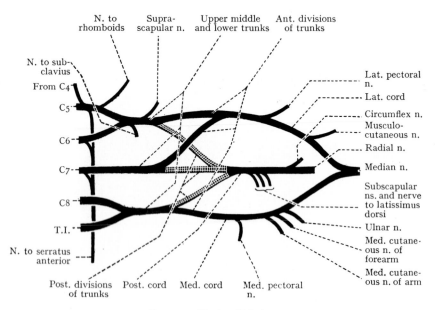

FIG. 175.—The brachial plexus.

The Nerve to Serratus Anterior (figs. 174 and 177) arises from the roots of C5, 6 and 7, runs down on the medial axillary wall with the lateral thoracic artery on the serratus anterior and supplies that muscle.

The Nerve to the Rhomboids arises from the root of C5 and runs along the medial border of the scapula beneath the levator scapulae, rhomboideus minor and major, and supplies all three muscles.

The Nerve to the Subclavius arises from the upper trunk (C5 and 6) and passes in front of the brachial plexus to the subclavius muscle.

The Suprascapular Nerve (fig. 176, facing p. 207) arises from the upper trunk (C5 and 6) and runs backwards above the main plexus to the suprascapular notch, descending on the posterior aspect of the scapula to supply the supraspinatus and infraspinatus muscles.

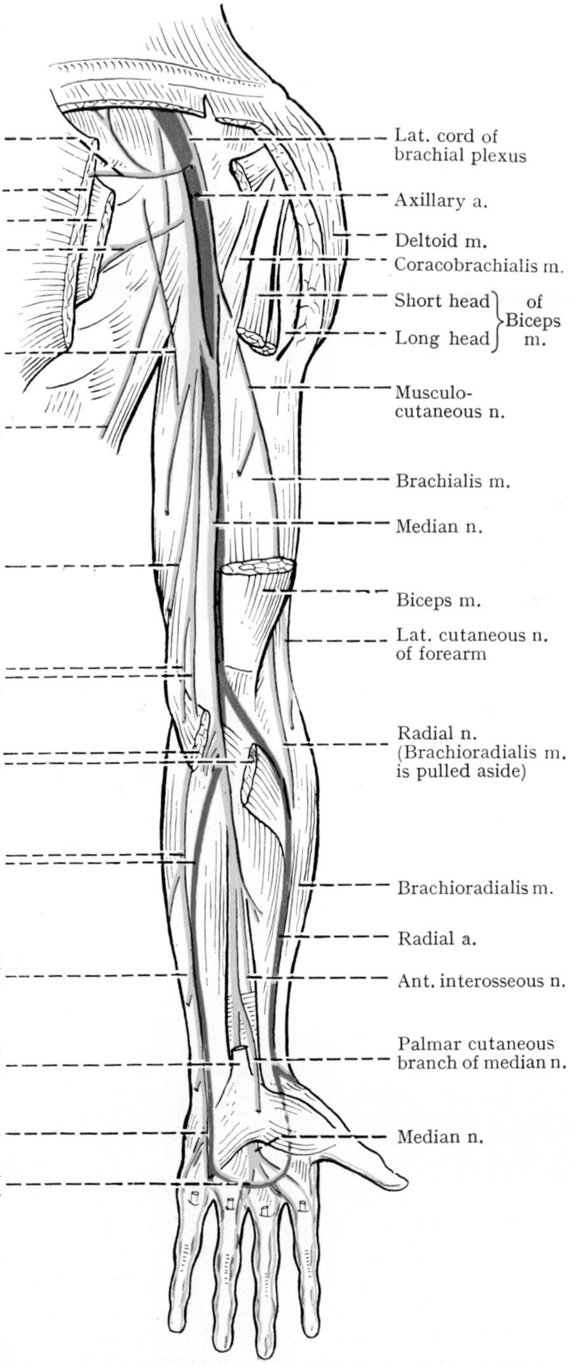

Lat. pectoral n.
Pectoralis major m.
Pectoralis minor m.
Med. pectoral n.
Intercosto-brachial n.
N. to serratus anterior
Ulnar n.
Med. cutaneous n. of forearm
Pronator teres m. (cut)
Ulnar a and n.
Flex. carpi ulnaris m.
Tendon of Palmaris longus m. (cut)
Ulnar n.
Superficial palmar arch
Lat. cord of brachial plexus
Axillary a.
Deltoid m.
Coracobrachialis m.
Short head
Long head
of Biceps m.
Musculo-cutaneous n.
Brachialis m.
Median n.
Biceps m.
Lat. cutaneous n. of forearm
Radial n. (Brachioradialis m. is pulled aside)
Brachioradialis m.
Radial a.
Ant. interosseous n.
Palmar cutaneous branch of median n.
Median n.

FIG. 177.—The arteries and nerves on the anterior aspect of the upper limb.

[*facing page 210*]

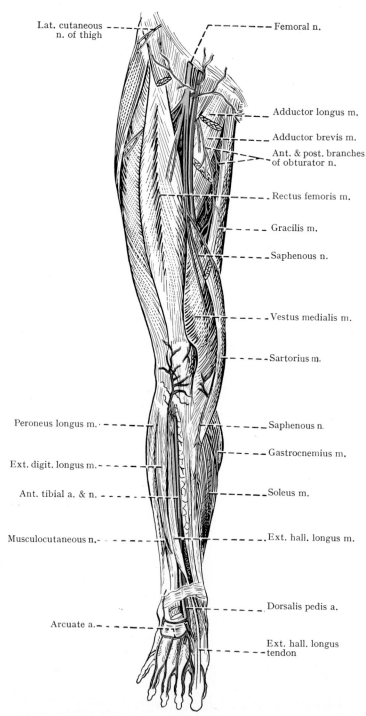

Lat. cutaneous
n. of thigh

Femoral n.

Adductor longus m.

Adductor brevis m.

Ant. & post. branches
of obturator n.

Rectus femoris m.

Gracilis m.

Saphenous n.

Vestus medialis m.

Sartorius m.

Peroneus longus m.

Saphenous n.

Gastrocnemius m.

Ext. digit. longus m.

Ant. tibial a. & n.

Soleus m.

Musculocutaneous n.

Ext. hall. longus m.

Dorsalis pedis a.

Arcuate a.

Ext. hall. longus
tendon

FIG. 183.—The arteries and nerves on the anterior aspect of the lower limb.
(Redrawn from Gray's "Anatomy.")

[facing page 211]

The **Lateral pectoral Nerve** (fig. 177) arises from the lateral cord (C5, 6 and 7) and pierces the clavipectoral fascia to supply pectoralis major.

The **Medial pectoral Nerve** (fig. 177) arises from the medial cord (C8 and T1) and pierces pectoralis minor to enter the pectoralis major. It supplies both these muscles.

The **Musculocutaneous Nerve** (fig. 177) arises from the lateral cord (C5, 6 and 7), pierces the coracobrachialis muscle and runs laterally and downwards on the front of the arm between biceps and brachialis. It pierces the deep fascia near the bend of the elbow and is then known as the *lateral cutaneous nerve of the forearm*. The musculocutaneous nerve gives *muscular* branches to the coracobrachialis, biceps and brachialis muscles and *articular* branches to the elbow joint.

The lateral cutaneous nerve of the forearm lies in the roof of the cubital fossa and supplies the skin on the lateral aspect of the front and back of the forearm extending down as far as the wrist, but is continued on to the ball of the thumb where it supplies a small area of skin.

The **Subscapular Nerves,** called the upper and lower, arise from the posterior cord. The *upper* subscapular nerve supplies the upper part of the subscapularis muscle and often the shoulder joint also. The *lower* subscapular nerve supplies the lower part of subscapularis and the teres major.

The **Nerve to Latissimus Dorsi** is a long nerve, arising from the posterior cord, and runs with the subscapular artery along the posterior axillary wall to end in the latissimus dorsi muscle.

The **Circumflex Nerve** (fig. 176)* arises from the posterior cord (C5 and 6), runs backwards through the quadrangular space (fig. 145) in close proximity to the capsule of the shoulder joint, supplies that joint, the deltoid and teres minor muscles and also an area of skin over the deltoid. Paralysis of the deltoid muscle causes a characteristic flattening of the shoulder (fig. 136).

The **Radial Nerve** (fig. 176)* arises from the posterior cord (C5, 6, 7, 8 and T1), winds round the back of the arm between the long and medial heads of triceps, runs in the spiral groove on the humerus beneath the lateral head of triceps, reaches the front of the arm between the brachialis and brachioradialis, and just above the elbow it gives off the *posterior interosseous* nerve.

It gives *muscular* branches to the three heads of triceps, anconeus, brachialis, brachioradialis and extensor carpi radialis longus—*articular* branches to the elbow joint—*cutaneous* branches to the posterior aspect of the arm called the posterior cutaneous and lower lateral cutaneous nerves of the arm and the posterior cutaneous nerve of the forearm which supplies the skin on the back of the forearm as far as the wrist.

The radial nerve (fig. 177, facing p. 210) continues into the forearm lateral to the radial artery and beneath the brachioradialis. In the lower third of the forearm it passes to the back of the limb where it gives *cutaneous* branches to the lateral half of the posterior aspect of the hand and to the lateral two-and-a-half digits, as far as the proximal interphalangeal joints (fig. 180).

The *posterior interosseous nerve* (fig. 176)* pierces the supinator, and winds

* Fig. 176 faces p. 207.

round the outer side of the radius to reach the posterior aspect of the interosseous membrane and on this structure it is carried to the wrist where it
gives *articular* branches to the wrist and carpal joints.

On the back of the forearm the posterior interosseous nerve gives off
muscular branches to the following nine muscles: supinator, extensor carpi
radialis brevis, extensor digitorum, extensor digiti minimi, extensor carpi
ulnaris, abductor pollicis longus, extensor pollicis longus, extensor pollicis
brevis, and extensor indicis.

The radial nerve is often injured in fractures of the humerus and as the
result of pressure in the axilla (crutch palsy). The result is a characteristic
dropping of the wrist due to paralysis of the extensor muscles.

The Median Nerve (fig. 177, facing p. 210) arises by two heads from
the medial and lateral cords of the brachial plexus (C5, 6, 7, 8 and T1). It
runs down the upper part of the arm on the lateral aspect of the axillary and
brachial arteries, crosses the latter vessel about the middle of the arm and
then lies on its medial aspect. It is seen in this position in the cubital
fossa which it leaves by passing between the two heads of the pronator teres.
In the forearm it is adherent to the under surface of the flexor digitorum
sublimis but becomes superficial at the wrist. It then enters the palm behind
the flexor retinaculum and divides into *medial* and *lateral terminal* branches.

On emerging from the cubital fossa it immediately gives off the
anterior interosseous nerve. This nerve runs down on the anterior aspect
of the interosseous membrane and gives *muscular* branches to the flexor
pollicis longus, the lateral half of flexor digitorum profundus and also the
pronator quadratus muscles. It gives *articular* branches to the wrist and
carpal joints.

The main trunk of the median nerve gives *muscular* branches to pronator
teres, flexor carpi radialis, palmaris longus and flexor digitorum sublimis,
articular branches to the elbow joint and a *cutaneous* branch to the central
and lateral aspects of the palm.

The *lateral terminal* branch of the nerve gives *muscular* branches to the
superficial short muscles of the thumb, viz., abductor, flexor and opponens
pollicis and the first lumbrical muscle. The *medial terminal* branch gives a
muscular branch to the second lumbrical muscle.

Both terminal branches give off *cutaneous* digital branches which supply
the outer $3\frac{1}{2}$ digits on their palmar aspect and the middle and distal phalanges
of these digits on their dorsal aspect (fig. 179 and 180).

The median nerve is responsible for the coarse movements of the hand
and has, therefore, been termed "the labourer's nerve." It is sometimes
severed in injuries at the wrist. This results in a loss of the pincer action
between the thumb and fingers, a wasting of the thenar muscles and anaesthesia of the cutaneous area supplied by the nerve.

The Medial Cutaneous Nerve of the Arm (fig. 179) arises from the
medial cord and is distributed to the skin on the medial aspect of the arm.

The Medial Cutaneous Nerve of the Forearm (figs. 179 and 180)
arises from the medial cord and pierces the deep fascia on the medial aspect
of biceps, appears in the roof of the cubital fossa and supplies an area of

skin on the front and back of the medial aspect of the forearm extending as far as the wrist.

The Ulnar Nerve (fig. 177) arises from the medial cord of the brachial plexus (C7, 8 and T1), runs down on the medial aspect of the axillary and brachial arteries as far as the middle of the arm, then on the medial head of triceps and thus reaches the back of the arm where it appears behind the medial epicondyle of the humerus and can be palpated with ease in that position (fig. 55). It enters the forearm between the two heads of flexor carpi ulnaris, is covered by this muscle in the upper part of the forearm, but

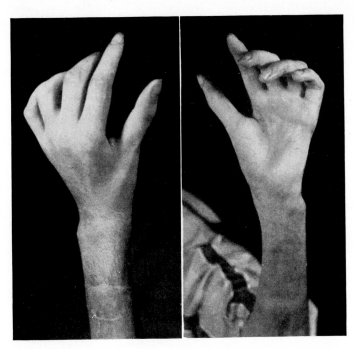

FIG. 178.—A case of ulnar nerve palsy showing partial claw hand.

Note the wasting of the intrinsic muscles of the hand—that of the first dorsal interosseus muscle is particularly well seen.

below it is covered only by skin and fascia. It enters the hand by passing over the flexor retinaculum, lateral to the pisiform bone and medial to the hook of the hamate. In the palm it divides into *superficial* and *deep terminal* branches.

The ulnar nerve gives off *articular* branches to the elbow joint and *muscular* branches to flexor carpi ulnaris and the medial half of flexor digitorum profundus.

A *palmar cutaneous* branch arises about the middle of the forearm and runs down on the ulnar artery to supply an area of skin on the medial aspect of the palm (fig. 179).

14—A.PH.

A *dorsal cutaneous* branch arises just above the wrist and passes beneath the flexor carpi ulnaris to reach the back of the hand supplying an area of skin on its medial aspect and also the posterior surface of the medial $2\frac{1}{2}$ digits (fig. 180).

The *superficial terminal* branch gives a *muscular* branch to palmaris brevis, a *cutaneous* branch to the medial aspect of the palm and the palmar surface of the medial $1\frac{1}{2}$ digits (fig. 179).

The *deep terminal* branch passes deeply into the palm between abductor and flexor digiti minimi and through opponens. In the palm it lies on the metacarpal bones and interossei in the concavity of the deep palmar arch. This nerve gives *muscular* branches to the abductor, flexor and opponens digiti minimi, the adductor pollicis, the two inner lumbricals and all eight interossei. It also gives an *articular* branch to the wrist joint.

The ulnar nerve is responsible for the finer movements of the hand and has thus been termed "the musician's nerve." When paralysed the metacarpophalangeal joints are extended and the interphalangeal joints flexed. This condition is known as "claw hand" and is accentuated if the median nerve is also involved (e.g., in wounds of the wrist).

The Intercostal Nerves

The intercostal nerves are the anterior rami of the thoracic nerves. There are twelve such nerves and each lies in an intercostal space with the exception of the 12th which lies below the last rib.

Each nerve lies in the subcostal groove on the under surface of a rib, together with the corresponding intercostal vessels. The position of the structures in a subcostal groove is vein, artery, nerve from above down. Each nerve gives off a *lateral* branch which pierces the thoracic muscles and divides into anterior and posterior cutaneous branches and also an *anterior* branch which divides into medial and lateral branches.

A typical intercostal nerve (fig. 181), after emerging from an intervertebral foramen, runs forwards between the pleura and the posterior intercostal membrane, then between intercostalis intimi and internal intercostal muscles and then between the latter muscle and the pleura. Just before its termination it lies on the sternocostalis muscle, where it crosses the internal mammary artery. Finally as an anterior cutaneous nerve it perforates the internal intercostal muscle, anterior intercostal membrane and pectoralis major and is distributed to the skin on the front of the chest. Near the angle of the rib an intercostal nerve gives off a collateral and a lateral cutaneous branch. The former runs along the upper border of the rib below and supplies the intercostal muscles. The *lateral cutaneous* branch perforates the internal and external intercostal muscles and the serratus anterior muscle and divides into branches which supply the lateral and posterior aspects of the chest ramifying posteriorly with branches from the posterior rami of the thoracic nerves and anteriorly with branches from the anterior branch of the intercostal nerve. In this way the skin over the whole of the thorax is innervated.

The first intercostal nerve makes a major contribution to the brachial

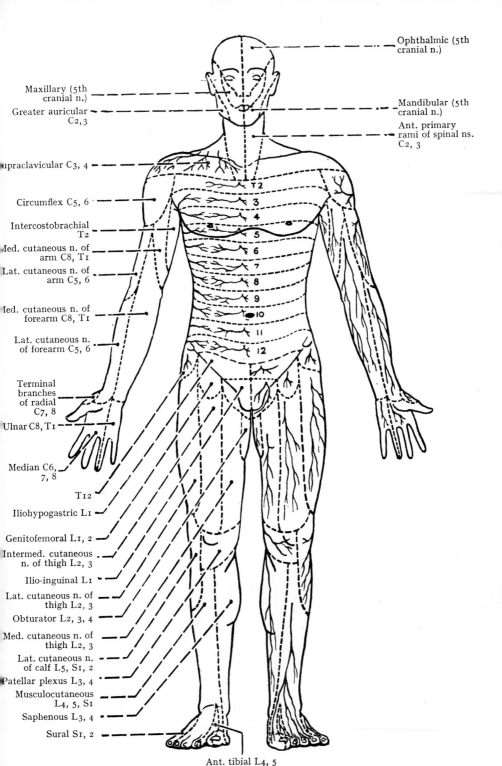

Ophthalmic (5th cranial n.)

Maxillary (5th cranial n.)

Greater auricular C2, 3

Mandibular (5th cranial n.)

Ant. primary rami of spinal ns. C2, 3

Supraclavicular C3, 4

Circumflex C5, 6

Intercostobrachial T2

Med. cutaneous n. of arm C8, T1

Lat. cutaneous n. of arm C5, 6

Med. cutaneous n. of forearm C8, T1

Lat. cutaneous n. of forearm C5, 6

Terminal branches of radial C7, 8

Ulnar C8, T1

Median C6, 7, 8

T12

Iliohypogastric L1

Genitofemoral L1, 2

Intermed. cutaneous n. of thigh L2, 3

Ilio-inguinal L1

Lat. cutaneous n. of thigh L2, 3

Obturator L2, 3, 4

Med. cutaneous n. of thigh L2, 3

Lat. cutaneous n. of calf L5, S1, 2

Patellar plexus L3, 4

Musculocutaneous L4, 5, S1

Saphenous L3, 4

Sural S1, 2

T2
3
4
5
6
7
8
9
10
11
12

Ant. tibial L4, 5

FIG. 179.—Cutaneous nerve supply to front of body.

215

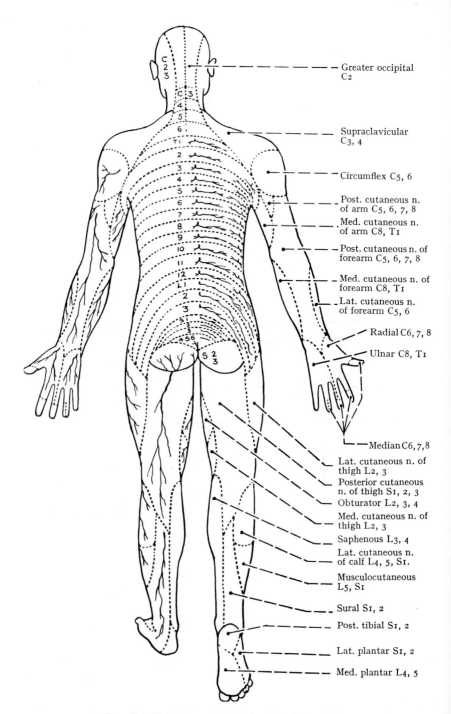

Greater occipital
C2

Supraclavicular
C3, 4

Circumflex C5, 6

Post. cutaneous n.
of arm C5, 6, 7, 8

Med. cutaneous n.
of arm C8, T1

Post. cutaneous n. of
forearm C5, 6, 7, 8

Med. cutaneous n. of
forearm C8, T1

Lat. cutaneous n.
of forearm C5, 6

Radial C6, 7, 8

Ulnar C8, T1

Median C6, 7, 8

Lat. cutaneous n. of
thigh L2, 3

Posterior cutaneous
n. of thigh S1, 2, 3

Obturator L2, 3, 4

Med. cutaneous n. of
thigh L2, 3

Saphenous L3, 4

Lat. cutaneous n.
of calf L4, 5, S1.

Musculocutaneous
L5, S1

Sural S1, 2

Post. tibial S1, 2

Lat. plantar S1, 2

Med. plantar L4, 5

FIG. 180.—Cutaneous nerve supply to back of body.

plexus and sends only a small branch to the first interspace while the lateral cutaneous branch of the second and sometimes the third passes to the arm as the *intercostobrachial nerve.*

It should be noted that the nerves of the thorax lie for the most part between the second and third layers of muscles on the thoracic wall and thus conform to the arrangement of the nerves on the abdominal wall.

The 7th to 11th thoracic nerves having run in the intercostal spaces descend behind the costal cartilages on to the abdominal wall where they branch in precisely the same way as the intercostal nerves. These nerves are, therefore, sometimes referred to as "the *thoraco-abdominal nerves.*"

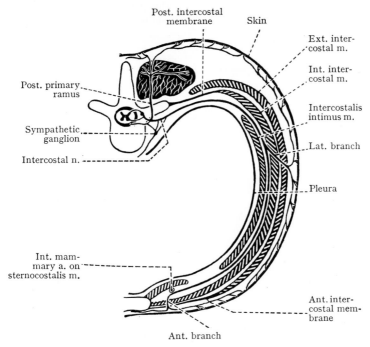

FIG. 181.—A typical intercostal nerve.

The 12th thoracic nerve lies below the 12th rib, descends beneath the lateral arcuate ligament into the abdomen, where it lies on the posterior abdominal wall behind the kidney. It then pierces the transversus muscle and runs forwards between that muscle and the internal oblique. It ends by supplying an area of skin just above the symphysis pubis. Its *lateral cutaneous* branch supplies an area of skin on the upper part of the lateral aspect of the thigh as far down as the greater trochanter.

The attention of the student is called to the fact that the skin in the region of the umbilicus is supplied by T10, in the region of the xiphoid process by T7 and in the region of the symphysis pubis by T12 and L1. The remaining nerves supply the intervening areas (fig. 179).

The intercostal nerves supply all the intercostal muscles; T7–12 supply also the muscles of the abdominal wall; T12 alone supplies the small vestigial pyramidalis muscle.

THE LUMBAR PLEXUS

The lumbar plexus is formed by the anterior rami of the first 5 lumbar nerves augmented by a small branch from the 12th thoracic and lies behind the psoas muscle.

The first lumbar nerve divides into the *iliohypogastric* and *ilio-inguinal* nerves, branches from L1 and L2 unite to form the *genitofemoral* nerve, branches from L2 and L3 form the *lateral cutaneous nerve of the thigh*, branches from L2, 3 and 4 form the *obturator* and *femoral* nerves and branches from

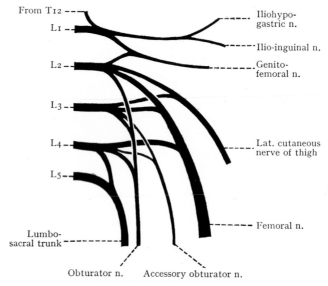

FIG. 182.—Lumbar plexus.

L3 and 4 form the *accessory obturator* nerve, while branches from L4 and L5 descend to join the sacral plexus as the *lumbosacral trunk*.

The **Iliohypogastric Nerve** arises from L1, passes over quadratus lumborum, behind the kidney, pierces transversus abdominis, runs forward between that muscle and internal oblique, pierces the internal oblique in front of the anterior superior spine of the ilium and pierces the external oblique above the external abdominal ring to supply the skin over the symphysis pubis. It gives off *muscular* branches to all the muscles of the anterior abdominal wall and a *lateral cutaneous* branch which supplies an area of skin on the buttock.

The **Ilio-inguinal Nerve** arises from L1, lies below the iliohypogastric nerve and runs a similar course. It pierces the internal oblique just above the middle of the inguinal ligament and runs in the inner half of the inguinal canal emerging through the external abdominal ring. It gives *muscular* branches to muscles on the abdominal wall (not pyramidalis or rectus abdominis) and *cutaneous* branches to the skin over the symphysis pubis, to the external genitalia and the upper part of the front of the thigh.

The **Genitofemoral Nerve** arises from L1 and 2, emerges from the middle of psoas and descends on that muscle to the lower abdomen where it divides into a *genital* branch which supplies the cremaster muscle on the spermatic cord and a *femoral* branch which supplies an area of skin on the upper part of the front of the thigh.

The **Lateral Cutaneous Nerve of the Thigh** (fig. 183)* arises from L2 and 3, emerges from the lateral border of psoas, crosses iliacus, lies in a groove below the anterior superior iliac spine where it pierces sartorius to supply an area of skin over the buttock and lateral aspect of the thigh.

The **Obturator Nerve** (fig. 183)* arises from the ventral branches of the anterior primary rami of L2, 3 and 4, emerges from the medial border of psoas, runs forward in front of the sacro-iliac joint, then along the lateral pelvic wall with the obturator vessels, emerges through the obturator canal in the obturator foramen and divides into an anterior and a posterior branch. These two branches lie at first on the obturator externus and are separated from each other as they descend in the thigh by the adductor brevis.

The *anterior* branch lies deep to adductor longus. It gives *muscular* branches to adductor longus, adductor brevis, gracilis and rarely to pectineus; *articular* branches to the hip joint and a *cutaneous* branch to the medial aspect of the thigh. The *posterior* branch lies deep to adductor brevis and gives *muscular* branches to obturator externus and adductor magnus. It also gives an *articular* branch which pierces adductor magnus and runs down on the popliteal artery to supply the knee joint.

The *accessory obturator nerve* is not constant. It arises from L3 and 4 and enters the thigh above the superior ramus of the pubis where it divides into three branches, a *communicating* branch to the obturator nerve, an *articular* branch to the hip joint and a *muscular* branch which supplies pectineus. When this muscle is supplied by the accessory obturator nerve it is not also supplied by the obturator nerve.

The **Femoral Nerve** (fig. 183)* arises from the dorsal branches of the anterior primary rami of L2, 3 and 4 and appears in the false pelvis, on the lateral border of the psoas, between that muscle and iliacus. It descends on the iliacus, behind the caecum on the right and the pelvic colon on the left and emerging from behind the inguinal ligament enters the thigh on the lateral aspect of the femoral vessels in the femoral triangle. The main trunk gives off the nerves to the iliacus muscle in the pelvis and the nerve to pectineus near the inguinal ligament and then divides into its terminal branches which commence as anterior and posterior divisions.

The *anterior division* gives off the *medial* and *intermediate cutaneous nerves of the thigh* which supply the skin on the medial and anterior aspects of the thigh respectively (fig. 179) and it also gives off *muscular* branches to the sartorius.

* Fig. 183 faces p. 211.

The *posterior division* gives off *muscular* branches to the muscles forming the quadriceps and also to the articularis genu. The branch to rectus femoris gives an *articular* branch to the hip joint, the other muscular branches give *articular* branches to the knee joint. The posterior division also gives off an important *cutaneous* nerve called the *saphenous* nerve (fig. 183, facing p. 211) which traverses the subsartorial canal and becomes superficial at the medial aspect of the knee. It descends on the medial aspect of the leg and foot as far as the ball of the great toe and supplies areas of skin in those regions.

The *subsartorial plexus* of nerves lie beneath the sartorius as it covers the subsartorial canal. It is formed by cutaneous branches from the femoral and obturator nerves.

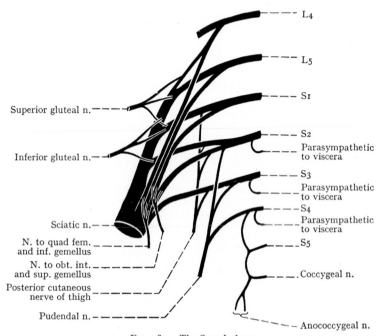

FIG. 184.—The Sacral plexus.

The *patellar plexus* (fig. 179) lies in front of the lower part of the patella and on the ligamentum patellae and is formed by cutaneous branches from the femoral nerve.

THE SACRAL PLEXUS

The sacral plexus is formed from the anterior rami of S1, 2 and 3, augmented by L4 and 5 from the lumbosacral trunk and by a branch from S4.

The nerves forming this plexus converge to form one large trunk which passes out of the pelvis through the greater sciatic foramen, below the piriformis muscle. From this trunk the following branches emerge:

The Nerve to Quadratus Femoris from L4, 5 and S1 supplies that muscle, the inferior gemellus and also the hip joint.

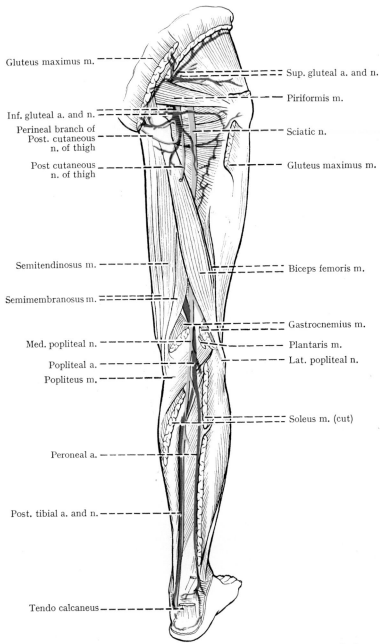

Gluteus maximus m.

Sup. gluteal a. and n.

Piriformis m.

Inf. gluteal a. and n.

Perineal branch of
Post. cutaneous
n. of thigh

Sciatic n.

Post cutaneous
n. of thigh

Gluteus maximus m.

Semitendinosus m.

Biceps femoris m.

Semimembranosus m.

Gastrocnemius m.

Med. popliteal n.

Plantaris m.

Popliteal a.

Lat. popliteal n.

Popliteus m.

Soleus m. (cut)

Peroneal a.

Post. tibial a. and n.

Tendo calcaneus

Fig. 185.—The arteries and nerves on the posterior aspect of the lower limb.
(Redrawn from "Gray's Anatomy.")

[facing page 220]

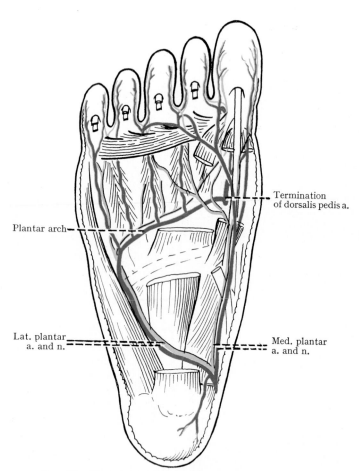

Termination
of dorsalis pedis a.

Plantar arch

Lat. plantar
a. and n.

Med. plantar
a. and n.

FIG. 186.—The arteries and nerves on the sole of the foot.

The Nerve to Obturator Internus from L5, S1 and 2 supplies superior gemellus and obturator internus.

The Superior Gluteal Nerve from L4, 5 and S1 emerges from the main trunk through the greater sciatic foramen above piriformis and supplies gluteus medius, minimus and tensor fasciae latae.

The Inferior Gluteal Nerve from L5, S1 and 2 supplies gluteus maximus.

The Nerve to Piriformis from S1 and 2 supplies that muscle.

The Posterior Cutaneous Nerve of the Thigh (fig. 185) arises from S1, 2 and 3, descends under cover of gluteus maximus into the thigh where it lies beneath the deep fascia and on the biceps femoris.   It pierces the deep fascia at the back of the knee and ends at the middle of the back of the calf of the leg.   The nerve is entirely cutaneous and supplies areas of skin over gluteus maximus, on the proximal part of the medial aspect of the thigh, on the back of the thigh and on the upper part of the leg.

The Sciatic Nerve (fig. 185) arises from L4, 5, S1, 2 and 3, descends under cover of gluteus maximus and passes into the thigh beneath the biceps femoris.   It lies first on the ischium near the acetabulum and then successively on superior gemellus, obturator internus, inferior gemellus, quadratus femoris and adductor magnus.   It ends just below the middle of the thigh (very variable) by dividing into *lateral* and *medial* popliteal nerves.

It gives *muscular* branches to the hamstrings, viz., biceps, semitendinosus, semimembranosus and the hamstring part of adductor magnus.   The branch to the short head of the biceps comes from the lateral popliteal portion of the nerve, while the remaining muscles are supplied from the medial popliteal portion.   It also gives an *articular* branch to the hip joint.

The sciatic nerve is a flat strap-like structure about 1 cm. wide.   It is the largest and strongest nerve in the body.

The Lateral Popliteal Nerve (fig. 185) is the smaller of the two terminal branches of the sciatic nerve.   It runs down on the lateral wall of the popliteal fossa in close proximity to the tendon of biceps and then winds round the neck of the fibula.   It can be palpated in both these regions.   It finally enters the substance of the peroneus longus muscle where it divides into its two terminal branches, viz., the *musculocutaneous* and *anterior tibial* nerves.   It gives off no muscular branches but gives *articular* branches to the knee joint and also *cutaneous* branches which supply the skin on the anterolateral aspect of the leg and joining a cutaneous branch from the medial popliteal nerve it forms the *sural* nerve which supplies the skin on the lateral aspect of the foot (fig. 179).

The Musculocutaneous Nerve (fig. 183) emerges from the peroneus longus and runs down the leg between that muscle and extensor digitorum longus, becomes cutaneous in the lower third of the leg and passes to the dorsum of the foot, giving *cutaneous* branches to these regions and also to the medial aspect of the great toe and the contiguous sides of the other toes with the exception of the cleft between the first and second toes (fig. 179).

The nerve gives *muscular* branches to the peroneus longus and brevis.

The Anterior Tibial Nerve (fig. 183, facing p. 211) runs deep to peroneus longus and extensor digitorum longus and reaches the anterior aspect of the interosseous membrane where it lies between tibialis anterior and extensor digitorum longus but is later crossed superficially by extensor hallucis longus. It then runs in front of the ankle joint to the dorsum of the foot where it divides into its two terminal branches—a *medial* branch which supplies the contiguous sides of the 1st and 2nd toes (fig. 179) the metatarsophalangeal joint of the great toe and the first dorsal interosseous muscle and a *lateral* branch which supplies extensor digitorum brevis, the second dorsal interosseous muscle and the tarsal and metatarsal joints.

The nerve gives *muscular* branches to the tibialis anterior, extensor digitorum longus, extensor hallucis longus and peroneus tertius. It also gives an *articular* branch to the ankle joint.

The Medial Popliteal Nerve (fig. 185) is the larger terminal branch of the sciatic nerve; it traverses the popliteal fossa, lying just beneath the deep fascia and crosses the popliteal vessels superficially from their lateral to their medial side. At the lower border of the popliteus muscle it becomes the *posterior tibial nerve.*

It gives off *muscular* branches to the gastrocnemius, plantaris, popliteus and soleus. It gives *articular* branches to the knee joint; *cutaneous* branches which supply the skin on the posteromedial aspect of the leg, one of which joins a branch from the lateral popliteal nerve to form the *sural nerve.*

The Posterior Tibial Nerve (fig. 185) is a continuation of the medial popliteal nerve and commences at the lower border of popliteus. It runs down beneath the calf muscles, but in the lower part of the leg is superficial, lying on the medial border of the tendo calcaneus. It descends between the medial malleolus and the heel and enters the sole beneath abductor hallucis where it divides into *medial* and *lateral plantar nerves.*

It gives *muscular* branches to soleus, tibialis posterior, flexor digitorum longus, flexor hallucis longus; *articular* branches to the ankle joint and a *cutaneous* branch to the skin on the back of the heel and the adjacent sole of the foot.

The Medial Plantar Nerve (fig. 186) runs forwards on the sole of the foot beneath abductor hallucis, giving *cutaneous* branches to the skin on the medial aspect of the sole and the inner 3½ toes; *muscular* branches to abductor hallucis, flexor digitorum brevis, flexor hallucis brevis and the first lumbrical muscle. It is comparable to the median nerve in the hand.

The Lateral Plantar Nerve (fig. 186) runs across the sole of the foot beneath flexor digitorum brevis to the base of the fifth digit and divides into a superficial and deep branch. The *superficial* branch gives *muscular* branches to the flexor digiti minimi and *cutaneous* branches to an area of skin on the sole and to the outer 1½ toes. The *deep* branch accompanies the plantar arch and gives *muscular* branches to the interossei, outer three lumbricals and the adductor hallucis. The *main trunk* of the lateral plantar nerve gives *muscular* branches to the flexor digitorum accessorius, abductor digiti minimi and a *cutaneous* branch to the lateral aspect of the sole. It is comparable to the ulnar nerve in the hand.

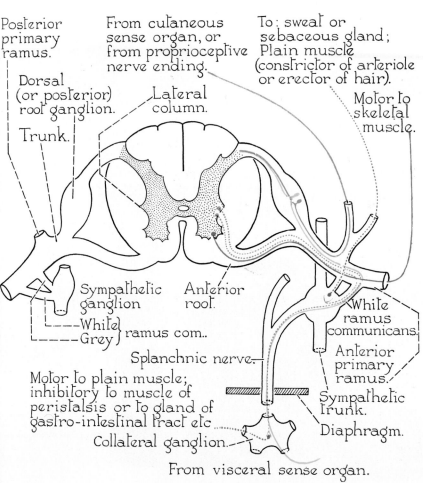

Posterior primary ramus.

From cutaneous sense organ, or from proprioceptive nerve ending.

To: sweat or sebaceous gland; Plain muscle (constrictor of arteriole or erector of hair).

Dorsal (or posterior) root ganglion.

Lateral column.

Motor to skeletal muscle.

Trunk.

Sympathetic ganglion

Anterior root.

White
Grey } ramus com..

White ramus communicans.

Anterior primary ramus.

Splanchnic nerve.

Sympathetic Trunk.

Motor to plain muscle; inhibitory to muscle of peristalsis or to gland of gastro-intestinal tract etc.

Diaphragm.

Collateral ganglion.

From visceral sense organ.

FIG. 187—A scheme of the sympathetic nervous system.

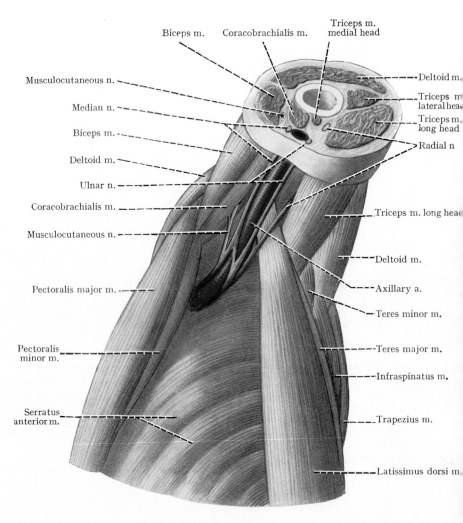

Biceps m.   Coracobrachialis m.   Triceps m. medial head

Musculocutaneous n.

Median n.

Biceps m.

Deltoid m.

Ulnar n.

Coracobrachialis m.

Musculocutaneous n.

Pectoralis major m.

Pectoralis minor m.

Serratus anterior m.

Deltoid m.

Triceps m. lateral head

Triceps m. long head

Radial n.

Triceps m. long head

Deltoid m.

Axillary a.

Teres minor m.

Teres major m.

Infraspinatus m.

Trapezius m.

Latissimus dorsi m.

Fig. 195.—The axillary artery in its relation to the brachial plexus.

THE AUTONOMIC OR INVOLUNTARY NERVOUS SYSTEM

This is really part of the general nervous system but its pharmacological reactions have caused it to be described separately. In the autonomic nervous system we include the sympathetic and parasympathetic systems. Probably all the organs of the body are supplied by both systems which,

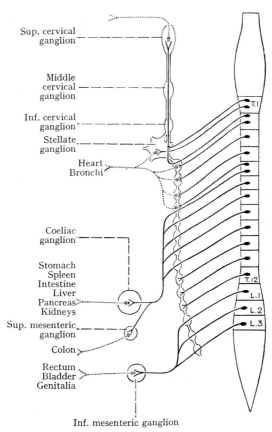

Sup. cervical ganglion

Middle cervical ganglion

Inf. cervical ganglion

Stellate ganglion

Heart
Bronchi

Coeliac ganglion

Stomach
Spleen
Intestine
Liver
Pancreas
Kidneys

Sup. mesenteric ganglion

Colon

Rectum
Bladder
Genitalia

T.I

T.12
L.I
L.2
L.3

Inf. mesenteric ganglion

FIG. 188.—A scheme of the sympathetic nervous system. (After Villiger.)
(see final paragraph, p. 224).

speaking generally, have opposing but complementary actions for when one is stimulated the other is inhibited.

It will have been understood that the central nervous system is concerned with receiving sensory impulses of which, with certain exceptions, the individual is made conscious, and as the result of these impressions it effects voluntary movements which are initiated by motor impulses sent from the brain to the voluntary muscles.

The autonomic nervous system innervates structures which are not controlled by the will and the individual is not conscious of its activities. It is a controlling factor in the movements of the heart, the bronchi, the pupil of the eye, the alimentary tract and the bladder and it governs the sphincters of the body. It is responsible for the tone of the blood vessels, especially the arterioles. It controls the small arrectores pilorum muscles of the skin and it regulates the secretions of the numerous glands throughout the body. The whole system is under the control of the brain, although many of the parent cells of its fibres are situated within cell stations which lie outside the central nervous system. The nerve fibres of the autonomic system are much more delicate than those of the spinal nerves, and when near their termination are distributed along, and are supported by, blood vessels going to the same parts.

In order to understand the autonomic nervous system the student should locate its cell stations and trace their connections with the central nervous system.

The cell stations of the sympathetic nervous system consist of a series of ganglia (nerve cells bound together by connective tissue) and inter-communicating trunks, which together constitute the *sympathetic chain*. This chain extends from the base of the skull to the coccyx, where it is united to its fellow of the opposite side. It is situated deeply at the side of the vertebral column. There are three ganglia in the neck, called the *superior*, *middle* and *inferior cervical ganglia*. The superior cervical ganglion is the largest in the body and is nearly 2·5 cm. long. In the thoracic region there are usually twelve ganglia, in the lumbar region four and in the sacral region four, but the numbers vary as fusion of adjacent ganglia is common.

Arising from the lower thoracic ganglia are the greater, lesser and least *splanchnic nerves* which pass into the abdomen and connect with further sympathetic ganglia called *collateral ganglia* which are to be found in close relation with the aorta and its branches. These comprise the *semilunar* or *coeliac ganglion* which supplies the stomach, small intestines, liver, spleen, pancreas and kidneys; the *superior mesenteric ganglion* which supplies the colon and the *inferior mesenteric ganglion* which supplies the rectum, bladder and the genital organs (fig. 188).

The fibres from the sympathetic ganglia form three large networks or nerve plexuses in the regions they supply. These are called the *cardiac plexus* which lies in the thorax at the base of the heart and receives fibres from the cervical as well as the upper six thoracic ganglia; the *solar plexus* which lies in the abdomen behind the stomach and receives its fibres from the coeliac ganglia; and the *hypogastric plexus* which lies in the pelvis in front of the sacral promontory. The solar plexus is by far the largest and from it a number of subsidiary plexuses arise which derive their names from the various organs innervated (e.g., renal, testicular, hepatic, etc.).

Connections with the central nervous system. Typically each ganglion is connected with a spinal nerve by two communicating branches called the *grey* and *white rami communicantes*.

In fig. 188 the spinal cord is represented on the right, certain collateral ganglia on the left and the sympathetic chain in the middle. The cervical ganglia are fused to form the superior, middle and inferior cervical ganglia.

The first thoracic ganglion is known as the stellate ganglion, because of its shape in man—in animals it is fused with the inferior cervical ganglion. Preganglionic fibres are seen issuing from the cord, some are relaying in the ganglia of the sympathetic chain whence postganglionic fibres emerge to be carried to the viscera (e.g., the heart and bronchi); others are passing directly through these ganglia to collateral ganglia whence postganglionic fibres emerge to be carried to other viscera (e.g., the stomach, intestine, liver, etc.). Postganglionic fibres are indicated by interrupted lines.

Each *white ramus* (fig. 187) conveys efferent fibres from the lateral column of grey matter in the spinal cord, which is confined to the thoracic and upper lumbar regions only and passing out via an anterior nerve root ends by arborising around cells in a ganglion in the sympathetic chain. Such nerves are, therefore, called *preganglionic* and are medullated.

From these ganglion cells a further set of nerve fibres carries the impulse back to the spinal nerve via a *grey ramus* (fig. 187), such nerves are, therefore, called *postganglionic* and are non-medullated. The composition of any spinal nerve, therefore, consists of sensory, motor and sympathetic nerve fibres.

Each spinal nerve throughout the body receives a grey ramus from the adjacent autonomic ganglion, yet only the spinal nerves from the thoracic and upper lumbar regions receive a white ramus (fig. 188). The sympathetic fibres which pass to the cervical ganglia to be distributed to the head and neck, upper limbs and heart all arise from the thoracic portion of the spinal cord.

The splanchnic nerves pass without interruption through the ganglia of the sympathetic chain to end in collateral ganglia. They consist of pre-ganglionic fibres which having arborised around the cells in these ganglia emerge as postganglionic fibres for distribution to the viscera and abdominal blood vessels (figs. 187 and 188).

The parasympathetic nervous system is confined to the head and trunk. Parasympathetic fibres are carried in the oculomotor, facial, glossopharyngeal and vagus nerves and in the 2nd, 3rd and 4th sacral nerves. Their cells stations are not in sympathetic ganglia but with a few exceptions lie within discrete ganglia in the walls of the organs innervated. It follows, therefore, that the postganglionic fibres of the parasympathetic nervous system are usually exceedingly short, e.g., the terminal fibres of the vagus, known as Auerbach's plexus, which are to be found in the walls of the alimentary canal. In addition there are vaso-dilator fibres which pass out by all the posterior nerve roots. These have now been shown to be para-sympathetic and to liberate acetylcholine like the vagus.

The action of the sympathetic, augmented by the action of adrenaline (from the suprarenal gland) which it immediately summons to its aid, is to accelerate the heart, to dilate the coronary vessels thus ensuring an adequate blood supply for the more active myocardium, to constrict the vessels of the skin and intestine and thus raise the blood pressure, to dilate the bronchi thus allowing adequate respiration, to dilate the blood vessels supplying active muscles, to increase the blood sugar from which the body will derive energy, to retard glandular secretion (except sweat), to inhibit the movements of the alimentary tract and the bladder and to close the sphincters. The sympathetic may, therefore, be looked upon as catering for the needs of the active body and its action is vital for the performance of any extra physical effort which may be needed in an emergency. It prepares the body for such effort and is immediately activated by any mental stress.

The action of the parasympathetic is the opposite to that of the sympathetic. Through the activities of the vagus it slows the heart, increases peristalsis, dilates the sphincters, increases glandular secretion (except sweat), mobilises insulin and, therefore, lowers the blood sugar. The parasympathetic, most active in physical and mental rest, is associated with the conservation of energy and in that sense it is complementary to the sympathetic, for the more energy we conserve the less readily do we succumb to fatigue, the greater our range of activity and the more effectively can we respond to a sudden emergency. There is, however, complete reciprocity between the two systems such as might be compared to that between the extensor and flexor muscles of a limb. In a trained athlete, for example, the action of the vagus is increased and the heart at rest beats very slowly, therefore, in exercise, when vagal activity is reduced, the heart has a greater range of activity which is still further enhanced by sympathetic action.

There is good reason to believe from the study of the effects of sensory stimulation on anaesthetised animals that massage or anything that stimulates the skin, e.g., baths, cold winds or exercise, all increase the action of the autonomic nervous system and generally "tone up" the individual, promoting a feeling of good health.

The pathway of visceral sensation. The fibres which carry impulses from the internal organs run with the efferent fibres of the autonomic nervous system but pass into the posterior nerve roots like ordinary sensory nerves. Their points of entrance are, however, not confined to any special region. The vagus is the afferent pathway from the lungs and stomach and irritation of its fibres may give rise to reflex coughing or vomiting.

Sympathectomy. The sympathetic is sectioned for the relief of excessive contraction of blood vessels. This condition may cause great discomfort especially in the legs during walking (intermittent claudication). When the sympathetic is sectioned either at operation, or by injury, the vessels of the part dilate and there is greatly increased blood flow. Unfortunately, the benefit is not always sustained, probably because the denervated vessels become abnormally sensitive to any vasoconstrictor substances which may circulate in the blood.

CHAPTER VI
THE CIRCULATORY SYSTEM

The heart will be described with the thoracic viscera, so that under the heading "Circulatory System" a description of the arterial, venous and lymphatic systems alone will be given.

THE ARTERIAL SYSTEM

The Pulmonary Trunk (fig. 189)

This vessel arises from the right ventricle and conveys venous blood to the lungs where it is oxygenated. It is the foremost structure on the

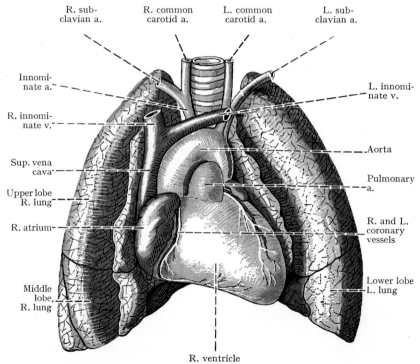

FIG. 189.—The lungs, heart and great vessels. (Redrawn from Gray's "Anatomy.")

surface of the heart running upwards and slightly to the left in front of the ascending aorta to end beneath the aortic arch by dividing into right and left branches. The pulmonary trunk is about 5 cm. long and is wholly contained within the pericardium.

The Right Pulmonary Artery is much shorter than the left. It passes

227

to the right lung root behind the ascending aorta, superior vena cava and pulmonary veins, in front of the right bronchus.

The Left Pulmonary Artery passes in front of the descending aorta and left bronchus and behind the left pulmonary veins to reach the left lung root.

Within the lung substance the pulmonary arteries divide and subdivide, accompanying the subdivisions of the bronchi, into the lobes and lobules of the lungs.

The Ascending Aorta (fig. 189)

This vessel emerges from the left ventricle at the left border of the sternum opposite the third costal cartilage. It passes upwards and to the right behind the sternum, ending at the level of the sternal angle (second costal cartilage), where it becomes the aortic arch.

Near its commencement there are three dilatations, one situated anteriorly and two posteriorly, called *the aortic sinuses*. From the anterior sinus, the right coronary artery and from the left posterior sinus, the left coronary artery, emerges. These vessels supply the heart wall.

The right coronary artery is distributed to the right margin and diaphragmatic surface of the heart.

The left coronary artery is distributed to the sternocostal (anterior) surface and apex of the heart.

The Aortic Arch (fig. 189)

The aortic arch commences at the second right costal cartilage and arching upwards, backwards and to the left over the root of the left lung and in front of the trachea, ends in the plane of Louis posteriorly, at the level of the disc between the fourth and fifth thoracic vertebrae, where it becomes the descending thoracic aorta.

It gives off three large branches called (from right to left) the *innominate, left common carotid* and *left subclavian arteries.*

The Innominate Artery

This artery arises from the aortic arch opposite the centre of the manubrium sterni. It is about 4 cm. long, runs obliquely upwards and to the right and ends behind the right sternoclavicular joint, where it divides into right subclavian and right common carotid vessels.

The Common Carotid Arteries (fig. 190)

The right common carotid artery is a terminal branch of the innominate artery and arises in the lower part of the neck. The left common carotid arises in the thorax.

The thoracic portion of the left common carotid artery arises from the aortic arch on the left of the innominate artery immediately behind the manubrium sterni. It runs upwards and to the left for 4 cm. and passing behind the left sternoclavicular joint enters the neck. In the thorax the vessel lies first on the trachea and then the oesophagus and is also in close relation with the left recurrent laryngeal nerve which lies between these structures. It is overlapped by the left lung and pleura.

The cervical portion of the common carotid arteries (fig. 190) run an almost similar course on the two sides of the body.

Each vessel ascends in the *carotid sheath*, which is part of the deep cervical fascia enclosing the internal jugular vein laterally, the common carotid (later the internal carotid) artery medially, with the vagus nerve behind

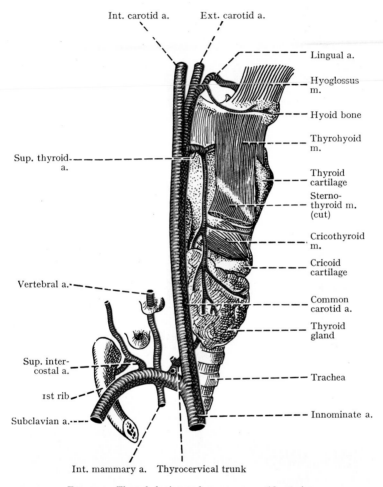

Int. carotid a.   Ext. carotid a.

Lingual a.

Hyoglossus m.

Hyoid bone

Thyrohyoid m.

Sup. thyroid. a.

Thyroid cartilage

Sterno-thyroid m. (cut)

Cricothyroid m.

Cricoid cartilage

Vertebral a.

Common carotid a.

Thyroid gland

Sup. inter-costal a.

Trachea

1st rib

Innominate a.

Subclavian a.

Int. mammary a.   Thyrocervical trunk

FIG. 190.—The subclavian and common carotid arteries.

and between the two. The common carotid arteries end at the upper border of the thyroid cartilage (which is on a level with the disc between the third and fourth cervical vertebrae) by dividing into internal and external carotids. This division takes place within the carotid triangle (fig. 228). Each common carotid artery lies behind the sternomastoid and infrahyoid muscles and behind the lateral lobe of the thyroid gland. It lies on the pre-

15—A.PH.

vertebral muscles in this region, viz., the longus capitis and longus cervicis. Immediately behind the carotid sheath is the cervical portion of the sympathetic chain.

The External Carotid Artery (fig. 191)

The external carotid artery arises in the carotid triangle as a terminal branch of the common carotid. It ascends for 7 cm. first behind the sterno-mastoid and then behind the posterior belly of the digastric and stylohyoid

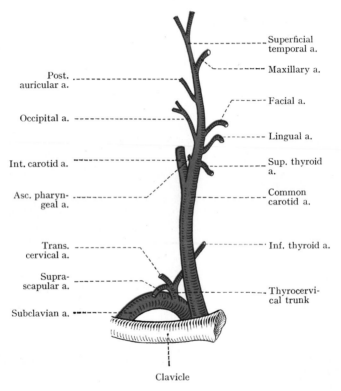

Superficial temporal a.

Maxillary a.

Post. auricular a.

Facial a.

Occipital a.

Lingual a.

Int. carotid a.

Sup. thyroid a.

Asc. pharyn-geal a.

Common carotid a.

Trans. cervical a.

Inf. thyroid a.

Supra-scapular a.

Thyrocervi-cal trunk

Subclavian a.

Clavicle

FIG. 191.—The common carotid, external carotid and subclavian arteries and their main branches.

muscles and finally enters the substance of the parotid gland. At the level of the lobe of the ear it divides into the superficial temporal and maxillary arteries. Before entering the parotid gland it lies in contact with the pharyngeal wall.

The Branches of the vessel from below upwards are: *ascending pharyngeal, superior thyroid, lingual, facial, occipital, posterior auricular, maxillary* and *superficial temporal arteries* (fig. 191).

These vessels hardly concern the student of physiotherapy and only the briefest description will be given.

The ascending pharyngeal artery is a small vessel which ascends on the pharyngeal wall supplying the muscles in that region and giving small branches to the meninges and middle ear cavity.

The superior thyroid artery. The course of this vessel is characteristic for it runs downwards, forwards and medially, thus it can be easily identified. It enters the superior border of the lateral lobe of the thyroid gland. Besides supplying a large part of this gland it gives branches to the adjacent muscles (sternomastoid especially) and to the mucous membrane in the upper part of the larynx.

The lingual artery is a vessel of some size which arises opposite the tip of the hyoid bone and is the main blood supply to the musculature of the tongue. It also helps to supply the tonsil. The lingual artery is characteristically looped at its origin, the loop being convex upwards and lying on this loop is the hypoglossal nerve.

The facial artery is, as its name implies, the main blood supply to the muscles and integument of the face. It also supplies the submandibular salivary gland, the muscles in the digastric triangle (submental branch) and contributes to the blood supply of the tonsil and palate.

It arises just above the hyoid bone in the digastric triangle (fig. 228), ascends in the substance of the submandibular gland, then over the body of the mandible (where it can be felt to pulsate as it lies on the antero-inferior angle of the masseter muscle), the buccinator and the deeper muscles of expression. It lies in close proximity to the angle of the mouth and the lateral aspect of the nose, and ends at the inner angle of the eye.

The vessel is conspicuously tortuous, a characteristic necessitated by the fact that the vessel is constantly being placed on the stretch by the muscles of expression.

The occipital artery arises opposite the facial artery, runs upwards and backwards beneath the posterior belly of digastric to the occipital region. It supplies the integument on the back of the scalp, the sternomastoid muscle and the deep muscles on the back of the neck. Some small branches from this vessel reach the meninges.

The posterior auricular artery is a small vessel which supplies the muscles and skin behind the ear. It gives off a branch which ascends to the middle ear by passing through the stylomastoid foramen.

The maxillary artery (fig. 192) is much the larger terminal branch of the external carotid. It arises within the parotid gland and runs forward on the lateral pterygoid muscle to the pterygopalatine fossa which it enters by passing between the two heads of the lateral pterygoid muscle.

It gives branches to the external ear, middle ear, the meninges (middle meningeal artery), the teeth of the upper and lower jaws, the muscles of mastication, the nasal cavity, palate and pharynx.

Many of its branches have the same name as, and accompany, the branches of the maxillary and mandibular divisions of the trigeminal nerve.

The superficial temporal artery is the smaller terminal branch of the external carotid. It ascends over the zygomatic arch and in front of the ear (where it can be felt to pulsate) to the temporal region where it supplies muscles and integument.

The Internal Carotid Artery

Arises in the carotid triangle as a terminal branch of the common carotid. It passes upwards to the base of the skull within the carotid sheath, where it lies in close contact with the internal jugular vein and the vagus nerve.

It ascends deep to the posterior belly of the digastric and stylohyoid muscles, and deep to the parotid gland and styloid process of the temporal bone. It lies in close contact with the pharyngeal wall which is medial to it, and on the vertebral column and longus capitis muscle. At the base of the

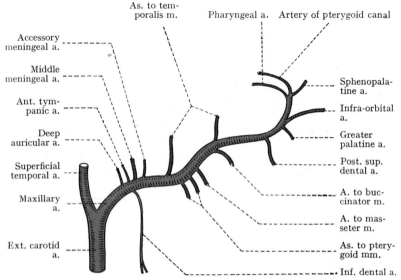

FIG. 192.—The maxillary artery and its branches.

skull the last four cranial nerves lie between it and the internal jugular vein. It gives off no branches until it reaches the interior of the skull.

At the base of the skull it runs in the carotid canal surrounded by the carotid plexus of sympathetic nerves (from the superior cervical ganglion) and enters the middle cranial fossa. It next lies on the cartilaginous plate which fills the foramen lacerum and running forward enters the cavernous blood sinus. Here, surrounded by venous blood, it is in close relation with the 3rd, 4th, 6th and the ophthalmic and maxillary divisions of the 5th cranial nerves (fig. 193). Emerging from the sinus near the superior orbital fissure it gives branches to the brain, the eye and structures within the orbit.

In the carotid canal it gives branches to the middle ear.

In the cavernous sinus it gives branches to the hypophysis which lies adjacent to it and also branches to the adjacent cranial nerves (fig. 193).

At the superior orbital fissure it gives off the *middle cerebral artery* which is almost a direct continuation of the main vessel and passes to the lateral aspect of the cerebral hemisphere, extending as far back as the occipital lobe; the *anterior cerebral artery* which runs a similar course to the middle cerebral on the medial aspect of the hemisphere; the *posterior communicating artery* which, besides supplying structures in the interpeduncular space, completes the circulus arteriosus (of Willis) (fig. 194); and the *ophthalmic artery* which supplies the eye and the structures within the orbit.

The Subclavian Arteries (fig. 190)

The left subclavian artery arises in the thorax, the right one arises in the neck as a terminal branch of the innominate. Except for this the two vessels run a similar course.

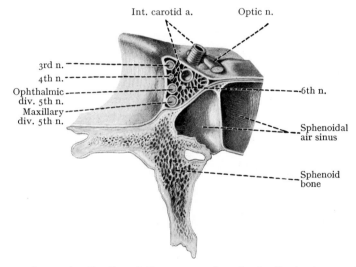

Fig. 193.—A coronal section through the cavernous sinus showing the structures contained within it.

The thoracic portion of the left subclavian artery (fig. 189) arises from the aortic arch on the left of and behind the left common carotid. It ascends into the root of the neck lying on the oesophagus, thoracic duct and longus cervicis. Between the left subclavian and left common carotid arteries the vagus and phrenic nerves descend to reach the anterolateral aspect of the aortic arch.

The cervical portion of the subclavian arteries run a similar course on each side of the body. Each vessel arches over the first rib and at the outer border of that bone becomes the axillary artery. A portion of the subclavian artery lies behind scalenus anterior, in direct contact with the apex of the lung and the dome of the pleura which are deeply grooved by the vessel. It is usual to describe the artery as consisting of three parts, the *first part* ending at the medial border of scalenus anterior, the *second part* lying behind that muscle, and the *third part* extending from the lateral border of that muscle to the outer border of the first rib.

All the important branches arise from the first part and include the *vertebral, thyrocervical trunk, internal mammary* and *superior intercostal arteries* (fig. 190).

The vertebral artery (fig. 190) ascends within the foramina in the transverse processes of the upper six cervical vertebrae. It passes through the foramen magnum to the ventral aspect of the brain stem where it meets its

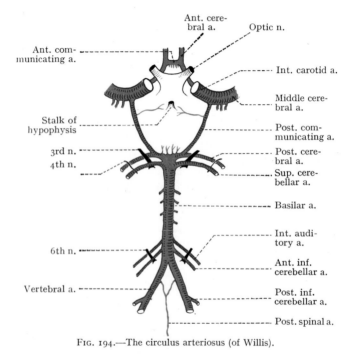

FIG. 194.—The circulus arteriosus (of Willis).

The circulus arteriosus lies at the base of the brain. Compare with fig. 160.

fellow of the opposite side to form the *basilar artery* (fig. 194). The vertebral artery gives off branches to the spinal cord and to the posterior aspect of the cerebellum. The basilar artery gives branches to the anterior aspect of the cerebellum, to the pons, internal ear, the superior aspect of the cerebellum (superior cerebellar) and to the medial and lateral aspects of the occipital lobe of the cerebral hemisphere (posterior cerebral). The latter vessel is joined by the posterior communicating artery from the internal carotid which completes the circulus arteriosus (of Willis) (fig. 194).

The thyrocervical trunk (fig. 191) is a short vessel. It quickly divides into three terminal branches—the *inferior thyroid* artery which enters the lower pole of the thyroid gland; the *transverse cervical* artery which crosses the root of the neck in front of the phrenic nerve and brachial plexus to supply the muscles in this region—one branch from this vessel descends on the vertebral border of the scapula deep to levator scapulae and the rhomboids; and the *suprascapular* artery which crosses the third part of the subclavian artery, reaches the dorsum of the scapula by passing over the suprascapular notch and is distributed to the supraspinatus, infraspinatus and adjacent muscles.

The internal mammary artery descends behind the costal cartilages 1 cm. from the lateral border of the sternum, and at the 6th intercostal space divides into the *musculophrenic* artery which supplies the lower intercostal spaces and part of the diaphragm and the *superior epigastric* artery which enters the rectus sheath to anastomose with the inferior epigastric artery.

The internal mammary artery supplies the pericardium, the upper intercostal spaces, pectoralis major and the integument which covers that muscle.

The superior intercostal artery not only supplies the first two intercostal spaces but also gives off a branch which ascends in the neck to supply the deep muscles in that region.

The Axillary Artery (fig. 195, facing p. 223)
The axillary artery is a continuation of the subclavian and extends from the outer border of the first rib to the lower border of the teres major which marks the inferior boundary of the axillary space. At this level the artery becomes the brachial.

The axillary artery is crossed by the pectoralis minor. For topographical purposes this muscle can be said to divide the artery into three segments: the *first part* extends from the outer border of the first rib to the upper border of the pectoralis minor; the *second part* lies behind pectoralis minor; and the *third part* lies below pectoralis minor and between it and the lower border of teres major.

The vessel is enveloped with its vein and the brachial plexus in a fascial sheath, which is continuous with the deep cervical fascia. Nearly the whole of this vessel lies under cover of the pectoralis major, the first part also under cover of the clavipectoral fascia, and the second part also under cover of the pectoralis minor. In the first interspace the artery lies on the serratus anterior and afterwards on the muscles forming the posterior axillary wall, viz., subscapularis, latissimus dorsi and teres major.

The medial cord of the brachial plexus lies behind and the lateral and posterior cords above the first part of the artery. The cords surround the second part of the artery and are named lateral, medial and posterior, according to their relations to this part of the vessel. The median nerve lies on the outer side, the ulnar nerve on the inner side and the radial and circumflex nerves behind the third part of the artery.

The axillary vein is medial to the artery throughout.

The axillary artery gives off the following *branches*: the *superior thoracic*, a small branch to the first interspace; the *acromiothoracic*, a vessel of some size which pierces the clavipectoral fascia and supplies the adjacent muscles; the *lateral thoracic*, a branch which runs down on the lateral thoracic wall with the nerve to serratus anterior; the *subscapular*, a large vessel which descends along the lower border of subscapularis, supplies adjacent muscles and gives a branch to the infraspinous fossa (the circumflex scapular artery); the *anterior humeral circumflex*, which runs in front of the surgical neck of the humerus; the *posterior humeral circumflex*, a much larger vessel which passes through the quadrangular space with the circumflex nerve and winds round the neck of the humerus under cover of the deltoid.

The Brachial Artery

The brachial artery extends from the lower border of teres major to the cubital fossa in front of the elbow where it divides into radial and ulnar arteries. As it descends it inclines laterally to reach the front of the lower part of the arm. The vessel is superficial but biceps and coracobrachialis overlap it to a variable extent while the bicipital aponeurosis covers it at the bend of the elbow. The vessel lies on the long and medial heads of triceps, the coracobrachialis (at its insertion) and the brachialis.

The median nerve is lateral and the ulnar nerve medial to it at first, but the ulnar nerve soon leaves the front of the arm by piercing the medial intermuscular septum and at this point the median nerve crosses the brachial artery either superficially or deeply and for the rest of its course descends on its medial aspect.

The brachial artery gives off the *profunda brachii* branch which accompanies the radial nerve to the back of the arm, an *ulnar collateral* branch which accompanies the ulnar nerve, *muscular* branches to the adjacent muscles and the *supratrochlear* branch which is distributed to the front and back of the elbow where it takes part in the anastomosis in that region.

The Radial Artery

The radial artery arises in the cubital fossa and inclines laterally, lying successively on the biceps tendon, supinator, pronator teres, flexor digitorum sublimis (radial head), flexor pollicis longus, pronator quadratus and the lower end of the radius. In the upper two-thirds of the forearm it is overlapped by the brachioradialis but in the lower third it is conveniently superficial and here, by gently compressing the radial artery against the lower end of the radius, the pulse can be felt.

On leaving the forearm the radial artery passes to the back of the hand by running deep to abductor pollicis longus and extensor pollicis brevis. It thus enters the anatomical "snuff-box" (fig. 242), where it is covered only by integument and lies on the lateral ligament of the wrist joint. It leaves the "snuff-box" by passing deep to extensor pollicis longus and enters the palm of the hand by passing between the two heads of the first dorsal interosseous muscle and between the transverse and oblique heads of adductor pollicis. In the palm it lies deeply, forming the major part of the deep palmar arch.

The radial artery gives off *in the forearm* a *radial recurrent* branch which takes part in the anastomosis around the elbow joint, *muscular* branches to the adjacent muscles, a *superficial palmar* branch which supplies the muscles of the thenar eminence and completes the superficial palmar arch and an *anterior carpal* branch which contributes to the carpal network at the wrist.

The radial artery gives off *at the wrist* a *posterior carpal* branch which joins the dorsal carpal network on the back of the wrist and the *first dorsal meta-carpal* artery which supplies the contiguous sides of the thumb and index finger.

The radial artery gives off *in the hand* the *princeps pollicis* artery which divides into two branches to supply both sides of the thumb and the *radialis indicis* artery which supplies the lateral side of the index finger.

The Ulnar Artery

The ulnar artery arises in the cubital fossa and runs deeply beneath the deep head of pronator teres and the muscles arising from the common flexor tendon.   It lies on brachialis and flexor digitorum profundus.   About the middle of the forearm it becomes more superficial and is overlapped only by the flexor carpi ulnaris.   At this point it is joined by the ulnar nerve which lies medial to it and this relationship is maintained for the remainder of its course.

It enters the palm by passing over the flexor retinaculum, lateral to the pisiform bone and medial to the hook of the hamate.   In this part of its course the vessel lies beneath palmaris brevis.   In the palm it divides into *superficial* and *deep terminal* branches which contribute to the superficial and deep palmar arches respectively.

The ulnar artery gives off the following branches:

At the elbow—the *anterior* and *posterior ulnar recurrent* arteries which take part in the anastomosis around the elbow joint.

In the forearm—the *common interosseous* artery which divides almost at once into anterior and posterior interosseous branches.   These vessels descend on the front and back of the interosseous membrane respectively. The posterior interosseous artery ends about two-thirds of the way down the forearm and at that point the anterior interosseous artery pierces the membrane and runs to the dorsum of the wrist.   Both branches, besides supplying adjacent muscles, also contribute to the anterior and posterior carpal networks.

At the wrist—the *anterior* and *posterior carpal arteries* which form a network on the front and back of the wrist respectively.

The Superficial Palmar Arch (figs. 196 and 243) is formed chiefly by

the ulnar artery which is joined by the superficial palmar branch of the radial artery on the lateral aspect of the thenar eminence.   The arch gives off three *palmar digital* branches which are joined by the three palmar metacarpal arteries from the deep arch.   They then divide into branches which supply the contiguous sides of the fingers and the ulnar side of the little finger (fig. 243).

The superficial palmar arch lies on a level with the medial border of the base of the fully abducted thumb.   It is covered by the palmar aponeurosis and lies on the flexor tendons, lumbricals and branches of the median nerve.

The Deep Palmar Arch (fig. 243) is formed chiefly by the radial artery which joins the deep branch of the ulnar artery on the inner aspect of the hypothenar eminence. The arch gives off three *palmar metacarpal* branches which communicate with the dorsal metacarpal arteries from the dorsal carpal network and join the palmar digital branches at the webs of the fingers (fig. 196).

The arch lies on the bases of the metacarpal bones and the interossei. It is covered by the flexor tendons and lumbrical muscles.

The Posterior Carpal Arch (fig. 196) lies on the dorsal aspect of the carpal bones and is formed by branches from the radial and ulnar arteries. It gives off three dorsal metacarpal arteries which communicate with similar branches from the deep palmar arch and these arteries divide at the webs of the fingers into digital branches which supply the contiguous sides of the second and third, third and fourth, and fourth and fifth digits. The first dorsal metacarpal artery which supplies the contiguous sides of the thumb and index fingers arises directly from the radial artery.

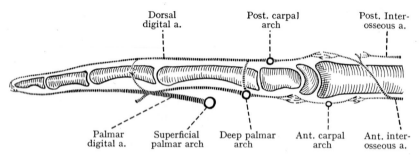

FIG. 196.—The scheme of the blood supply to the hand. (After Grant.)

There is an *anterior carpal arch* on the front of the wrist corresponding to the posterior network, but beyond communicating with the deep palmar arch it gives off no branches and is insignificant.

The Descending Thoracic Aorta

The descending aorta is a continuation of the aortic arch and commences at the plane of Louis. It is a vessel of large calibre, slightly wider than the thumb, and it descends in the posterior mediastinum.

Commencing on the left of the mid-line it gradually inclines medially and at its termination in the thorax it lies on the centre of the vertebral column.

It ends at the level of the 12th thoracic vertebra by passing through the aortic opening in the diaphragm.

The heart and pericardium lie in front of the aorta, while just before its termination, the oesophagus crosses it superficially from right to left. It is in close contact with the left lung and pleura which it grooves deeply, and it lies on the lower eight thoracic vertebrae and the anterior longitudinal ligament of the vertebral column.

The descending aorta gives off the following *branches* in the thorax: nine pairs of *posterior intercostal* arteries which run forward in the lower nine spaces between the ribs and anastomose with the anterior intercostals from the internal mammary artery; one pair of *subcostal* arteries which pass beneath the 12th rib and accompany the 12th thoracic nerve on to the anterior abdominal wall; *diaphragmatic, bronchial, oesophageal* and *pericardial* arteries.

The Abdominal Aorta (fig. 197)

The abdominal aorta is a continuation of the descending thoracic aorta.

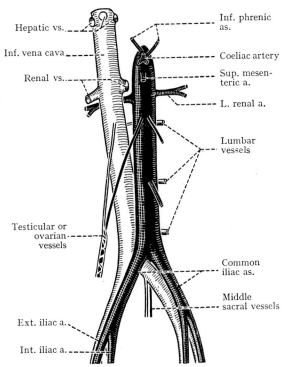

Hepatic vs.

Inf. vena cava

Renal vs.

Inf. phrenic as.

Coeliac artery

Sup. mesenteric a.

L. renal a.

Lumbar vessels

Testicular or ovarian vessels

Common iliac as.

Middle sacral vessels

Ext. iliac a.

Int. iliac a.

FIG. 197.—The abdominal aorta and inferior vena cava.

Commencing at the aortic opening in the diaphragm at the level of T12, it ends at the level of the fourth lumbar vertebra by dividing into the common iliac arteries.

It lies behind the pancreas, the third part of the duodenum, the root of the mesentery and coils of small intestine. It lies on the vertebral column and the anterior longitudinal ligament.

It gives off numerous **branches** (unpaired unless otherwise stated) which, however, need not be described in detail, viz.:

The inferior phrenic arteries (paired) pass to the under surface of the diaphragm. Each gives a small branch to the suprarenal gland.

The coeliac artery divides almost immediately into three branches, viz., the *left gastric* artery, which runs from left to right along the lesser curvature of the stomach; the *hepatic* artery, which passes to the porta hepatis in the liver giving off a right gastric branch which runs from right to left along the lesser curvature of the stomach and anastomoses with the left gastric, and a gastroduodenal branch which divides into right gastro-epiploic and superior pancreaticoduodenal branches, the former passing to the greater curvature of the stomach and the latter to the head of the pancreas and the adjacent duodenum; and the *splenic* artery, which runs along the upper border of the pancreas to the spleen supplying both these organs and gives off small branches to the fundus of the stomach and a branch which runs from left to right along the greater curvature called the left gastro-epiploic.

The **middle suprarenal arteries** (paired) pass to the suprarenal glands.

The **superior mesenteric artery** runs in the mesentery, dividing into branches which supply the whole of the small intestine except the commencement of the duodenum. It also supplies the caecum, ascending colon, appendix and the greater part of the transverse colon.

The **renal arteries** (paired) run almost horizontally to the hilum of each kidney. The right vessel passes behind the inferior vena cava and right renal vein; the left, behind the left renal vein. Each artery gives a branch to the suprarenal gland.

The **testicular (or ovarian) arteries** (paired) run to the testes via the spermatic cords or to the ovaries via the broad ligaments.

The **lumbar arteries** (four pairs) arise from the back of the aorta and pass laterally to the abdominal wall.

The **inferior mesenteric artery** arises on the left of the aorta and descends in the pelvic mesocolon, giving branches to the terminal part of the transverse colon and to the remainder of the large intestine as far as the anal canal.

The **middle sacral artery** arises at the bifurcation of the aorta and descends on the front of the sacrum.

The Common Iliac Artery

Each common iliac artery runs downwards and outwards to end at the sacro-iliac joint where it bifurcates into external and internal iliac arteries.

The Internal Iliac Artery

The internal iliac arteries supply the pelvic organs but some branches pass out of the pelvis into the buttock (superior and inferior gluteal arteries) and supply the muscles in that region.

The External Iliac Artery

The external iliac artery commences at the level of the sacro-iliac joint, runs downwards and laterally on the psoas and ends behind the middle of the inguinal ligament by becoming the femoral.

The Femoral Artery

The femoral artery commences at the middle of the inguinal ligament and traverses the femoral triangle and the subsartorial canal. It ends by passing through an opening in adductor magnus, where it descends into the popliteal fossa as the popliteal artery.

In the femoral triangle the artery lies on psoas, pectineus and adductor longus from above down and is covered only by skin and fascia. In the subsartorial canal it lies on adductors longus and magnus and is covered by vastus medialis and sartorius.

In the upper part of the femoral triangle it is enclosed in the *femoral sheath* (fig. 198). This sheath is formed by the fascia transversalis in front and the

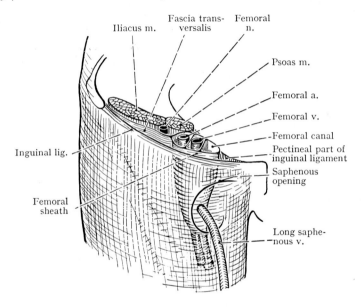

Fig. 198.—The femoral sheath (schematic). (After Grant.)

fascia iliaca behind, and is divided into three compartments by two septa. The lateral compartment contains the femoral artery, the middle compartment the femoral vein, while the medial compartment is known as the *femoral canal* (fig. 198). This canal is triangular with its base above and its apex below. It is about 2 cm. long and is empty except for the presence of an occasional lymph node. The base of the canal, called the *femoral ring*, is bounded anteriorly by the inguinal ligament, posteriorly by the fascia covering the pectineus muscle, laterally by the femoral vein and medially by the pectineal part of the inguinal ligament. The importance of the canal lies in the fact that a femoral hernia, when present, passes through it, and since the canal communicates with the saphenous opening the hernia protrudes beneath the skin in that region.

The femoral vein, which is medial to the artery in the upper part of the femoral triangle, is posterior to the artery in the lower part of the triangle, while in the lower part of the subsartorial canal the vein is lateral to the artery. The saphenous nerve is first lateral, then superficial and finally medial to the artery.

The femoral artery gives off a number of small branches to the lower part of the abdominal wall, to the external genitalia and to adjacent muscles. It also gives off a large branch known as the profunda femoris.

The profunda femoris artery arises from the lateral aspect of the femoral artery and, passing deeply beneath adductor longus, ends by dividing into branches which are distributed to the hamstring muscles and to the hip joint.

The Popliteal Artery (fig. 185, facing p. 220)

The popliteal artery commences at the opening in the adductor magnus and traversing the centre of the popliteal fossa ends at the lower border of the popliteus muscle by dividing into anterior and posterior tibial arteries. It lies on the popliteal surface of the femur, the capsule of the knee joint and the popliteus, and is crossed superficially from without in by the popliteal vein and the medial popliteal nerve. It gives branches to the adjacent muscles and to the knee joint.

The Anterior Tibial Artery

The anterior tibial artery arises at the lower border of the popliteus, pierces the interosseous membrane and so reaches the anterior compartment of the leg. It descends on that membrane with the anterior tibial nerve which lies superficial or lateral to it. At first the artery lies between the extensor digitorum longus and tibialis anterior, but extensor hallucis longus crosses the artery superficially and in the lower part of the leg the artery lies between the extensor hallucis longus medially and the extensor digitorum longus laterally. It descends in front of the capsule of the ankle joint and enters the foot as the dorsalis pedis artery.

It supplies adjacent muscles and takes part in the formation of arterial networks around the knee and ankle joints.

The dorsalis pedis artery is a continuation of the anterior tibial and runs forward on the inner group of tarsal bones to the first intermetatarsal space. Here it dips between the two heads of the first dorsal interosseous muscle to enter the sole of the foot where it ends by joining the plantar arch (fig. 186, facing p. 221).

It gives branches to the arterial network at the ankle joint, to adjacent muscles and, forming an arch at its termination on the dorsum of the foot, gives cutaneous branches to the toes.

The Posterior Tibial Artery (fig. 185, facing p. 220)

The posterior tibial artery commences at the lower border of popliteus and runs down on tibialis posterior, flexor digitorum longus and the lower end of the tibia. It is covered by soleus and gastrocnemius above and by integument below. On the deltoid ligament of the ankle joint midway between the medial malleolus and the heel, the artery divides into medial and lateral plantar arteries.

The **medial plantar artery*** is the smaller terminal branch of the posterior tibial and descends into the sole deep to the abductor hallucis and ends by supplying the inner side of the great toe.

The **lateral plantar artery*** is the larger terminal branch of the posterior tibial and descends into the sole deep to the abductor hallucis and flexor digitorum brevis. Coursing laterally to the base of the fifth metatarsal bone it turns medially at this point and ends at the first intermetatarsal space by joining the deep branch of the dorsalis pedis. In this way the plantar arch is formed from which cutaneous branches to the toes arise.

The lateral plantar artery gives branches to the skin and the muscles on the sole.

THE VENOUS SYSTEM

Most arteries have companion veins. In certain parts of the body (e.g., the distal parts of the limbs) these take the form of two small vessels which accompany each artery (venae comitantes), elsewhere there is one vessel which lies adjacent to each artery.

The veins can be divided into the *pulmonary system*, consisting of four veins draining the lungs; the *systemic system*, which is by far the largest since it drains almost the whole of the body into the superior and inferior venae cavae; the *cardiac system*, consisting of veins draining the heart wall into the coronary sinus; and the *portal system* by which blood is drained from the stomach, spleen, pancreas and intestines into the liver.

The Pulmonary Veins (fig. 211)

The pulmonary veins are four in number, two on each side of the body, which commence at the hilum of the lung and carry *arterial* blood from the lungs to the left atrium of the heart.

The Superior Vena Cava (fig. 189)

The superior vena cava drains the head, neck, upper limbs, thorax and the greater part of the anterior and posterior abdominal walls into the right atrium of the heart. It is a large vessel almost as wide as the thumb, which lies in the superior mediastinum on the right side of the body in contact with the apex of the right lung. It is formed by the union of the right and left innominate veins and receives near its termination the *vena azygos* (fig. 211).

The *azygos venous system* consists of the azygos vein and the superior and inferior hemiazygos veins. They lie on or adjacent to the vertebral column, the azygos vein on the right of the mid-line and the hemiazygos veins on the left. The superior hemiazygos vein drains into the azygos vein at the level of T7 and the inferior hemiazygos at the level of T8. The azygos system drains the upper two lumbar veins on each side, all the posterior intercostal veins (except the first on the right side and the first three on the left side), the bronchial vein on the right side and the oesophageal, pericardial and mediastinal veins. The vena azygos commences in the abdomen at the level

* Fig. 186 facing p. 221.

of L2, and ascends into the thorax through the aortic opening in the dia-phragm where it lies behind the oesophagus and on the right of the thoracic duct. It ends by arching over the root of the right lung and entering the superior vena cava in the plane of Louis.

The Innominate Veins (fig. 189)

Each innominate vein is formed by the union of the internal jugular and subclavian veins. The right innominate vein is a short trunk, but the left vein is much longer and extends from the left sternoclavicular joint to the first right costal cartilage. Here the two innominate veins unite to form the superior vena cava.

The Internal Jugular Vein

The internal jugular vein commences at the base of the skull as a con-tinuation of the lateral sinus. It passes down the neck within the carotid sheath lying lateral to the internal carotid (later the common carotid) artery and with the vagus nerve lying behind and medial to it.

In addition to draining the transverse sinus it drains most of the structures in the head and neck. At its termination it unites with the subclavian vein to form the innominate vein.

There is a smaller *external jugular* vein which commences in the region of the parotid gland and descends downwards and backwards over the sterno-mastoid to end in the subclavian vein. A tributary of the external jugular vein drains the front of the neck and is called the *anterior jugular* vein.

The Venous Sinuses of the Dura Mater (fig. 168) drain the brain, the eye, the inner parts of the ear and the meninges. They also communicate with veins draining the scalp and the deeper regions of the face. The cavernous sinus because it envelops two of the main divisions of the tri-geminal nerve, and the lateral sinus because it is continued as the internal jugular vein, have already been mentioned. The rest hardly come within the scope of the student of physiotherapy.

The Subclavian Vein

The subclavian vein is a continuation of the axillary vein. It commences at the outer border of the first rib and ends at the sternoclavicular joint by uniting with the internal jugular to form the innominate vein. It lies below the subclavian artery but otherwise runs a similar course to that vessel.

The Axillary Vein

The axillary vein commences at the lower border of the teres major and ends at the outer border of the first rib, where it becomes the subclavian. It is formed by the union of the basilic vein with the companion veins of the brachial artery.

The brachial, ulnar and radial arteries each have a pair of companion veins (venae comitantes) which accompany them.

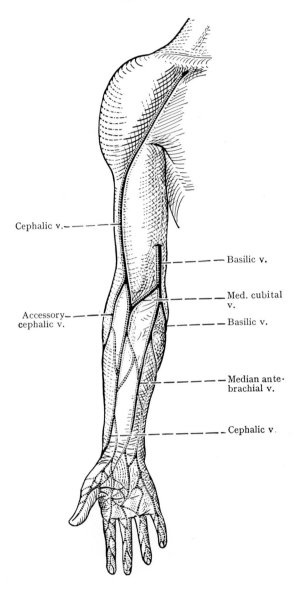

Cephalic v.

Accessory cephalic v.

Basilic v.

Med. cubital v.

Basilic v.

Median antebrachial v.

Cephalic v.

FIG. 199.—The superficial veins of the upper extremity.

The superficial veins of the upper limb are of importance but are subject to great variation (fig. 199).

The fingers are drained by dorsal digital veins which are connected with plexuses on the palmar aspect of the digits. These drain into the dorsal venous plexus situated on the back of the hand from which the cephalic

16—A.PH.

and basilic veins arise. A venous plexus on the superficial aspect of the palmar aponeurosis drains into the median vein.

The median cubital vein (fig. 199) commences in the palm and ascends in the superficial tissues in the middle of the forearm when at the bend of the elbow it enters the basilic vein but its termination is variable.

The cephalic vein (fig. 199) commences on the back of the hand where it drains the outer part of the dorsal venous plexus. It crosses to the front of the forearm in the roof of the anatomical snuff-box, and ascends in the superficial tissues on the lateral aspect of the forearm. It gives off the median cubital vein which joins the basilic vein in front of the elbow, ascends in the arm on the outer side of biceps and then between the deltoid and pectoralis major. It ends by piercing the clavipectoral fascia in the infraclavicular fossa, where it enters the axillary or subclavian veins.

The basilic vein (fig. 199) commences on the back of the hand, where it drains the inner part of the dorsal venous plexus. It ascends in the superficial tissues on the back of the forearm but curls round to the front of the forearm at the elbow where it is joined by the median cubital vein. It ascends on the inner side of biceps and enters the axillary vein by piercing the deep fascia at the lower border of teres major.

The Inferior Vena Cava (fig. 197)

The inferior vena cava commences at the body of the fifth lumbar vertebra by the union of the common iliac veins. It ascends on the vertebral column on the right of the aorta, pierces the central tendon of the diaphragm at the level of the eighth thoracic vertebra and almost immediately enters the right atrium. Only a very small fraction of this vessel lies within the thorax (less than 0·5 cm.).

The inferior vena cava receives the following tributaries: the *lower lumbar veins*, the *right testicular* (or *ovarian*) *veins*, both *renal veins*, the *right suprarenal vein*, the *right inferior phrenic vein* and both *hepatic veins*.

The left testicular, left suprarenal and left inferior phrenic veins drain into the left renal vein.

The Common Iliac Veins (fig. 197)

The common iliac veins commence at the pelvic brim, by the union of the internal and external iliac veins, and end at the fifth lumbar vertebra by uniting to form the inferior vena cava.

The Internal Iliac Vein (fig. 197)

The internal iliac vein lies on the posterior pelvic wall and drains the pelvic viscera.

The External Iliac Vein (fig. 197)

The external iliac vein commences at the inguinal ligament as a continuation of the femoral vein, runs upwards on the psoas muscle and ends at the sacro-iliac joint by uniting with the internal iliac to form the common iliac vein.

The Femoral Vein (fig. 198)

The femoral vein commences at the opening in the adductor magnus in the lower part of the thigh as a continuation of the popliteal vein. It ascends in the subsartorial canal, where it lies first lateral and then posterior to the femoral artery, passes through the femoral triangle and at its termination it lies on the medial aspect of the femoral artery. Behind the inguinal ligament it is continued as the external iliac vein.

It receives veins corresponding to the branches of the femoral artery and also near its termination, the long saphenous vein.

The Popliteal Vein

The popliteal vein is formed at the lower border of the popliteus muscle by the union of the anterior and posterior tibial veins. It ascends in the middle of the popliteal fossa with the popliteal artery lying on its deep aspect and the medial popliteal nerve lying on its superficial aspect and ends at the opening in the adductor magnus by becoming the femoral vein.

It receives tributaries corresponding to the branches of the popliteal artery and also the short saphenous vein.

Companion veins accompany the anterior and posterior tibial, the dorsalis pedis and the medial and lateral plantar arteries.

The toes are drained by dorsal digital veins which pass into the dorsal venous arch. This arch extends across the heads of the metatarsal bones and from it medial and lateral marginal veins pass towards the ankle and mark the commencement of the saphenous veins. These marginal veins are united on the dorsum of the foot by a dorsal venous plexus and are connected with the plexus which drains the sole.

The Long Saphenous Vein (fig. 200)

The long saphenous vein commences on the medial aspect of the dorsal venous network. It passes upwards in front of the medial malleolus, ascends on the inner side of the leg, enters the thigh behind the medial condyle of the femur, ascends on the inner aspect of the thigh and ends by passing through the saphenous opening 4 cm. below and lateral to the inner end of the inguinal ligament, where it joins the femoral vein.

The long saphenous vein is cutaneous throughout its extent and drains the skin of the thigh and the medial aspect of the leg and foot. It is accompanied during the distal part of its course by the saphenous nerve. Near its termination it usually receives a large branch (or branches) known as the *accessory saphenous* vein and also smaller branches which drain the external genitalia and lower abdominal wall.

The long saphenous vein has a very long and dependent course and is much more liable to become varicose than any other vein in the body. Varicose ulcers are a common sequel to varicose veins.

The Short Saphenous Vein

The short saphenous vein commences on the lateral aspect of the dorsal venous network. It passes upwards behind the lateral malleolus and

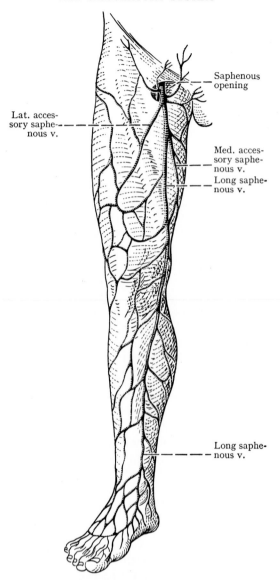

Lat. acces-
sory saphe-
nous v.

Saphenous
opening

Med. acces-
sory saphe-
nous v.

Long saphe-
nous v.

Long saphe-
nous v.

FIG. 200.—The long saphenous vein and tributaries.

ascends on the posterior aspect of the leg. It ends by perforating the fascia covering the popliteal fossa where it joins the popliteal vein. It drains areas of skin on the posterolateral aspect of the leg and the lateral aspect of the foot.

In the foot and lower part of the leg the sural nerve lies alongside it, while in the upper part of the leg the posterior cutaneous nerve of the thigh is adjacent to it.

The Coronary Sinus (fig. 211)

The coronary sinus drains the heart wall into the right atrium. Its opening is adjacent to that of the inferior vena cava, and its mouth is guarded by a rudimentary valve.

The Portal Vein (fig. 201)

The portal vein drains the stomach, spleen, pancreas and almost the whole of the intestinal tract. Some of its tributaries commence as small capillaries

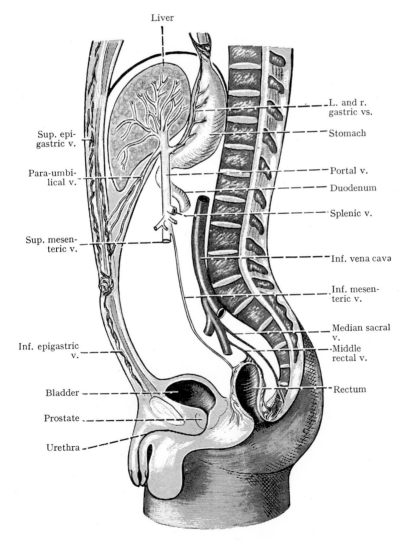

FIG. 201.—The portal vein. (After Tandler.)

in the villi of the small intestine (fig. 291). It arises in the transpyloric plane by the union of the superior mesenteric and splenic veins, behind the neck of the pancreas. It ascends in the right free border of the lesser omentum in front of the aditus to the lesser sac, behind and between the common bile duct and hepatic artery. It enters the hilum of the liver, where it breaks up into right and left branches which further subdivide and eventually break up into capillaries (sinusoids) which are common to the portal vein and the hepatic artery. The portal system, therefore, both starts and ends as capillaries.

The portal vein carries highly nutritious blood from the small intestine to the liver. The major part of the products of digestion are transported along this route.

At the lower end of the anal canal the portal and systemic systems of veins anastomose (fig. 201). Because of this and because the veins have such a long course in the body before they reach their termination, the veins in the anal region are very liable to become varicose giving rise to the condition known as haemorrhoids (piles).

CHAPTER VII

THE LYMPHATIC SYSTEM

The lymphatic system consists of a series of small nodular vessels containing valves, called *lymph vessels* (*vide* p. 16) interposed along the course of which are nodules of lymphoid tissue called lymph glands or *lymph nodes* (fig. 25). The latter term will be used throughout this book since the term gland suggests secretion and these nodes have no secretory function but act as filters.

Lymphatic vessels follow the course of the veins and can be divided into superficial and deep sets. The superficial set lies in the superficial fascia immediately beneath the skin, a fact that can be verified easily, when these vessels become inflamed (lymphangitis) and appear as red streaks on the surface of the skin. The lymphatic vessels convey the lymph which is derived from the blood into relatively large ducts, called the *thoracic duct* (since it lies principally within the thorax) and the much smaller *right lymphatic duct*. These ducts open into the venous system at the root of the neck, and there is no doubt that, in the limbs especially, some lymphatic vessels open directly into adjacent veins.

A large percentage of the digested fats are carried into the thoracic duct via the intestinal lymphatics in the form of a milky fluid called *chyle*.

Lymph nodes are aggregated in groups throughout the body; thus we speak of the cervical group (or chain), the axillary group, the mediastinal group, the aortic group, the iliac group, the inguinal group and the popliteal group. When the nodes become inflamed the condition is known as lymphadenitis.

The Cranio-Cervical Lymph Nodes (fig. 202)

The lymph nodes in the head are small and inconstant.

An *anterior auricular* group lies on the parotid gland in front of the ear and drains the forehead and side of the scalp. There is a *posterior auricular group* which lies behind the ear on the base of the mastoid process and drains the side of the scalp; an *occipital group* which lies lateral to the external occipital protuberance and drains the back of the scalp; a *buccal group* which lies on the buccinator muscle and drains the nose and part of the face; a *parotid group* which lies in the substance of the parotid gland and drains that structure and a *deep facial group* which lies on the pterygoid muscles and drains the deeper parts of the face. Efferents from all these nodes pass into the deep cervical chain.

The cervical lymph nodes consist of superficial and deep chains.

The *superficial chain* lies on the sternomastoid alongside the external jugular vein and receives afferents from the superficial structures in the neck. Their efferents drain into the deep cervical chain.

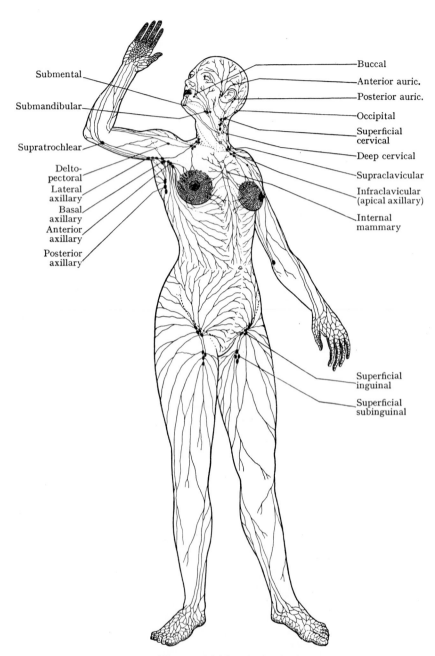

Submental

Submandibular

Supratrochlear

Delto-
pectoral

Lateral
axillary

Basal
axillary

Anterior
axillary

Posterior
axillary

Buccal

Anterior auric.

Posterior auric.

Occipital

Superficial
cervical

Deep cervical

Supraclavicular

Infraclavicular
(apical axillary)

Internal
mammary

Superficial
inguinal

Superficial
subinguinal

Fig. 202.—The superficial lymphatics of the body.

Two deep groups, the internal mammary and deep cervical have been included for convenience.

The *deep chain* is much more extensive. The chief nodes in this chain are the *submental group* which lies immediately beneath the symphysis menti and drains the incisor teeth and the middle of the lower lip; the *submandibular group* which lies adjacent to the submaxillary gland and drains the face, the greater part of the lips, the tongue and interior of the mouth; the *deep cervical group* which lies beneath the sternomastoid muscle and alongside the internal jugular vein. The *superior deep cervical group* drains the preceding cranio-cervical lymph nodes and also the tonsil. The *inferior deep cervical* or *supraclavicular group* drains all the cranio-cervical nodes and also the axillary nodes. A relatively large vessel (the jugular trunk) passes from these nodes direct into the thoracic duct on the left and the right lymphatic duct on the right.

The Axillary Lymph Nodes (fig. 202)

The axillary lymph nodes drain the upper limb and the outer half of the breast. There are five groups of nodes—a *lateral* group lying alongside the axillary vein, a *posterior* group lying on the posterior axillary wall, an *anterior* group lying on the inferior border of the pectoralis minor, a *basal* group lying in the base of the axilla, and an *apical* group lying in the infra-clavicular fossa in the apex of the axilla.

A *supratrochlear lymph node* is usually present on the medial aspect of the bend of the elbow. This drains the inner half of the forearm and hand. Occasionally small nodes are present on the upper lateral aspect of the arm between the deltoid and pectoralis major (*deltopectoral lymph nodes*). These nodes drain the lateral aspect of the upper limb and their efferents pass into the apical group.

The Mediastinal Lymph Nodes

The mediastinal lymph nodes include the *internal mammary* group which lies behind the sternum in close relation with the internal mammary vessels and drains the greater part of the inner half of the breast and the upper part of the anterior abdominal wall (fig. 202). Deep to these are the tracheal and bronchial groups, the latter including the nodes in the lung root which are important since they are sometimes the seat of primary disease, e.g., tubercle and carcinoma. Deep to these, the *posterior mediastinal* group lies alongside the aorta, near the vertebral ends of the ribs (fig. 203).

The Abdominal Aortic Lymph Nodes

The lymph nodes alongside the abdominal aorta are some of the largest and most numerous in the body. They consist of the *lateral aortic* lymph nodes which drain the pelvic viscera and lower limbs and the *pre-aortic* nodes which drain the alimentary tract. The former drain into the lumbar trunks and the latter into the intestinal trunks. These trunks open directly into the cisterna chyli.

The Iliac Group of Lymph Nodes

The iliac group of nodes surrounds the common iliac, internal and external iliac vessels and drains the pelvic organs and also the lower limbs.

The Inguinal group of Lymph Nodes (fig. 202)

The inguinal group of nodes is made up of three subdivisions. The *superficial inguinal* group which lies in the superficial fascia immediately below the inguinal ligament and drains the skin of the adjacent regions, notably the external genitalia, lower abdominal wall, buttock and anal orifice; the *superficial subinguinal* group which lies alongside the termination of the long saphenous vein and drains the skin on the medial aspect of the thigh and leg, and the *deep inguinal* group which lies alongside the femoral vein and receives efferents from both superficial inguinal groups, from the popliteal group and from the deep vessels in the thigh. Efferents from the deep inguinal group pass into the external iliac nodes.

The Popliteal group of Lymph Nodes

The popliteal lymph nodes lie within the popliteal fossa. The *superficial* group is related to the termination of the short saphenous vein and drains the skin on the postero-lateral aspect of the leg and foot. The *middle* group lies alongside the popliteal vein and drains the deeper structures in the leg and foot. The *deep* group lies on the capsule of the knee joint, deep to the popliteal artery and drains the knee joint.

Efferents from the popliteal group drain into the deep inguinal group usually, but they may end in the superficial subinguinal group.

The Thoracic Duct (fig. 203)

The thoracic duct commences as a dilatation known as the *cisterna chyli*, which lies on the bodies of the second and third lumbar vertebrae. The cistern receives tributaries from the intestines (the intestinal trunk), from the aortic nodes (the lumbar trunks) and from the posterior mediastinum (the posterior mediastinal trunks).

The thoracic duct ascends through the aortic opening in the diaphragm and runs upwards on the posterior thoracic wall behind the oesophagus. At the level of the plane of Louis it inclines to the left by passing behind the aortic arch. In the superior mediastinum it lies behind the subclavian artery and on the left of the oesophagus.

In the neck at the level of the seventh cervical vertebra it passes behind the carotid sheath, then in front of the scalenus anterior and phrenic nerve and ends by arching in front of the first part of the subclavian artery to join the junction of the left subclavian with the left innominate veins.

The thoracic duct, which is about 45 cm. long, drains the abdomen and lower limbs, the left half of the thorax, the left side of the head and neck and the left upper limb.

The remainder of the body drains into the *right lymphatic duct* (fig. 203). This duct is slender and short (4. cm.) and corresponds on the right side to the terminal part of the thoracic duct.

There are no lymphatics in the central nervous system and the cerebrospinal fluid may be looked upon as taking its place.

Lymphatic drainage of the head and neck. Vessels from the front of the scalp (forehead) pass into the anterior auricular group of nodes chiefly, but a few pass into the submandibular group direct. Vessels from the side of the scalp pass into the anterior and posterior auricular groups, while those from the back of the scalp pass into the occipital group. Vessels from the eyelids and posterior part of the cheek pass into the anterior auricular group,

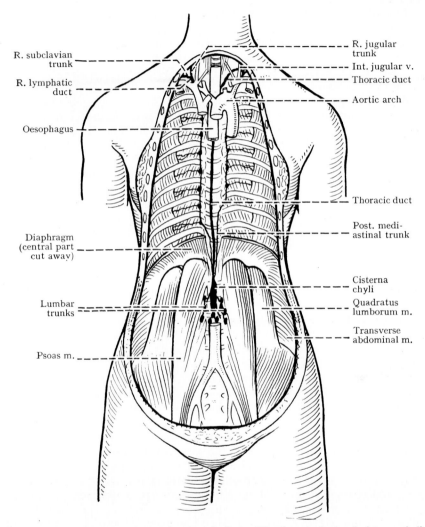

R. subclavian trunk
R. lymphatic duct
Oesophagus
Diaphragm (central part cut away)
Lumbar trunks
Psoas m.

R. jugular trunk
Int. jugular v.
Thoracic duct
Aortic arch
Thoracic duct
Post. medi- astinal trunk
Cisterna chyli
Quadratus lumborum m.
Transverse abdominal m.

FIG. 203.—The origin and course of the thoracic duct. (The thoracic duct and cisterna chyli have been drawn slightly out of proportion to give clarity.)

while those from the nose, upper lip and lateral part of the lower lip pass into the submandibular nodes via the small buccal group. Those from the centre of the lower lip pass into the submental group. The deeper lymphatic vessels from the head and neck drain into the deep facial group which lies on the pterygoid muscles whence they pass into the deep cervical chain.

The superficial vessels of the neck drain into the superficial group of nodes which lies on the sternomastoid, the deep vessels drain into the deep group of nodes which lies deep to the sternomastoid in close proximity with the internal jugular vein.

Lymphatic drainage of the upper extremity. A pair of lymphatic vessels drains each digit and passes to the dorsum of the hand. There is a dense network of lymphatic vessels in the palm which communicates with the digital lymphatics and passes round the margins of the palm to the dorsum of the hand. From here vessels ascend alongside the tributaries of the cephalic and basilic veins. Some from the medial aspect of the hand and forearm pass to the supratrochlear node before entering the lateral axillary group which lies alongside the axillary vessels on the lateral axillary wall. A few vessels from the lateral aspect of the upper limb pass to the deltopectoral nodes and thence to the apical group of axillary nodes or to the deep cervical (supraclavicular) nodes. The deep lymphatics accompany the main blood vessels and pass to the lateral axillary group of nodes into which the majority of the upper limb drains.

Lymphatic drainage of the trunk. The anterior wall of the trunk above the umbilicus, including the breast, drains chiefly into the anterior axillary group of nodes but some vessels pass into the internal mammary group. The posterior wall above the umbilicus drains into the posterior axillary (subscapular) group. The anterior and posterior walls of the trunk below the umbilicus drain into the superficial inguinal group in the groin.

In two regions of the body the superficial lymphatics run in different directions and these are known as the *lymphatic watersheds* of the skin. A reference to fig. 202 will show that these regions are situated around the body at the level of the umbilicus where the lymphatic vessels may pass downwards into the inguinal region or upwards into the axilla, and at the level of the clavicle where the lymphatics may pass upwards into the deep cervical chain or downwards to the axilla.

The deep lymphatics of the trunk tend to follow the superior epigastric vessels to the internal mammary group and the inferior epigastric vessels to the external iliac group.

Lymphatic drainage of the lower extremity. A pair of lymphatic vessels drains each digit and passes to the dorsum of the foot as in the hand. There is a plexus in the sole which also drains into the dorsum. From the dorsal network a large medial group follows the course of the long saphenous vein and running in front of the medial malleolus and behind the medial condyle of the femur, drains into the superficial subinguinal group in the groin. A smaller lateral group follows the course of the short saphenous vein and running behind the lateral malleolus, ascends on the back of the calf to the superficial group of nodes in the popliteal fossa. There are communications between the medial and lateral groups just below the knee.

Superficial lymphatics from the buttocks pass almost horizontally around the upper and outer part of the thigh to drain into the superficial inguinal group in the groin.

The deep lymphatics of the lower extremity follow the course of the main blood vessels and are thus divided into anterior and posterior tibial and peroneal groups which drain into the middle group of nodes in the popliteal fossa and a femoral group which drains into the deep subinguinal group lying within the femoral sheath.

CHAPTER VIII

THE THORACIC AND ABDOMINAL VISCERA

THE THORACIC VISCERA

The thoracic viscera include the lungs and heart lying in the cavity of the thorax. The cavity of the thorax is separated from the cavity of the abdomen by the diaphragm.

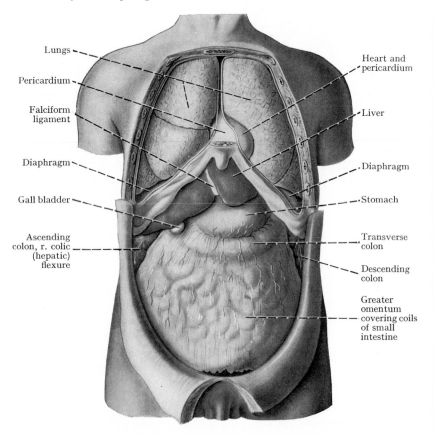

Fig. 204.—The thoracic and abdominal viscera. (Redrawn from Gray's "Anatomy.")

The Respiratory Passages

Air may be drawn into either the nasal or mouth cavity. The nasal cavity is divided into two by a central septum and at the entrance there are coarse hairs which act as a filter. In the lateral wall of the cavity are three *conchae* (fig. 33). These are perforated scroll-like bones which further filter the air.

The nasal cavity is very vascular and in this way the air is warmed before coming into contact with the delicate mucous membrane of the lower respiratory passages. This defensive mechanism is short-circuited when air is drawn through the mouth.

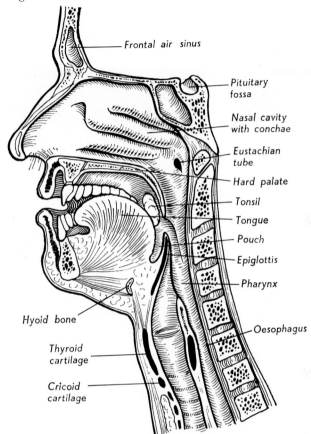

Frontal air sinus

Pituitary fossa

Nasal cavity with conchae

Eustachian tube

Hard palate

Tonsil

Tongue

Pouch

Epiglottis

Pharynx

Hyoid bone

Oesophagus

Thyroid cartilage

Cricoid cartilage

FIG. 205.—A median sagittal section through the head and neck showing the upper respiratory passages.

From the nasal cavity the air passes into the *nasopharynx* (a space above the soft palate) before entering the *oral pharynx* (a space behind the mouth cavity). The pharynx leads into two tubes, one placed anteriorly called the *larynx*, which is continuous with the trachea or windpipe, and the other placed posteriorly called the *oesophagus* or gullet (fig. 205).

The Larynx is the voice box and consists of a series of cartilages and muscles which regulate the pitch of the voice. The largest of these cartilages, called the *thyroid cartilage*, forms a prominence in the mid-line of the neck, called the pomum Adami (Adam's apple). Below the thyroid cartilage is the *cricoid cartilage* which is continuous with the trachea. The larynx is guarded by a cartilage called the *epiglottis* which helps to close the air passages during swallowing and guides the food into the oesophagus. The inspired air passes into the larynx, trachea and bronchi before entering the lungs. The upper end of the larynx is called the glottis. This closes at the very commencement of expiration, thereby regulating the passage of air from the lungs.

The Trachea commences at the lower border of the cricoid cartilage at the level of the 6th cervical vertebra and ends by bifurcating into right and left bronchi at the sternal angle. The trachea is a muscular tube reinforced

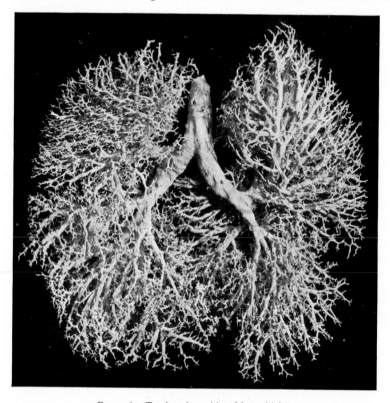

Fig. 206.—Trachea, bronchi and bronchioles.

Injected by the celluloid corrosion technique. (Bacsich and Smout.)

by a series of 18 to 20 U-shaped cartilaginous rings which keep the tube patent.

The Bronchi commence at the sternal angle and end at the lung roots. The right bronchus is wider and more vertical than the left, a point of some importance since foreign bodies entering the trachea almost invariably pass into the right bronchus. The bronchi end as small tubes called *bronchioles* (fig. 206) which have relatively thick muscular walls but are devoid of cartilage. They contract during expiration and spasmodic contraction of the bronchioles manifests itself in the form of asthma.

The Lungs are two large pyramidal-shaped, spongy organs which lie on either side of the heart within the thoracic cavity. Each lung is divided into two *lobes*—*upper* and *lower*—by an *oblique fissure*, while a third lobe, called the *middle lobe*, is usually present in the right lung due to the presence of a *transverse fissure*. A feature of the left lung is the *cardiac notch* on the anterior border; here the lung recedes from the mid-line for about 4 cm., leaving the heart, covered by its pericardium, exposed to the chest wall (fig. 204).

Each lung has an *apex* which extends upwards into the neck for 4 cm. above the clavicle and a *base* which is concave and rests upon the diaphragm. The posterolateral surface of each lung is grooved by the ribs. The medial surface presents a shallow depression for the heart and grooves for the great vessels.

The bronchi enter the lung *roots* and in each root there are also two pulmonary veins, carrying oxygenated blood from the lungs, and one artery, the pulmonary artery, carrying venous blood to the lungs. Also within the lung root are some lymph nodes which are important since they are some-

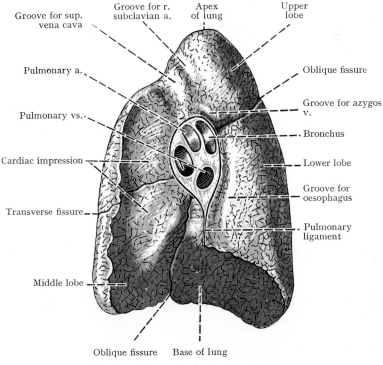

Groove for sup. vena cava   Groove for r. subclavian a.   Apex of lung   Upper lobe

Pulmonary a.

Pulmonary vs.

Cardiac impression

Transverse fissure

Middle lobe

Oblique fissure

Groove for azygos v.

Bronchus

Lower lobe

Groove for oesophagus

Pulmonary ligament

Oblique fissure   Base of lung

FIG. 207.—The mediastinal surface right lung.

times the seat of primary disease, e.g., tuberculosis or carcinoma. Tuberculosis often commences in the apex of the lung, pneumonia usually in the base.

The main subdivisions of the bronchi are as follows (fig. 208):

When each main bronchus enters the substance of the lung it divides like the branches of a tree and each division passes to a definite segment of lung tissue.

The Right Main Bronchus divides into a right superior lobe bronchus to the upper lobe, a right middle lobe bronchus to the middle lobe and a right inferior lobe bronchus to the lower lobe.

The right superior lobe bronchus divides into (i) an apical segmental bronchus which passes upwards to the apex, (ii) an interior segmental bronchus which passes forwards and (iii) a posterior segmental bronchus which passes backwards.

The right middle lobe bronchus divides into (i) a lateral segmental bronchus and (ii) a medial segmental bronchus.

The right inferior lobe bronchus divides into (i) a superior segmental bronchus to the upper part of the lower lobe, (ii) an anterior basal segmental bronchus, (iii) a posterior basal segmental bronchus, (iv) a lateral basal segmental bronchus and (v) a medial basal segmental bronchus.

The Left Main Bronchus divides into a left superior lobe bronchus to the upper lobe and a left inferior lobe bronchus to the lower lobe.

The left superior lobe bronchus divides into (i) an anterior segmental bronchus and (ii) an apico-posterior segmental bronchus and to the lower part of the superior lobe which is called the lingula; (iii) a superior lingular bronchus and (iv) an inferior lingular bronchus.

The left inferior lobe bronchus divides into (i) a superior segmental bronchus, (ii) an anterior basal segmental bronchus, (iii) a posterior basal segmental bronchus and (iv) a lateral basal segmental bronchus.

The Pleura is a serous membrane which lines the cavity of the thorax and covers the surface of the lungs, dipping into the fissures. These two layers of the pleura are, therefore, known as the parietal and visceral layers respectively. There is normally just sufficient moisture between the two layers to facilitate the excursions of the lungs without friction. Should the pleura become inflamed, the pleuritic fluid is likely to increase and this is spoken of as "pleurisy with effusion."

The Mediastinum is the space between the two pleural cavities. The mediastinum is divided for purposes of description into superior and inferior mediastina by the imaginary *plane of Louis*. This is a horizontal plane extending backwards from the sternal angle (p. 33) to the disc between the 4th and 5th thoracic vertebrae.

The *superior mediastinum* contains the trachea and bronchi, the oesophagus, aortic arch and great vessels, viz., the innominate, left common carotid and left subclavian arteries, the left and right innominate veins and the superior vena cava. It also contains the upper part of the thoracic duct and the terminal part of the azygos vein.

The *inferior mediastinum* is divided into anterior, middle and posterior mediastinal cavities by the heart which lies centrally in the middle mediastinum. The space in front of the heart is known as the anterior mediastinum and the space behind it, the posterior mediastinum.

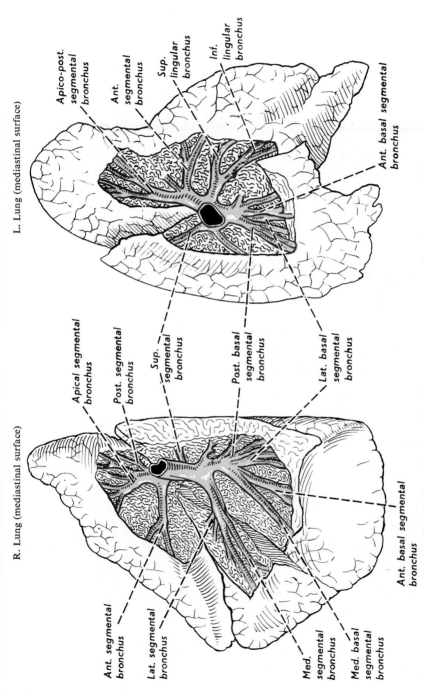

FIG. 208.—The Division of the Bronchi. (Redrawn from Zuckerman's " A New System of Anatomy.")

L. Lung (mediastinal surface)

R. Lung (mediastinal surface)

Apico-post. segmental bronchus

Ant. segmental bronchus

Sup. lingular bronchus

Inf. lingular bronchus

Ant. basal segmental bronchus

Apical segmental bronchus

Post. segmental bronchus

Sup. segmental bronchus

Post. basal segmental bronchus

Lat. basal segmental bronchus

Ant. basal segmental bronchus

Ant. segmental bronchus

Lat. segmental bronchus

Med. segmental bronchus

Med. basal segmental bronchus

The *anterior mediastinum* is a small space containing lymph nodes (fig. 209). The *middle mediastinum* contains the heart, pericardium and phrenic nerves.

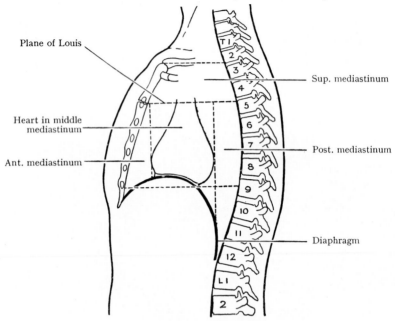

Fig. 209.—The mediastinal cavities (schematic).
Note that the suprasternal notch lies at the level of the lower border of T2 and the base of the xiphoid process at the level of T9.

The *posterior mediastinum* contains the oesophagus, surrounded by the oesophageal plexus of nerves (branches of the vagus nerve), the descending aorta, thoracic duct, azygos vein, and the sympathetic chain giving off the greater, lesser and least splanchnic nerves and some lymph nodes. The oesophageal plexus (branches of the vagus nerve) surrounds the oesophagus (fig. 172, facing page 206).

The Heart and Pericardium

The Heart is a muscular pump, conical in shape, with an apex below and anteriorly, and a base above and posteriorly. It lies within the mediastinal cavity, almost completely overlapped by the lungs, and is surrounded by a serous membrane called the *pericardium*. The heart is in contact with the thin central tendon of the diaphragm which alone separates it from the fundus of the stomach. Thus when the stomach becomes over-distended with gas or food it cramps the heart and by interfering with its blood supply may cause sudden death. The heart is not likely to be affected in this way unless it is already the seat of disease.

The Pericardium is an invaginated serous sac with an outer covering of fibrous tissue. Thus we speak of a serous pericardium and a fibrous pericardium.

The *serous pericardium* consists of two layers, one covering the surface of the heart, called the visceral layer, and the other lining the fibrous peri-cardium called the parietal layer. Normally there is just sufficient fluid between these two layers to facilitate the movement of the heart without friction. In pericarditis with effusion the amount of fluid is increased.

The visceral layer of serous pericardium is reflected around the great vessels in the form of two tubes; the aorta and pulmonary artery are enclosed in one tube and the superior and inferior venae cavae and the four pulmonary veins are enclosed in another tube. There is a space bounded by the pulmonary artery and aorta in front and the left atrium behind, known as the *transverse sinus of the pericardium*, while the space behind the left

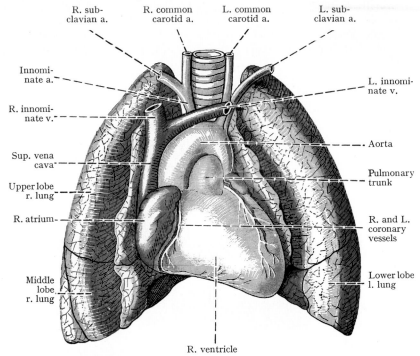

FIG. 210.—The lungs, heart and great vessels. (Redrawn from Gray's "Anatomy.")

atrium, limited above by the reflection of pericardium between right and left pulmonary veins, is known as the *oblique sinus of the pericardium*.

The *fibrous pericardium* blends with the adjacent pleura externally and with the parietal layer of serous pericardium internally. It is adherent to the central tendon of the diaphragm and is attached to the sternum.

The Heart Chambers. The heart contains four *chambers*, two atria and two ventricles with interatrial and interventricular septa and atrio-ventricular valves dividing them.

Into the *right atrium* the great veins open, viz., the superior vena cava bringing blood from the head and neck, upper extremities and thorax, and the inferior vena cava bringing blood from the abdomen, pelvis and lower extremities. Also opening into the right atrium is the coronary sinus, a large vein which drains the heart wall (fig. 211).

A small appendage attached to each *atrium* is known as the *auricle*.

The right atrium leads into the *right ventricle*, the opening being guarded by a valve with three triangular cusps forming the *tricuspid valve*. The cusps are attached to the interior of the right ventricle by *tendinous cords* (chordae tendineae) which support the valve when the heart contracts.

The walls of the atrial cavities are smooth, but the walls of the ventricular cavities are ridged by the *trabeculae carneae* (fig. 212). Some of the trabeculae are especially large, forming pillars known as the *papillary muscles*. There are usually two or three papillary muscles in each ventricular cavity and to these the tendinous cords of the valves are attached. A muscular band is sometimes present in the right ventricle running from the interventricular septum to the anterior papillary muscle. It is believed to prevent over-distension of the ventricle during atrial systole and is called the *moderator band*.

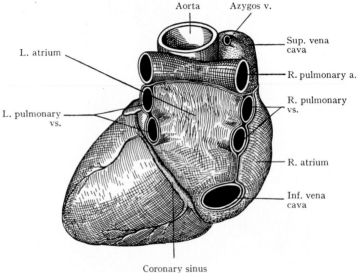

FIG. 211.—Posterior surface of heart. The serous pericardium is seen reflected around the veins. (Redrawn from Gray's "Anatomy.")

The pulmonary artery emerges from the right ventricle and this is guarded by a valve with three semilunar cusps which prevent the blood regurgitating towards the heart (fig. 212).

The *left atrium* (fig. 211) forms almost the whole of the base of the heart and is directed backwards. It extends from the 5th to the 8th thoracic vertebra. This cavity receives the four pulmonary veins and leads into the left ventricle, the opening into this cavity being guarded by the *mitral valve* which consists of two triangular cusps. Tendinous cords anchor these cusps to papillary muscles.

The interior of the *left ventricle* has an appearance similar to that of the right ventricle but its walls are much thicker, the ratio being 2/1. The left ventricle pumps the blood into the aorta which arises from it and its thickness is explained by the fact that it is responsible for the propelling force of the systemic circulation. The aorta, like the pulmonary artery, is guarded by a valve with three semilunar cusps which similarly prevent the blood regurgitating towards the heart.

The pericardium has already been described as covering the surface of the heart and this must be distinguished from the *endocardium* which is the lining membrane of the interior of the heart and the tissue which with a few fibres from the heart muscle forms the valves. The heart muscle is called the *myocardium*.

The term *pericarditis* thus means an inflammation of the membrane on the surface of the heart; *myocarditis* means an inflammation (often a degeneration) of the heart muscles; *endocarditis* means an inflammation of the valves of the heart (valvular disease of the heart or V.D.H.).

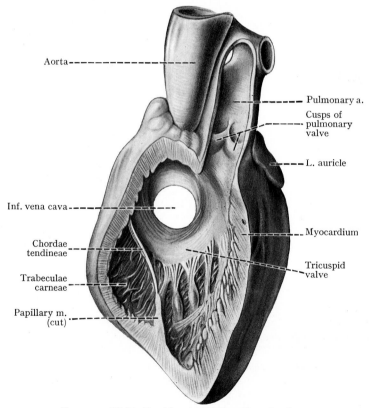

FIG. 212.—Right side of heart opened to show chambers.

THE ABDOMINAL VISCERA

The abdominal viscera include the alimentary tract, the liver, spleen, pancreas, kidneys and suprarenal glands. These all lie within the abdominal cavity and are partly or wholly covered by peritoneum.

The Peritoneum is comparable to the pericardium and pleura in that it is composed of serous membrane consisting of two layers which have been invaginated by the contained organs. Thus again we describe a *parietal layer*, which lines the abdominal wall and a *visceral layer* which is reflected over the surface of the contained viscera. The potential space bounded by the two layers is called the *peritoneal cavity*. This is divided into a larger space called the *greater sac* and a smaller space, which is a diverticulum of the larger, called the *lesser sac*. The two sacs communicate with each other via the aditus to the lesser sac.

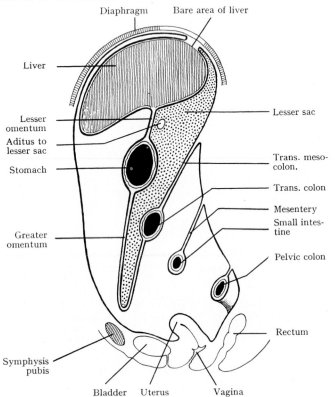

FIG. 213.—The peritoneum as seen in a median sagittal section through the abdominal cavity in the female (diagrammatic).

In the male the peritoneal cavity is a closed sac but in the female it communicates with the exterior, since the uterine tubes open into it. In the female, therefore, the peritoneum may be attacked by a direct infection spreading upwards from the exterior via the vagina, uterus and tubes.

The peritoneum is thrown into a series of folds by which the viscera are slung to one another and more particularly to the posterior abdominal wall. Some of these folds are large and of importance. They will be described in some detail.

The greater omentum (fig. 204) is a double fold of peritoneum extending from the greater curvature of the stomach to the transverse colon. It is made up of two layers of peritoneum folded back upon themselves and, therefore, is described as consisting of four layers. A reference to fig. 213 will show that these layers bound the lower part of the lesser sac. The greater omentum is suspended in front of the small intestines, like an apron. When the abdominal cavity is opened it is usually the first thing seen. It is extremely mobile and is impregnated with fat. The greater omentum plays an important defensive role and has earned the title of "the abdominal policeman." It is "summoned" to the seat of any disturbance within the abdominal cavity (e.g., an inflamed appendix) and tends to keep the trouble localised. A perforated appendix may, by the enfolding of the great omentum, become "walled off," resulting in a localised appendix abscess rather than a generalised peritonitis.

The lesser omentum (fig. 213) is a double fold of peritoneum extending from the lesser curvature of the stomach to the porta hepatis of the liver. It has a right free border which contains the common bile duct, portal vein and hepatic artery. This free border forms the anterior boundary of the aditus to the lesser sac.

The transverse mesocolon (fig. 213) is a double layer of peritoneum by which the transverse colon is slung to the posterior abdominal wall.

The mesentery (fig. 213) is a double layer of peritoneum by which the greater part of the small intestines is slung to the posterior abdominal wall. The mesentery is fan-shaped with a root about 15 cm. long and a base 6 metres long which envelops the small intestine. In order to conserve space the mesentery is thrown into a series of pleats. Between its two layers are the important vessels which carry the products of digestion to the liver and a number of lymphatic nodes and vessels. The latter are known as *lacteals*.

Before commencing a description of the abdominal viscera it is expedient to start by briefly describing the upper part of the alimentary tract at its origin within the mouth cavity.

The Alimentary Tract

The *mouth cavity* is bounded above by the hard and soft palates and below by a muscular floor in which the *tongue* occupies a central and dominant position. The mucous membrane on the dorsum of the tongue is covered with papillae some of which are tactile, others gustatory. Between the mouth cavity and the pharynx is the *cavity of the fauces* bounded on each side by anterior and posterior pillars between which is the *palatine tonsil*. The pharynx is continuous with the oesophagus.

The Oesophagus (fig. 172)* commences at the cricoid cartilage at the level of the 6th cervical vertebra. It is a tube about 25 cm. long which pierces the diaphragm at the level of the 10th thoracic vertebra and ends in the abdomen at the level of T11 where it opens into the stomach. The tube is not straight but curves antero-posteriorly in conformity with the curve of the vertebral column. It also curves to the left slightly, soon after its commencement, regaining the mid-line in the upper part of the thorax but

* Fig. 172 faces p. 206.

it takes a much wider sweep to the left just before its termination and here crosses in front of the aorta. It lies on the vertebral column, behind the trachea above, and the heart and pericardium below. It is constricted in three places viz.: at its commencement, where the left bronchus crosses it and where it perforates the diaphragm. The commencement of the oesophagus is the narrowest part of the alimentary tract except for the sphincters.

The abdominal portion of the oesophagus is very short—usually about 1·5 cm.—and lies behind the liver (oesophageal notch, fig. 219).

The Stomach (fig 214) is a hollow muscular organ lined by mucous membrane. It is freely mobile, especially its lower part, and its shape, size and position vary greatly. It has two borders called the *greater* and *lesser curvatures* and two surfaces. When the stomach is empty one surface faces upwards and forwards and the other downwards and backwards. To the greater curvature the greater omentum and to the lesser curvature the

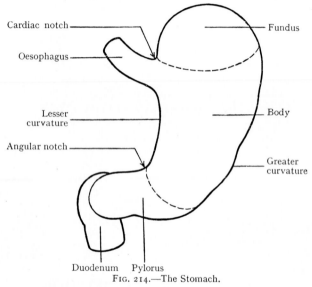

FIG. 214.—The Stomach.

lesser omentum are attached (fig. 213). Running along these borders are the main blood vessels supplying the organ. The antero-superior surface is in contact with the liver and the anterior abdominal wall, the postero-inferior surface lies on the *stomach bed* which is constituted by the pancreas, diaphragm, left kidney, left suprarenal gland, spleen and part of the transverse mesocolon. The lesser sac intervenes between these structures and the stomach (fig. 213).

Although the stomach is by no means constant in shape two notches can usually be seen on its borders; one is situated at the junction of the oesophagus with the greater curvature and is known as the *cardiac notch*, while the other is situated on the lesser curvature and is known as the *angular notch*. For the purpose of description the stomach is divided into three areas; the *fundus* which lies above an imaginary line drawn horizontally from the cardiac notch, the *body* which lies below the fundus and terminates at an imaginary line drawn vertically from the angular notch (fig. 214), and the *pylorus* which extends from the pyloric antrum to the pyloric sphincter.

The fundus of the stomach is separated from the heart only by the thin central tendon of the diaphragm. It is a reservoir for gas; no digestion takes place in this region. The body is principally a reservoir for food; digestion takes place chiefly in the pylorus.

The *pyloric sphincter* is formed by a thickening of the circular muscle fibres of the stomach wall.

The Small Intestine succeeds the stomach and is about 6 metres long. It commences as the C-shaped *duodenum* (fig. 215) which is about 25 cm. long and is the widest and most fixed part of the small intestine. Commencing at the pyloric sphincter the duodenum ends at the duodenojejunal flexure. It lies on the right kidney and the great vessels, on the posterior abdominal wall and behind the liver, transverse colon and coils of small intestine. A feature of the duodenum is that it has no mesentery.

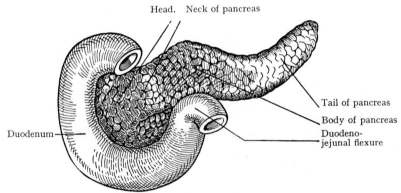

Head. Neck of pancreas

Tail of pancreas

Body of pancreas

Duodenum

Duodeno-jejunal flexure

FIG. 215.—The duodenum and pancreas.

The head of the pancreas lies in its concavity and opening into this part of the gut about 10 cm. from the pylorus is the fusion of the common bile and pancreatic ducts. This union forms a swelling which projects into the lumen of the duodenum as the *duodenal papilla* (fig. 220).

The duodenum is continued into the jejunum and the junction between these two parts of the small intestine is marked by a kink called the *duodeno-jejunal flexure* (fig. 215).

The *jejunum* passes imperceptibly into the *ileum* which ends by joining the large intestine at the *ileocolic valve*.

The jejunum and ileum are slung to the posterior abdominal wall by the mesentery and are thus extremely mobile. This part of the small intestine is surrounded above and laterally by the large intestine while below it tends to migrate into the pelvic cavity where it comes to lie in the rectovesical pouch of peritoneum in the male and in the rectovaginal pouch in the female (fig. 132, facing p. 141).

The external appearance of the jejunum differs from that of the ileum in that it is redder, thicker and more vascular. When the jejunum is opened its mucous membrane is seen as a series of transverse folds, called the *circular folds*. On these folds there are a very large number of finger-like processes hardly visible to the naked eye called *villi* (fig. 291). The villi are concerned with the absorption of the food, while the folds are so arranged as to hold up the food until such time as the villi have an opportunity of absorbing nourishment resulting from its digestion.

As jejunum passes to ileum, these folds and villi become less numerous and the smooth mucous membrane of the ileum is seen to be studded at intervals by islands of lymphoid tissue termed the *aggregated lymphatic nodules*. These islands have a protective function and it is here that the typhoid bacillus may commence excavations which culminate in the formation of a typhoid ulcer.

The entrance from small intestine to large intestine is guarded by the *ileocolic valve* formed by a reduplication of the circular muscle fibres at the termination of the ileum.

The Large Intestine differs considerably in appearance from the small

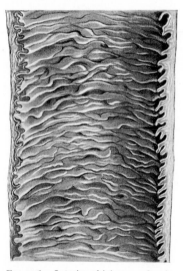

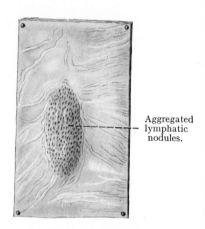

Aggregated lymphatic nodules.

FIG. 216.—Interior of jejunum, showing circular folds.

FIG. 217.—Interior of ileum showing aggregated lymphatic nodules.

intestine, for it is larger in calibre and more fixed. The longitudinal muscle fibres in its wall are aggregated into bands called *taeniae* and these pucker the gut so that the large intestine is sacculated. Another characteristic feature is the appendages of fat enveloped in peritoneum called the *appendices epiploicae* which are scattered over the surface of this part of the alimentary tract (fig. 218). There are no taeniae or appendices epiploicae on the walls of the rectum and anal canal.

The *caecum* is the commencement of the large intestine. It is a blind pouch about 7 cm. long which lies in the false pelvis above the middle of the inguinal ligament and behind the anterior abdominal wall, greater omentum and sometimes coils of small intestine. It lies on the iliacus and psoas muscles and on the femoral nerve which emerges between those muscles. The caecum is covered by peritoneum but has no mesentery, while lying behind it there is often a fossa, variable in size, extending up towards the kidney called the *retrocaecal fossa*. This is of some importance because the appendix not infrequently migrates into it, and should it become inflamed the condition is known as "a retrocaecal appendix."

The *vermiform appendix* is a narrow worm-like tube also blind, which communicates with the caecum about 2·5 cm. below and behind the ileocolic valve. It is about 10 cm. long and is anchored to the caecum and the termination of the ileum by a double fold of peritoneum called the *mesentery of the appendix* (meso-appendix).

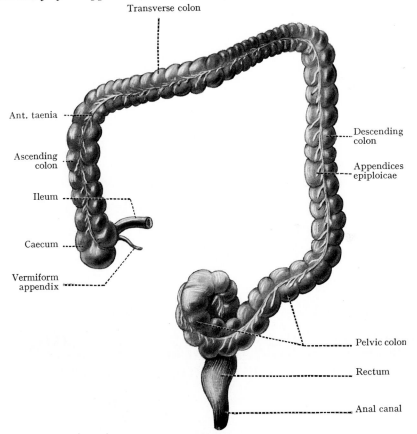

FIG. 218.—The large intestine.

The appendix usually lies below and to the left of the caecum. It may, however, extend over the pelvic brim (pelvic appendix) and may come into relation with the right tube and ovary.

The *ascending* colon (fig. 218) succeeds the caecum at the ileocolic valve. It passes upwards behind the anterior abdominal wall, lying on the muscles of the posterior abdominal wall, viz., psoas, quadratus lumborum, transversus abdominis and diaphragm (a very little) until it reaches the lower pole of the right kidney and the under surface of the liver where it turns to the left to become the transverse colon. This kink in the large intestine is known as the *right colic (hepatic) flexure.*

The *transverse colon* (fig. 218) runs across the abdomen just above the umbilical plane, behind the lesser sac of peritoneum; lying on the duodenum, root of mesentery, duodenojejunal flexure and coils of small intestine. On reaching the lower pole of the left kidney, it turns downwards beneath the spleen forming the *left colic (splenic) flexure.*

The *descending colon* (fig. 218) succeeds the transverse colon and has almost exactly similar relations on the left side as has the ascending colon on the right.

Reaching the pelvic brim the descending colon becomes the *pelvic colon* which runs transversely across the pelvic cavity and turning back upon itself in an S-formation reaches the level of the 3rd sacral vertebra to become the *rectum.* The rectum terminates in the *anal canal* and the large intestine ends at the *anal orifice.*

While the greater part of the large intestine is fixed to the posterior aspect of the trunk, the transverse colon and the pelvic colon are suspended by mesenteries called the *transverse mesocolon* and the *pelvic mesocolon* respectively. These two parts of the large intestines are, therefore, mobile.

The Liver is the largest gland in the body and weighs about 1·4 kilogm. It lies chiefly on the right side of the upper part of the abdomen immediately beneath the diaphragm, only a small part crosses the mid-line and lies on the left. It is almost entirely under cover of the ribs for its lower border usually corresponds with the right costal margin. The gland is wedge-shaped, the base of the wedge being directed to the right and the small apex to the left.

It is divided into lobes by an *H-shaped* "fossa," the left limb of the H separating the larger *right lobe* from the smaller *left lobe*; the right limb of the H and the transverse limb separate the *caudate lobe* from the *quadrate lobe.* The vertical limbs of the H are known as the *right* and *left sagittal fossae*; the transverse limb is known as the *porta hepatis.*

The left sagittal fossa transmits certain foetal remnants, viz., the ligamentum teres below and the ligamentum venosum above. The right sagittal fossa lodges the gall bladder below and the inferior vena cava above. The porta hepatis transmits the portal vein, common hepatic duct and the hepatic artery.

The liver is covered by peritoneum except for a triangular *bare area* on its postero-superior surface (fig. 219). It is attached to the anterior abdominal wall as far down as the umbilicus by the *falciform ligament* (fig. 204); to the diaphragm by the *right* and *left triangular* and the superior and inferior layers of the *coronary ligament* (fig. 219).

The *superior surface* of the liver is marked by a shallow depression upon which the diaphragmatic surface of the heart rests—the thin central tendon of the diaphragm intervening. The *postero-inferior* surface of the liver is in contact from left to right with the oesophagus and stomach; the pylorus and first part of duodenum (in contact with the quadrate lobe); the descending part of the duodenum, right kidney, right suprarenal gland and the hepatic flexure of the colon (fig. 219).

On this surface just above the impression for the stomach there is a rounded prominence called the *papillary process* which is in contact with the lesser sac of peritoneum.

The liver secretes the bile which passes down the *right* and *left hepatic ducts* within the substance of the liver. At the porta hepatis these ducts fuse to form the *common hepatic duct* which is joined by the duct of the gall bladder—the *cystic duct*—to form the common bile duct.

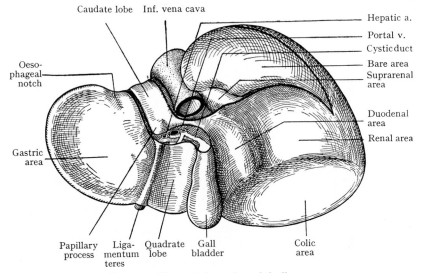

FIG. 219.—The posterior surface of the liver.

The bare area is bounded above by the superior and below by the inferior layers of the coronary ligament (black lines). These layers fuse at the apex of the bare area forming the right triangular ligament.

The Common Bile Duct descends in the right free border of the lesser omentum, then behind the first part of the duodenum and the head of the pancreas to open in conjunction with the duct of the pancreas into the descending limb of the duodenum. The fusion of the two ducts forms the ampulla of the bile duct which opens on the duodenal papilla which lies in the interior of the duodenum about 10 cm. from the pylorus (fig. 220).

The Gall Bladder is a green, pear-shaped sac which lies for the most part in the fossa for the gall bladder on the under surface of the right lobe of the liver. It consists of a fundus, body and neck. The *fundus* is the most dependent part and lies just below the lower border of the liver (fig. 204). It can be palpated at the level of the 9th costal cartilage where the lateral border of the right rectus muscle crosses the lower border of the thorax.

The *body* lies behind the liver and on the transverse colon, while the *neck* lies on the duodenum and is continuous with the cystic duct.

The hepatic and cystic ducts are each about 4 cm. long; the common bile duct and gall bladder are each about 8 cm long.

Within the cystic duct there is a spiral valve. The common bile duct is usually guarded by a sphincter (the *sphincter of Oddi*). It has been pointed out (Gordon Taylor) that the common bile duct passes through the duodenal wall obliquely, thus preventing regurgitation of the duodenal contents into the duct.

Bile is secreted continually and passes down the hepatic and common bile ducts. If the ampulla is closed, the bile is diverted via the spiral valve into

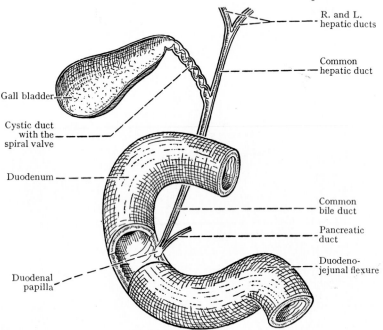

FIG. 220.—The excretory apparatus of the liver.

the gall bladder which acts as a reservoir. The ampulla is relaxed when fats pass into the duodenum and at the same time a hormone causes the gall bladder to contract and thus bile is poured into the duodenum. It follows, therefore, that the gall bladder is likely to be full and distended before a meal and empty soon afterwards.

The Pancreas (fig. 215) is a tongue-shaped gland with a head, neck, body and tail. The head lies in the concavity of the duodenum on the inferior vena cava and behind the transverse colon and coils of small intestine. The neck is formed by a bulging forward of the gland as it lies in front of the portal vein. The body stretches across the posterior abdominal wall behind the peritoneum lying on the aorta, left psoas muscle, left kidney and left suprarenal gland while the tail rests on the hilum of the spleen. The stomach, duodenojejunal flexure, coils of small intestine and the splenic flexure of the colon are in contact with the anterior surface of the body.

The main duct of the pancreas opens with the common bile duct into the second part of the duodenum.

The Spleen (figs. 221 and 222) lies in the left upper quadrant of the abdominal cavity beneath the 9th, 10th and 11th ribs. Its long axis corresponds with the long axis of the 10th rib, while its anterior border which is characteristically notched does not extend beyond the mid-axillary line in normal circumstances. A normal spleen cannot, therefore, be palpated but if for any reason it becomes enlarged, it extends beyond the left costal margin and can be readily felt.

It is entirely covered by peritoneum except at the hilum where the vessels enter and leave the gland. From the spleen the peritoneum is reflected on to the left kidney and stomach.

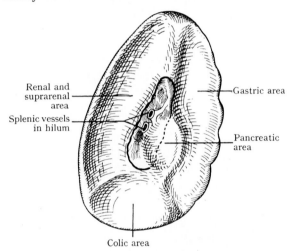

Fig. 221.—The visceral surface of the spleen.

The spleen has much the same consistency as the liver and is normally about the size of the clenched fist.

It has a convex parietal surface which is separated by the diaphragm from the base of the lungs and the 9th, 10th and 11th ribs. It has a concave visceral surface which is in contact with the stomach and pancreas anteriorly; the left kidney and left suprarenal gland posteriorly; and the splenic flexure of the colon inferiorly.

The Kidneys lie behind the peritoneum on the posterior abdominal wall. Each gland is covered by a capsule surrounding which is a large quantity of fat enclosed in a fascial sheath. Each kidney weighs about 150 gm. and is about 11 cm. long.

The *posterior surfaces* of the kidneys are in contact with the diaphragm above, which separates them from the 11th and 12th ribs on the left and from the 12th rib on the right, for the right kidney lies slightly below the left.   Below the diaphragm the kidneys lie on the psoas, quadratus lumborum and transversus abdominis muscles (fig. 223).

The *anterior surface of the right kidney* is in contact with the right suprarenal gland above and medially, the liver laterally, the duodenum medially and the hepatic flexure of the colon and coils of small intestine inferiorly (fig. 224).

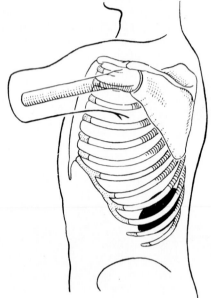

FIG. 222.—The spleen in situ.   (After Corning.)

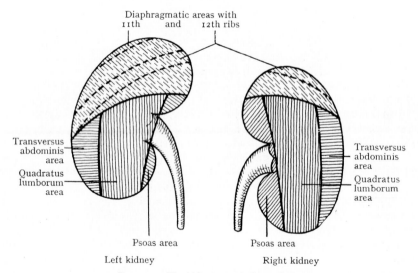

Diaphragmatic areas with
11th   and   12th ribs

Transversus
abdominis
area

Quadratus
lumborum
area

Transversus
abdominis
area

Quadratus
lumborum
area

Psoas area   Psoas area

Left kidney   Right kidney

FIG. 223.—The kidneys, posterior surface.

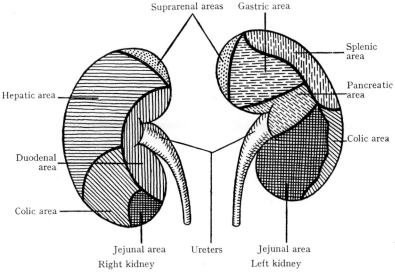

Suprarenal areas   Gastric area

Splenic area

Pancreatic area

Hepatic area

Colic area

Duodenal area

Colic area

Jejunal area   Ureters   Jejunal area
Right kidney   Left kidney

FIG. 224.—The kidneys, anterior surface.

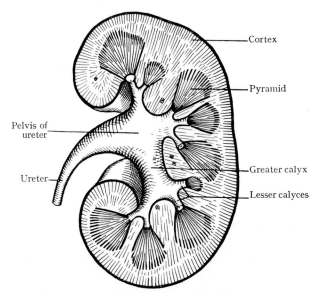

Cortex

Pyramid

Pelvis of ureter

Greater calyx

Ureter

Lesser calyces

FIG. 225.—A sagittal section through the kidney.

The *anterior surface of the left kidney* is in contact with the left suprarenal gland above and medially, the spleen laterally, the stomach and pancreas medially, the splenic flexure of the colon and coils of small intestine inferiorly (fig. 224).

The blood vessels and the ureter enter or leave the gland at the renal sinus, the ureter lying usually behind the vessels.

When the kidney is sectioned it is seen to be composed of a *cortex* at the periphery and a *medulla* centrally. The medulla is composed of a number of pyramids, at the apex of which there is a small opening which is the termination of a collecting tubule. These *collecting tubules* open into larger tubes called the *lesser calyces* and these open into the *greater calyces* which in turn open into the *pelvis* of the ureter (fig 225).

The Ureters are narrow tubes connecting the kidneys with the bladder. Each ureter runs obliquely over the psoas muscle, behind the peritoneum and, reaching the pelvis, enters the trigone of the bladder.

The Suprarenal Glands (fig. 226). The right gland is pyramidal in shape (resembles a "cocked hat"), the left gland is semilunar (resembles a

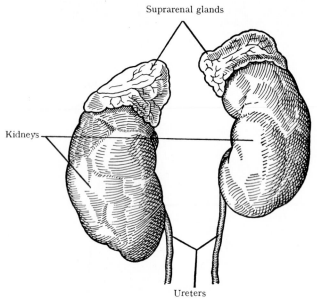

Suprarenal glands

Kidneys

Ureters

Fig. 226.—The kidneys and suprarenal glands from a child aged 6 months.

brazil nut). Each gland lies on the corresponding kidney and on the adjacent surface of the diaphragm.

The right gland is in contact anteriorly with the inferior vena cava and the liver and the left gland with the pancreas, stomach and spleen. The suprarenal glands are almost as large at birth as in the adult.

THE PELVIS AND PELVIC ORGANS

The pelvic cavity lies below the pelvic brim and is bounded inferiorly by the muscular pelvic floor.

The male pelvic organs (fig. 227) consist of the urinary *bladder* and *prostate gland* anteriorly; the *pelvic colon, rectum* and *anal canal* posteriorly.

The *urethra* which leads from the bladder to the exterior perforates the prostate gland and penis.

The *seminal vesicles* lie behind the base of the bladder and act as reservoirs for the semen which is secreted by the testes. The *vasa deferentia* are ducts which convey the semen into the seminal vesicles or directly into the urethra.

The female pelvic organs (fig. 132, facing p. 141) consist of the bladder and urethra anteriorly; the reproductive organs comprising the ovaries, tubes, uterus and vagina centrally; the pelvic colon, rectum and anal canal posteriorly.

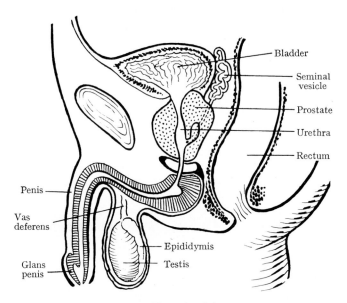

FIG. 227.—The male pelvic organs.

The ovaries are two oval glands, each about the size of the distal phalanx of the thumb. In a nullipara each gland lies in a small fossa on the lateral pelvic wall, situated at the bifurcation of the common iliac artery. It is attached at its upper pole to the lateral pelvic wall by a double fold of peritoneum conveying the ovarian vessels and nerves called the *infundibulo-pelvic fold*; by its lower pole to the body of the uterus by the *ovarian ligament*; and by its anterior border to the broad ligament by a double fold of peritoneum called the *mesovarium*. During pregnancy it rises with the uterus into the abdomen and after parturition may never regain its normal position. This displacement of the ovary does not cause any inconvenience as a rule.

The uterine tubes open at one end into the abdominal cavity, the opening being called the *abdominal ostium*, and at the other into the cavity of the uterus. The abdominal ostium is surrounded by a number of finger-like processes called fimbriae, one of which, larger than the rest, is called the *ovarian fimbria*. This fimbria lies in contact with the surface of the ovary and is believed to direct the extruded ovum at ovulation into the tubal cavity.

The uterus is a thick walled, fibro-muscular organ, about 7 cm. long and 5 cm. wide. Its walls are about 1·5 cm. thick. The uterine tubes open into it above, whilst below it opens into the vagina at the external os. It is divided into a *fundus*, the part above the opening of the uterine tubes; a *body* which lies between the tubes and a constricted part called the isthmus; and a *cervix* which perforates the anterior vaginal wall. It is somewhat hard because it contains a large amount of fibrous tissue in addition to muscle fibres. The cavity of the body is triangular in shape with its base above and its apex below, the cavity of the cervix is fusiform ending below at the external os.

The uterus is normally anteflexed (flexed forwards) and anteverted (tilted forwards) and is held in this position by the round ligaments. The cervix of the uterus is relatively fixed but the body is mobile, and its position in the pelvis varies with the degree of distension of the surrounding viscera, especially the bladder.

The uterus is almost completely covered by peritoneum which is reflected from its lateral walls on to the lateral pelvic wall as the **broad ligaments of the uterus**. Each ligament extends down as far as the pelvic floor and between its two peritoneal layers there is some pelvic connective tissue called the **parametrium**. Inflammation of this tissue is, therefore, known as parametritis. The peritoneum is reflected from the posterior surface of the uterus on to the vagina and thence to the rectum. The large potential space between these organs, bounded in this way by peritoneum, is known as the **rectovaginal pouch of Douglas**.

The uterus has a rich blood supply from the uterine, ovarian and vaginal arteries (see also p. 467).

The **round ligaments of the uterus** are attached to the body of that organ. Each ligament passes through the deep inguinal ring and turning at right angles through the inguinal canal on the anterior abdominal wall, passes out of the canal at the superficial inguinal ring, to end just beneath the skin of the labium majus. Their function is to keep the uterus anteflexed and anteverted.

The vagina is a fibro-muscular sheath about 7 cm. long. It commences at the cleft between the labia minora called the vestibule and ends above as a vault, the anterior wall of which is perforated by the cervix of the uterus. In this way the upper end of the vagina is divided into four arches or fornices—an *anterior fornix* in front of the cervix, in contact with the base of the bladder, a *posterior fornix* behind the cervix, in contact with the rectovaginal pouch and two *lateral fornices*, in contact with part of the uterine arteries and the termination of the ureters. The female urethra is embedded in the anterior vaginal wall.

CHAPTER IX

ANATOMICAL REGIONS

The neck is divided into anterior and posterior triangles by the sterno-mastoid muscle, the anterior triangle lying in front and the posterior triangle behind that muscle.

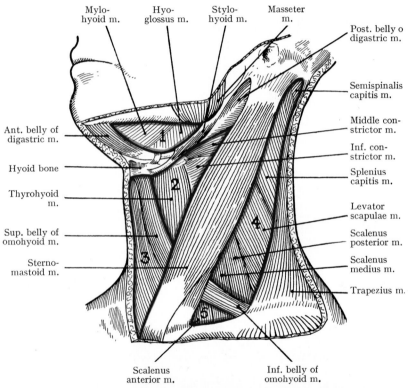

Mylo-hyoid m.	Hyo-glossus m.	Stylo-hyoid m.	Masseter m.

Post. belly o digastric m.

Semispinalis capitis m.

Ant. belly of digastric m.

Middle con-strictor m.

Inf. con-strictor m.

Hyoid bone

Splenius capitis m.

Thyrohyoid m.

Levator scapulae m.

Sup. belly of omohyoid m.

Scalenus posterior m.

Sterno-mastoid m.

Scalenus medius m.

Trapezius m.

Scalenus anterior m.

Inf. belly of omohyoid m.

FIG. 228.—The triangles of the neck.

1. The astricdig triangle.　2. The carotid triangle.　3. The muscular triangle.
4. The ipitalocc triangle.　5. The subclavian triangle.

The Anterior Triangle of the Neck (fig. 228)
The anterior triangle of the neck is bounded as follows:

Anteriorly by the mid-line of the neck.
Posteriorly by the anterior border of the sternomastoid.
Superiorly by the lower border of the mandible which forms the base of the triangle.

Its *roof* is formed by skin, superficial fascia, platysma and deep fascia. In the roof are the cervical branch of the facial nerve, the cervical cutaneous nerve and the anterior branch of the supraclavicular nerve. Its *floor* is further subdivided into triangles by the digastric and omohyoid muscles. These triangles are known as the submental, digastric, carotid and muscular triangles.

The submental triangle (fig. 229) lies just below the symphysis menti. It is small and unimportant.   Its boundaries are as follows:

Its *apex* and *lateral borders* by the anterior bellies of the digastric muscle.

Its *base* by the hyoid bone.

Its *floor* is formed by the muscular diaphragm of the mouth, viz., the mylohyoid muscle.

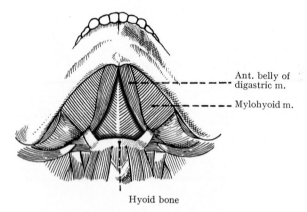

Ant. belly of digastric m.

Mylohyoid m.

Hyoid bone

FIG. 229.—The submental triangle.

It contains the submental lymph nodes which readily become infected in septic conditions of the lower lip and lower incisor teeth.

The digastric triangle (fig. 228) lies just below the body of the mandible. Its boundaries are as follows:

Anteriorly by the anterior belly of the digastric muscle.

Posteriorly by the posterior belly of the digastric and stylohyoid muscles.

Its *apex* by part of the hyoid bone.

Its *base* by the body of the mandible.

Its *floor* is formed by the mylohyoid, hyoglossus and superior constrictor muscles.

The triangle contains the submandibular salivary gland with the facial artery embedded within it and the submandibular lymph nodes lying on it; the hypoglossal nerve lying deep to the gland, between it and the hyoglossus muscle; the nerve and vessels to the mylohyoid muscle.

The **carotid triangle** (fig. 228) is relatively small but contains a number of important structures. Its boundaries are as follows:
Superiorly by the posterior belly of the digastric and stylohyoid muscles.
Antero-inferiorly by the superior belly of the omohyoid muscle.
Its *apex* by the greater cornu of the hyoid bone.
Its *base* by part of the anterior border of the sternomastoid muscle.
Its *floor* is formed by the thyrohyoid muscle and the middle and inferior constrictors of the pharynx.

The triangle contains the common carotid artery, bifurcating into internal and external carotids, the vagus nerve, the internal jugular vein, all within the carotid sheath and lying deep to the sternomastoid muscle; numerous branches of the external carotid artery; the common facial vein; the hypoglossal nerve with the descendens hypoglossi lying on the carotid sheath; the accessory nerve crossing the transverse process of the atlas at the upper angle of the triangle (fig. 235); the nerves to the larynx and some important lymph nodes belonging to the deep cervical chain.

The **muscular triangle** (fig. 228) is bounded as follows:
Anteriorly by the mid-line of the neck.
Superiorly by the omohyoid muscle.
Inferiorly by the anterior border of the sternomastoid muscle.
Its *floor* is formed by the infrahyoid muscles.

The contents of this triangle are insignificant but deep to its floor are such important structures as the thyroid gland, the larynx, trachea and oesophagus.

The **Posterior Triangle of the Neck** (fig. 228) is bounded as follows:
Anteriorly by the posterior border of sternomastoid.
Posteriorly by the anterior border of the trapezius.
Its *base* by the middle third of the clavicle.
Its *roof* is formed by skin, superficial fascia, platysma, deep fascia, in which ramify the anterior, middle and posterior supraclavicular nerves.

The omohyoid muscle divides the posterior triangle into a larger occipital triangle and a smaller subclavian triangle.

The **occipital triangle** (fig. 228) is bounded as follows:
Anteriorly by the posterior border of the sternomastoid.
Posteriorly by the anterior border of the trapezius.
Its *base* by the inferior belly of the omohyoid.
Its *floor* is formed by the following muscles from above down: semispinalis capitis (sometimes) splenius capitis, levator scapulae, scalenus posterior, scalenus medius and sometimes by scalenus anterior, but this muscle may be entirely hidden by sternomastoid.

The triangle contains the accessory nerve which lying on the levator scapulae crosses the space as it passes to the trapezius muscle; branches of the 3rd and 4th cervical nerves to levator scapulae and trapezius below this; and the nerve to the rhomboids from C5 below these. In addition, the cutaneous branches of the cervical plexus curl round the posterior border of the sternomastoid immediately below the point of emergence of the accessory nerve, viz., the lesser occipital nerve from C2, the great auricular and the cervical cutaneous nerves from C2 and 3 (fig. 174).

The upper trunks of the brachial plexus, and the transverse cervical artery may penetrate into the lower part of the triangle.

The subclavian triangle (fig. 228) is bounded as follows:
Anteriorly by part of the posterior border of the sternomastoid.
Superiorly by the omohyoid.
Inferiorly by the middle third of the clavicle.
Its *floor* is formed by the scalenus anterior (sometimes), the scalenus medius and the first serration of the serratus anterior.

The triangle contains the third part of the subclavian artery and vein and the lowest trunk of the brachial plexus, all of which lie on the first rib, the upper and middle trunks of the brachial plexus crossed by the transverse cervical and suprascapular vessels and the nerve to subclavius from C5 and 6.

The Axilla (fig. 195, facing p. 223)
The axilla is pyramidal in shape with its apex above and its base below. It should be noted that its apex is bony for it protects the axillary sheath which contains the vessels and nerves passing to the upper limb. Its boundaries are as follows:

Anterior wall by pectorales major et minor. The latter muscle is ensheathed by the clavipectoral fascia and this fills a gap on the anterior axillary wall between the clavicle and the upper border of the pectoralis minor (fig. 134).
Posterior wall by subscapularis, teres major and latissimus dorsi muscles in that order from above down. The posterior wall extends beyond the anterior wall.
Medial wall by the upper 4 or 5 ribs covered by the serratus anterior.
Lateral wall by the coracobrachialis and short head of biceps.
Apex by the middle of the posterior border of clavicle, the outer border of the first rib and the superior border of the scapula.
Base by the integument stretching between anterior and posterior walls.

The axilla contains the axillary artery surrounded by the cords of the brachial plexus, the branches of the artery, the axillary vein lying medial to the artery, the intercostobrachial nerve from T2, numerous lymph nodes and a large quantity of fat. The nerves arising from the cords of the brachial plexus in the axilla are:

from the *lateral cord* the lateral pectoral and musculocutaneous nerves (fig. 175);

from the *posterior cord* the upper and lower subscapular, nerve to latissimus dorsi, circumflex and radial nerves (fig. 175);

from the *medial cord* the medial pectoral nerve, the medial cutaneous nerve of the arm, the medial cutaneous nerve of the forearm, the ulnar nerve, and the median nerve from the union of the medial and lateral cords (fig. 175).

In addition to these the nerve to serratus anterior from the roots of C5, 6 and 7 descends along the medial axillary wall on the serratus anterior.

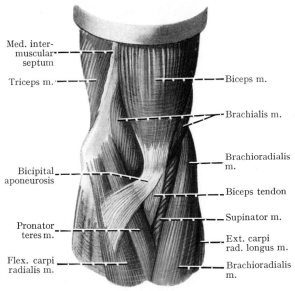

Med. inter-
muscular
septum

Triceps m.

Bicipital
aponeurosis

Pronator
teres m.

Flex. carpi
radialis m.

Biceps m.

Brachialis m.

Brachioradialis
m.

Biceps tendon

Supinator m.

Ext. carpi
rad. longus m.

Brachioradialis
m.

FIG. 230.—The cubital fossa (left side).

The Cubital Fossa (fig. 230)
This fossa lies at the bend of the elbow and is triangular in shape.

Its *lateral boundary* is formed by the brachioradialis muscle.

Its *medial boundary* by the pronator teres muscle.

Its *base* is formed by an imaginary line drawn between the two condyles of the humerus.

Its *floor* is formed chiefly by the brachialis muscle, but includes part of the supinator laterally.

Its *roof* is formed by skin and fascia reinforced medially by the tendinous slip from the biceps muscle called the *bicipital aponeurosis* which blends with the fascia of the forearm. In the roof are the medial and lateral cutaneous nerves of the forearm and usually the median cephalic and median basilic veins.

The fossa contains the tendon of biceps with the brachial artery lying medial to it and the median nerve lying medial to the artery. The median nerve leaves the fossa between the two heads of the pronator teres muscle and in the fossa the brachial artery divides into its two terminal branches, viz., radial and ulnar. The former leaves the fossa by passing laterally on supinator and pronator teres and beneath the brachioradialis muscle. The latter leaves the fossa deep to the deep head of pronator teres, so that this head separates the median nerve from the ulnar artery in this region.

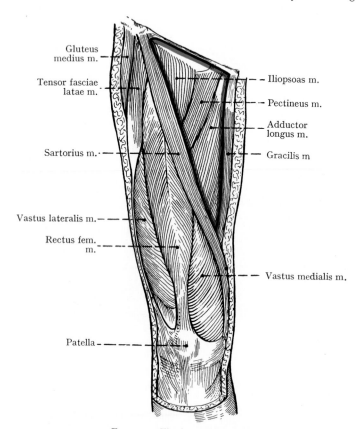

Gluteus medius m.

Tensor fasciae latae m.

Sartorius m.

Vastus lateralis m.

Rectus fem. m.

Patella

Iliopsoas m.

Pectineus m.

Adductor longus m.

Gracilis m

Vastus medialis m.

FIG. 231.—The femoral triangle.

The Femoral Triangle (fig. 231)

The femoral triangle is situated in the upper part of the medial aspect of the thigh. Its boundaries are as follows:

Its *lateral* boundary is formed by the medial border of the sartorius muscle.

Its *medial* boundary is formed by the medial border of the adductor longus muscle.

Its *base* is formed by the inguinal ligament.

Its *roof* is formed by the skin, superficial fascia and fascia lata of the thigh which is pierced medially by the saphenous opening. In the roof are the long and accessory saphenous veins; some small blood vessels; cutaneous branches of the ilio-inguinal, genitofemoral, 12th thoracic and obturator nerves and the medial and intermediate cutaneous nerves of the thigh (fig. 179) and the superficial inguinal lymph nodes.

Its *floor* is formed from the medial to the lateral side by the adductor longus, pectineus, psoas and iliacus muscles.

Its *apex* is continuous with the subsartorial canal.

The triangle contains the femoral artery, which is the central and dominant structure, and the femoral vein medial to the artery. These two struc-

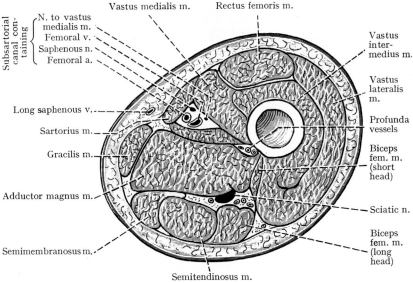

FIG. 232.—Transverse section through the middle of thigh, showing the subsartorial canal. (Redrawn from Gray's "Anatomy.")

tures together with the deep inguinal lymph nodes are enclosed within the femoral sheath (fig. 198). Other contents of the femoral triangle are the femoral nerve which lies lateral to the artery and outside the sheath and the lateral cutaneous nerve of the thigh which usually perforates sartorius to reach the lateral aspect of the thigh.

Within the triangle the femoral nerve breaks up into its constituent branches and the femoral artery gives off some small branches and one large one, viz., the profunda femoris.

The Subsartorial Canal (fig. 232)

The subsartorial lies on the medial aspect of the middle third of the thigh. It commences at the apex of the femoral triangle and ends at the opening in the adductor magnus. Its boundaries are as follows:

Its *lateral* boundary is formed by the vastus medialis muscle.

Its *anteromedial* boundary by the aponeurotic arch which connects adductors longus and magnus with the vastus medialis. The sartorius muscle lies on this arch (fig. 232).

Its *posteromedial* boundary is formed by the adductors longus and magnus.

The canal is triangular on cross-section and contains the femoral artery and vein, the saphenous nerve and the nerve to the vastus medialis muscle. The latter is the most lateral structure within the canal, the vein is at first posterior and then lateral to the artery, while the saphenous nerve crosses the artery superficially from the lateral to the medial side.

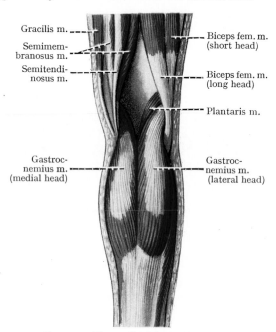

Gracilis m.

Semimembranosus m.

Semitendinosus m.

Biceps fem. m. (short head)

Biceps fem. m. (long head)

Plantaris m.

Gastrocnemius m. (medial head)

Gastrocnemius m. (lateral head)

FIG. 233.—The popliteal fossa (right side).

The Popliteal Fossa (fig. 233)

The popliteal fossa lies at the back of the knee. It is a diamond-shaped space having the following boundaries:

Its *superior* boundary by the biceps femoris tendon laterally and the tendons of semimembranosus and semitendinosus medially.

Its *inferior* boundary by the two heads of gastrocnemius muscle and also by the plantaris muscle laterally.

Its *roof* is formed by skin, superficial fascia and the fascia lata of the thigh which is perforated by the posterior cutaneous nerve of the thigh and by the termination of the short saphenous vein.

Its *floor* is formed above down by the popliteal surface of the femur the posterior oblique ligament, the upper end of the tibia and the popliteus muscle.

The fossa contains the popliteal artery and the genicular branch of the obturator nerve lying deeply on its floor, the popliteal vein which crosses the artery superficially from the lateral to the medial side, the medial popliteal nerve crossing the vein in a similar manner, the lateral popliteal nerve lying directly on the medial border of the biceps tendon and the popliteal group of lymph nodes. For an account of the arrangement of these nodes in the popliteal fossa the reader is referred to p. 254.

CHAPTER X

LIVING ANATOMY

A knowledge of anatomy is of no great value unless it is based upon and can be readily applied to the living body. To learn by heart a mass of detailed facts and to be able to repeat them "parrot-fashion" at the opportune moment is no indication of knowledge. A student who can write a good answer to an anatomical question and who is lost when confronted with the living model has missed the whole point of the subject.

Of all the chapters in this section of the book, this one should be the most carefully read. It cannot be too strongly emphasised that mere reading is valueless unless at the same time every point is verified systematically on the living body.

Living Anatomy of the Head and Neck

The bony points of the skull should first be verified (figs. 33 and 34).

The *nasion* is the depression at the root of the nose; just above it there is an elevation called the *glabella*. Running outwards from the glabella are two prominent ridges which lie above the margin of the orbit; these are the *superciliary arches* and they are of importance because they mark the position of the frontal air sinuses which lie on their deep aspect.

The *inion* corresponds to the nasion posteriorly and lies in the middle of the squamous portion of the occipital bone. It is identical with the external occipital protuberance and marks the uppermost point of origin of the trapezius muscle and the attachment of the ligamentum nuchae. From the inion the superior nuchal line runs laterally giving attachment to such muscles as the sternomastoid, occipitalis and splenius capitis.

On the lateral aspect of the skull is the *parietal eminence* which marks the termination of the lateral fissure on the brain.

Running forwards in front of the ear is the *zygomatic arch* which terminates anteriorly in the zygomatic bone and gives origin to the masseter muscle. Just above this arch is the *temporal fossa*, a depression in the skull which is filled by the temporalis muscle.

In examining this region, clench the teeth firmly and feel these powerful muscles of mastication—temporalis and masseter—stiffen and contract.

Above the zygomatic bone, along the lateral margin of the orbit, is the suture joining this bone to the frontal bone, indicated by an eminence known as the *zygomatic process* (fig. 235). A point 4 cm. behind this process and 4 cm. above the zygomatic arch marks the position of the middle meningeal artery and the stem of the lateral fissure on the brain.

Immediately behind the ear is the *mastoid process* of the temporal bone. This is not solid but contains numerous air cells, one of which, larger than the rest called the *mastoid antrum*, communicates with the middle ear cavity. The mastoid process is larger in the male than the female for it is produced by the pull of the sternomastoid muscle which is attached to it. Other and less familiar muscles attached to this process are the splenius capitis, longissimus capitis and the posterior belly of the digastric.

The *sternomastoid muscle* should be palpated throughout its course from below upwards. It is concerned with rotating the head and flexing it against resistance; thus if the hand be placed against the forehead and used to prevent flexion of the head, this muscle will be felt to contract firmly. The

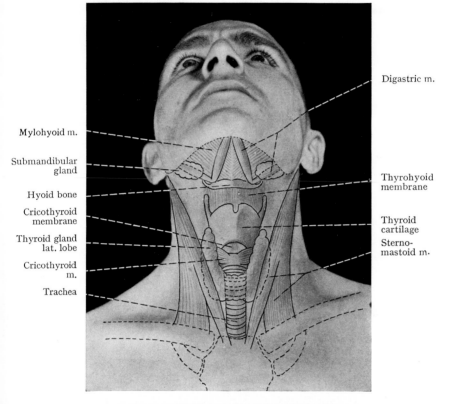

Mylohyoid m.

Submandibular gland

Hyoid bone

Cricothyroid membrane

Thyroid gland lat. lobe

Cricothyroid m.

Trachea

Digastric m.

Thyrohyoid membrane

Thyroid cartilage

Sterno-mastoid m.

FIG. 234.—The head and neck from the front.

sternomastoid overlies the carotid sheath, which contains the common carotid or internal carotid arteries, the internal jugular vein and the vagus nerve. If the fingers are inserted deeply beneath the anterior border of this muscle with the head slightly flexed, the artery will be felt to pulsate.

The sternomastoid muscle is the boundary between the anterior and posterior triangles of the neck. The former is bounded in front by the mid-line of the neck and the latter is bounded behind by the trapezius muscle.

In the anterior triangle are the structures which can be palpated in the mid-line of the neck, viz., the *laryngeal cartilages*, the *isthmus of the thyroid gland* and the cartilaginous rings of the *trachea*. The laryngeal cartilages

20—A.PH.

from above down are the *hyoid bone* at the base of the tongue, the *thyroid cartilage* (Adam's apple) and the *cricoid cartilage*. The upper part of the trachea lies in the neck and is crossed by the isthmus of the thyroid gland which is the connecting link between the two *lateral lobes of the gland*. These lobes can be palpated beneath the sternomastoid muscle.

In the posterior triangle there are some important nerves whose position should be marked on the living model. The middle of the posterior border of the sternomastoid marks their point of emergence (fig. 174) and here the

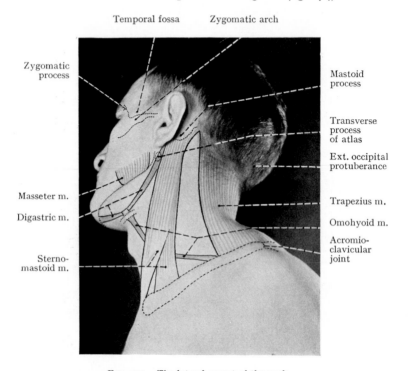

FIG. 235.—The lateral aspect of the neck.

accessory nerve passes downwards and backwards on the levator scapulae muscle to enter the trapezius. At this point also the *lesser occipital nerve* passes upwards and backwards to supply the skin of the scalp behind the ear; the **great auricular nerve**, upwards and forwards over the sternomastoid muscle to supply the skin in front of the ear; the *anterior cutaneous nerve* of the neck forwards over the sternomastoid to supply the skin of the neck; and the **supraclavicular nerves** downwards as three separate strands to supply the skin in the lower part of the neck and in the first intercostal space. Certain muscles in the floor of this triangle can be seen in certain circumstances, viz., the **scalenes** and **levator scapulae**.

A bony prominence worthy of notice can be palpated immediately below the lobe of the ear behind and above the angle of the jaw (fig. 235). It is the *transverse process of the atlas* and lying on it is the accessory nerve just before it descends behind the sternomastoid muscle.

The three salivary glands can be palpated: the *parotid gland* in front of the ear, the *submandibular gland* just below and in front of the angle of the jaw, and the *sublingual gland* from within the cavity of the mouth. The *duct of the parotid gland* is easy to locate when the teeth are firmly clenched. It can then be rolled over the anterior border of the contracted masseter muscle just beneath the zygomatic arch.

The upper border of the *sternum* should be palpated in the neck; it is marked by the suprasternal notch.

The Living Anatomy of the Thorax

The anterior part of the *first rib* can be palpated just below the inner end of the clavicle, the first intercostal space lies immediately below this and is

Supraclavicular fossa

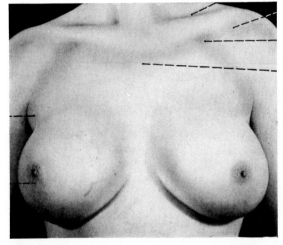

Deltoid m.

Deltopectoral triangle

Sternal angle

Axillary tail

Areola showing tubercles

FIG. 236.—The female virgin breasts of a girl aged 18 years.

bounded by the 2nd rib. The *second rib* is much more easily and extensively palpable than the first and is located at the *sternal angle*. This angle is prominently situated at the junction of the manubrium with the body, and so many things happen at this level that it is regarded as a landmark of great importance.

The sternal angle marks:
The level of the disc between vertebrae T/4 and T/5.
The division between the superior and inferior mediastinal cavities.
The bifurcation of the pulmonary artery.
The bifurcation of the trachea.
The termination of the aortic arch and the beginning of the descending aorta.

The position of the azygos vein as it arches over the root of the right lung. The position of the thoracic duct as it passes from right to left behind the oesophagus.

Where the pleura meets its fellow of the opposite side.

A prominent feature of the thorax is the presence of the *breast* or *mammary gland* (fig. 236). In the female after puberty it is usually a large pendulous organ extending from the 2nd to the 6th rib, and from the lateral margin of the sternum nearly to the axilla. It can be moved freely in all directions for it lies on the deep fascia covering the pectoralis major and serratus anterior muscles. A small but conspicuous part of the breast lies in the axilla beneath the deep fascia; this is known as the *axillary tail* and is easily located. The *nipple* lies in the 4th interspace but its position varies greatly if the breast is at all pendulous; it is not centrally situated but lies in the lower half of the organ. Around the nipple is the *areola*, a pigmented circular area upon which numerous small tubercles marking the openings of the ducts of sebaceous glands are seen. These glands secrete a lubricant which keeps the nipple supple.

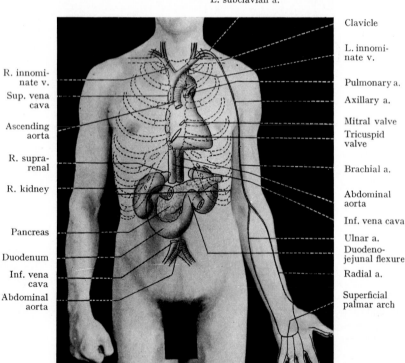

FIG. 237.—Heart and great vessels. Duodenum, pancreas, kidneys, etc.

The position of the *heart* should be marked on the chest.   A considerable part of this organ lies behind the sternum.   The apex beat should first be located; it lies in the fifth interspace 8 cm. from the mid-sternal line and can be felt pulsating about 1·5 cm. inside the nipple line.   The upper border of the heart is located by drawing a line from the lower border of the 2nd left costal cartilage 2·5 cm. from the mid-line to the upper border of the 3rd right costal cartilage 2·5 cm. from the mid-line.   The right border is indicated by a line from the 3rd right costal cartilage to the 6th right costal cartilage slightly convex to the right.   If now the apex beat be joined to this point on the 6th right costal cartilage and to the original point on the 2nd left costal cartilage the position of the heart in relation to the thoracic wall will be indicated.

The lines of *pleural reflection* (fig. 238) are located as follows: a point is taken 4 cm. above the centre of the clavicle, behind the sternomastoid muscle indicating the upper limit of the apex of the lung.   From here the position of the pleura is indicated by a line which crosses the sternoclavicular joint obliquely and meets its fellow of the opposite side behind the sternal

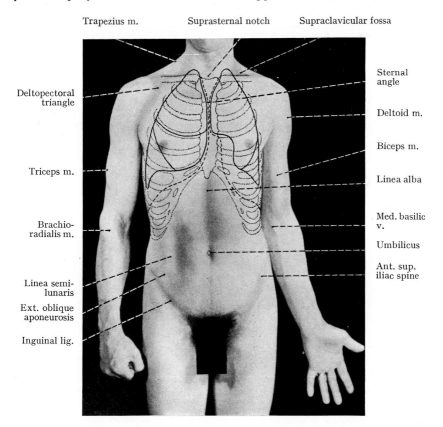

FIG. 238.—The lines of pleural reflection, the anterior abdominal wall, etc.

angle in the mid-line. From this level the two pleural sacs lie adjacent to each other as far as the 4th costal cartilage. Here the left pleura sweeps to the left for about 4 cm. exposing the pericardium to the chest wall. The lower boundary of the pleural sac lies at the level 'of the 8th rib in the nipple line, the 10th rib in the mid-axillary line, the 11th rib in the mid-scapular line and the 12th rib at the lateral margin of the sacrospinalis muscle.

In mapping out the *lungs* similar landmarks are taken, but the lower boundary of the lungs does not extend as far down as the pleura and the figures 6, 8, 10, 10 should be substituted for the figures 8, 10, 11, 12 given for the lower margin of the pleura.

The position of the *aortic arch* (fig. 237) in relation to the thoracic wall should be noted. The ascending aorta starts at the level of the 3rd left costal cartilage near the sternal margin and ascends obliquely for about 2 in. to the 2nd right costal cartilage. It then arches backwards to the left over the pulmonary artery and the left bronchus and in front of the trachea. It ends on the posterior thoracic wall in the plane of Louis at the level of the disc between the 4th and 5th thoracic vertebrae. The upper border of the arch from which the great vessels emerge lies about 2·5 cm. below the suprasternal notch.

Living Anatomy of the Abdomen

For descriptive purposes the abdomen is divided into nine zones as follows: a line is drawn across the body through a point midway between the suprasternal notch and the upper border of the symphysis pubis. This is known as the *transpyloric plane* since it bisects the pylorus of the stomach. A further line is drawn across the body level with the tubercle on the iliac crest and is called the *transtubercular plane*. This plane lies at the level of the superior border of the 5th lumbar vertebra. Two vertical lines are then drawn upwards from points midway between the mid-line and the anterior superior iliac spine. The zones thus mapped out are called the *right* and *left hypochondriac*, the *epigastric*, the *right* and *left lumbar*, the *umbilical*, the *right* and *left iliac* and the *hypogastric regions* (fig. 239). The *transpyloric plane* (of Addison) is particularly useful. It marks the level of the lower border of the 1st lumbar vertebra and thus the lowest limit of the spinal cord. The pylorus of the stomach lies at this level as does the fundus of the gall bladder, the 9th costal cartilage and the hilum of the left kidney. The portal vein originates on this plane.

The *umbilicus* in the normal individual lies at the level of the disc between the 3rd and 4th lumbar vertebrae, but as age advances and the abdomen tends to become pendulous it lies below this level.

The *rectus abdominis* muscle is very clearly seen and its boundaries are accentuated if the head is raised when the body is in the supine position. The lateral border of the rectus is easily demonstrable, as is the medial border forming the *linea alba* with the umbilicus situated rather below its centre. It should be noted that these muscles diverge as they ascend, thus the gap between them is much wider above than below. Evidence of the *tendinous intersections* formed by adhesions between the muscle and the front wall of the sheath can sometimes be seen in the living subject.

The *anterior superior iliac spines* are easily palpable and in most subjects the *iliac crests* can be followed along their whole length. The crest ends at the posterior superior spine, the position of which is conveniently indicated by a dimple which marks the position of the 2nd sacral vertebra and the centre of the sacro-iliac joint.

The *iliac tubercle*, a prominence on the iliac crest about 6 cm. behind the anterior superior spine, is a useful landmark.

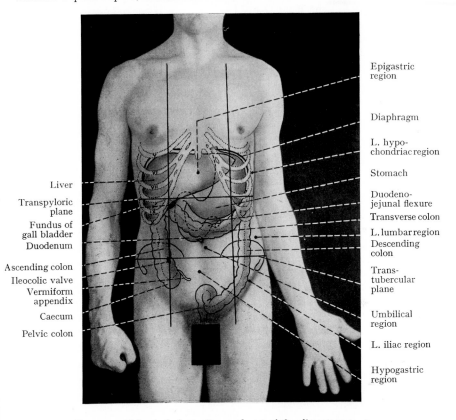

Epigastric region

Diaphragm

L. hypo-chondriac region

Stomach

Liver

Duodeno-jejunal flexure

Transpyloric plane

Transverse colon

Fundus of gall bladder

L. lumbar region

Duodenum

Descending colon

Ascending colon

Ileocolic valve

Trans-tubercular plane

Vermiform appendix

Caecum

Umbilical region

Pelvic colon

L. iliac region

Hypogastric region

FIG. 239.—Abdominal planes, liver and part of the alimentary tract.

The *inguinal ligament* should be palpated throughout its course. It commences at the anterior superior spine and ends at the pubic tubercle which forms the outer boundary of the pubic crest.

Just above the inner end of the inguinal ligament is the *superficial inguinal ring*—an opening large enough in the male to admit the tip of the index finger but rather smaller in the female. In the male it transmits the spermatic cord, in the female the round ligament of the uterus and in both sexes an inguinal hernia (rupture) may pass through this opening.

The *caecum* and *appendix* lie in the right iliac fossa just above the middle of the inguinal ligament.

The kidneys lie on the posterior abdominal wall and can be mapped out by drawing *Morris's parallelogram* on the posterior aspect of the trunk (fig. 240). Two horizontal lines are drawn, one at the level of the 11th thoracic vertebra and the other at the level of the 3rd lumbar vertebra, and two vertical lines are drawn 2·5 cm. and 9 cm. from the mid-line. If the kidneys are to be mapped out from the front it should be remembered that the hilum lies in the transpyloric plane about 2·5 cm. medial to the 9th costal cartilage. Thus, if the size of the kidney be borne in mind (12 cm. long), it is easy to map out its position with reasonable accuracy.

The *abdominal aorta* lying on the posterior abdominal wall can be felt to pulsate in thin subjects when the abdomen is palpated between the two recti muscles above the umbilicus. The vessel ends 1·5 cm. below the umbilicus by dividing into the two common iliac arteries.

The *liver* (fig. 239) can be mapped out by taking a point in the 5th intercostal space on the left side, 9 cm. from the mid-line—this corresponds to the apex beat of the heart but only the thin central tendon of the diaphragm separates heart from liver in this area—and by drawing a line from this point to the 9th right costal cartilage, and then following the costal margin. The upper border of the liver runs to the right forming a slightly upward convexity and at the back of the trunk it lies about 1·5 cm. below the inferior angle of the right scapula when the arm is in contact with the side of the body.

The *fundus of the gall bladder* (fig. 239) can be accurately located at the point where the lateral border of the right rectus muscle crosses the 9th costal cartilage.

The *spleen* lies deeply in the left hypochondrium. Its anterior border does not normally extend beyond the mid-axillary line. It lies obliquely and is separated by the diaphragm from the 9th, 10th and 11th ribs, its long axis corresponding to the long axis of the 10th rib (fig. 222).

At the end of a normal inspiration the right dome of the *diaphragm* corresponds to the 4th intercostal space and the left dome to the 5th rib anteriorly. The diaphragm is highest when the patient is in the recumbent position, is lower when standing and is lower still when sitting. This fact emphasises the importance of keeping the patient in "the Fowler position" in all cases where breathing is laboured.

Living Anatomy of the Upper Extremity

The bony points around the shoulder region should be located.

The *clavicle* can be palpated throughout its entire extent. Its inner two-thirds are round and convex forwards, its outer third is flat and concave forwards. The positions of the *sternoclavicular* and *acromioclavicular joints* should be located (fig. 235).

Beneath the outer third of the clavicle there is a triangular depression, bounded by the pectoralis major and the deltoid called the *deltopectoral triangle* (fig. 236). Its floor is formed by the *clavipectoral fascia*, which is pierced in this region by the cephalic vein, the acromiothoracic vessels and the lateral pectoral nerve. In the lateral angle of this triangle there is a bony projection lying under cover of the deltoid muscle. This is the *coracoid process* of the scapula and should be located, as it is a landmark of some importance. Lateral to this, the *head of the humerus* can be felt. This is overhung by the *acromion* of the scapula which is subcutaneous throughout its extent and easily located. The acromion is the lateral extremity of the spine of the scapula. Certain other parts of the scapula will be palpated without difficulty, especially the *inferior angle* and the student should not fail to notice the movement of the bones of the shoulder girdle when the arm is rotated above the head.

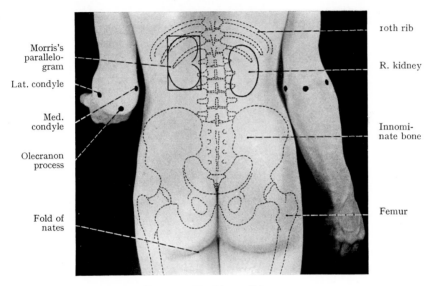

Fig. 240.—Morris's parallelogram.

To examine the *axilla* the forearm should be supported and the pectoral muscles relaxed. The anterior axillary wall should be taken between the finger and thumb and the student should realise that he is holding the *pectoralis major* chiefly and to a lesser extent the *pectoralis minor*, a much smaller muscle lying deep to the major. Similarly, the posterior wall should be palpated with the flat of the hand and the muscles which present themselves for examination in that region are the *subscapularis* high up beneath the scapula, the *teres major* and *latissimus dorsi*. The medial wall presents the upper ribs covered by the *serratus anterior*, the serrations of which can be seen in a muscular subject. The lateral wall presents the *biceps* and *coracobrachialis*. High up in the axilla the *axillary artery* may be felt pulsating. Surrounding the artery are the cords of the brachial plexus. Also in the axilla there are numerous lymph nodes embedded in a quantity of fat. These nodes become involved in carcinoma (cancer) of the breast and not infrequently in septic conditions of the upper limb.

The bony points at the elbow should next be examined (fig. 240). The *medial* and *lateral condyles* of the humerus and the *olecranon process* of the ulna are easily defined. Note that they normally lie in the same straight line when the forearm is extended and that these three points form the boundaries of an equilateral triangle when the forearm is flexed.

The *cubital fossa* can be seen and felt. Palpate the *brachioradialis* forming its lateral boundary and the *pronator teres* forming its medial boundary. The *tendon of the biceps* can be located without difficulty in the fossa (fig. 241)

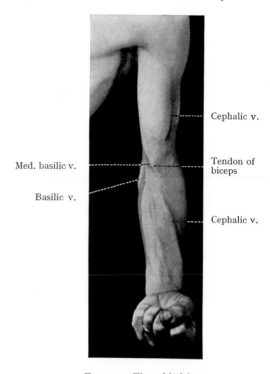

Cephalic v.

Med. basilic v.

Tendon of biceps

Basilic v.

Cephalic v.

Fig. 241.—The cubital fossa.

and on its medial aspect a further tendinous slip may be felt when the forearm is flexed—it is the *bicipital aponeurosis* which leaves the muscle to join the fascia of the forearm. Beneath this slip of fascia the *brachial artery* may be felt to pulsate and this vessel is also palpable in the middle of the arm as it lies on the medial aspect of the biceps (fig. 237).

In the roof of the fossa two veins are seen. They are the *median cephalic* and *median basilic veins,* the former ascending into the arm on the lateral aspect and the latter on the medial aspect of the biceps muscle.

In the lateral aspect of the fossa beneath the medial border of the brachio-radialis the *head of the radius* can be palpated and if the forearm be rotated, its precise position can be verified easily.

The *ulnar nerve* should be rolled beneath the finger as it lies behind the

Ext. poll. longus
tendon

Styloid process
of radius

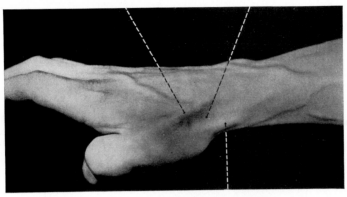

Abd. poll. longus and ext.
poll. brevis tendons

FIG. 242.—The anatomical snuff-box.

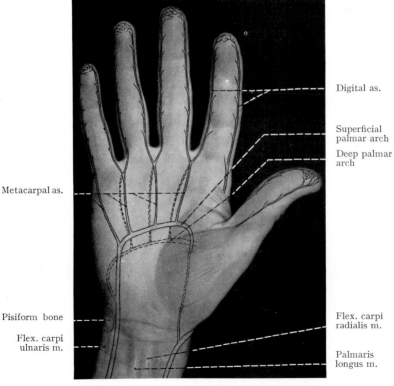

Digital as.

Superficial
palmar arch

Deep palmar
arch

Metacarpal as.

Pisiform bone

Flex. carpi
ulnaris m.

Flex. carpi
radialis m.

Palmaris
longus m.

FIG. 243.—The wrist and hand, showing superficial and deep palmar arches
and their branches.

303

medial condyle of the humerus (fig. 55). It feels like a rounded cord, and when compressed is likely to produce sensations (pins and needles) which will be felt on the inner aspect of the hand.

On the front of the medial condyle is a solitary but important lymph node, called the *supratrochlear lymph node* (fig. 202) scarcely palpable under normal circumstances but likely to enlarge from septic infections on the inner side of the hand.

The *styloid processes* of the radius and ulna should be palpated at the wrist. It should be noted that the styloid process of the radius lies 1·5 cm. distal to that of the ulna. The relative position of these two prominent points will be altered in fractures of the lower end of the forearm. This, therefore, is one of the crucial tests in a suspected case of Colles' fracture.

The *pisiform bone* is readily found on the medial aspect of the wrist between the two transverse creases and the *hook of the hamate* lies a finger's breadth distal and lateral to the pisiform but will be felt only on deep palpation. The *triquetral bone* is prominent on the dorsum of the wrist immediately distal to the styloid process of the ulna.

The *anatomical snuff-box* (fig. 242) lies on the lateral aspect of the wrist, below the styloid process of the radius. It is bounded *laterally* by the tendons of abductor pollicis longus and extensor pollicis brevis; *medially* by the tendon of extensor pollicis longus. In its *roof* is a branch of the radial nerve and the commencement of the cephalic vein; in its *floor* are the radial styloid process; the most lateral of the carpal bones, viz., the scaphoid and trapezium and the lateral ligament of the wrist joint. *Within the snuff-box* is the radial artery as it winds round the wrist to reach the dorsum of the hand.

The structures which can be located on the front of the wrist should be verified. The most conspicuous is the tendon of *flexor carpi radialis*. Medial to this the tendon of *palmaris longus* may be present overlying the *median nerve*. Medial to this a swelling will be seen when the wrist and fingers are flexed; this is the *flexor digitorum sublimis* muscle and on its medial aspect is the *flexor carpi ulnaris*.

The *proximal transverse crease at the wrist* corresponds to the level of the wrist joint, the *distal crease* corresponds to the proximal border of the flexor retinaculum.

On the back of the wrist, the radial *tubercle* can be felt at the lower border of the radius and it should be realised that this tubercle separates the tendon of *extensor pollicis longus* medially from those of *extensores carpi radialis longus et brevis* laterally.

The *superficial palmar arch* (fig. 243) is situated centrally and does not extend beyond a line drawn across the palm at the level of the fully abducted thumb. The *deep palmar arch* lies 1·5 cm. proximal to this.

It should be noted that the *metacarpophalangeal joints* lie approximately at the level of the distal palmar transverse crease and not at the level of the proximal crease of the fingers.

The *interphalangeal joints* correspond with the middle and distal finger creases.

The *knuckles* are formed by the heads of the metacarpal bones.

Living Anatomy of the Lower Limb

The position of the *greater trochanter* on the lateral aspect of the thigh can be verified by flexing and extending the hip joint.

The *ischial tuberosity* can be felt in the region of the buttock. In the standing position it is covered by the gluteus maximus, but in the sitting position it is covered only by a bursa and a pad of fat.

If a line be drawn from the anterior superior iliac spine to the ischial tuberosity it crosses the superior border of the greater trochanter of the femur. This is known as *Nélaton's line* (fig. 244), and is of great importance in determining pathological conditions of the hip joint.

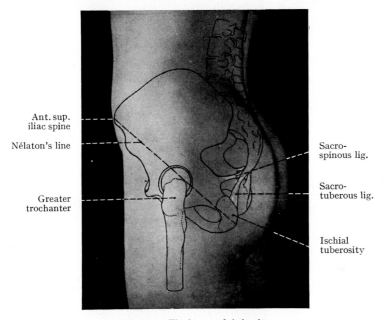

Ant. sup.
iliac spine

Nélaton's line

Greater
trochanter

Sacro-
spinous lig.

Sacro-
tuberous lig.

Ischial
tuberosity

FIG. 244.—The bony pelvis in situ.

There is normally a well-marked depression above and behind the greater trochanter.

The fold of the nates (fig. 240) does not correspond with the lower border of the gluteus maximus.

The Femoral Triangle lies immediately below the inguinal ligament on the upper part of the medial aspect of the thigh. It can be felt as a well-marked depression in this region and when the thigh is flexed, abducted and laterally rotated, its boundaries are readily seen. The *base* formed by the inguinal ligament, the *lateral boundary* by the sartorius and the *medial boundary* by the adductor longus should be verified. The *apex* leads into the subsartorial canal.

The *femoral artery* can be felt pulsating within the triangle near the centre of the inguinal ligament, the *femoral nerve* lies immediately lateral and the *femoral vein* immediately medial to the artery.   In the *roof* of the triangle are the important *inguinal lymph nodes* and the *saphenous opening*.

The *sartorius muscle* should be palpated as it descends obliquely from the anterior superior iliac spine to the medial aspect of the leg.   To demonstrate this muscle the thigh should be abducted, flexed and laterally rotated.

The *tendon of adductor longus* is an important landmark which should be located.   It forms the extreme medial boundary of the upper part of the thigh and can be palpated just below the groin as a rounded cord when the lower limb is abducted.   This tendon when traced upwards leads to the *pubic tubercle*, a landmark which is of paramount importance in defining a

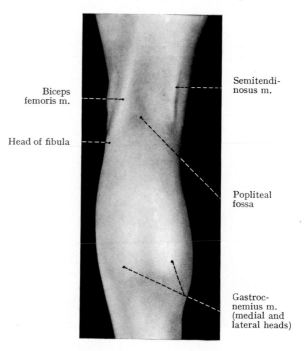

Biceps
femoris m.

Head of fibula

Semitendi-
nosus m.

Popliteal
fossa

Gastroc-
nemius m.
(medial and
lateral heads)

FIG. 245—Popliteal fossa (left side).

hernia, since the *superficial inguinal ring* lies above and medial to the tubercle and the *saphenous opening* 4 cm. below and lateral to the tubercle.   It follows, therefore, that when the neck of a hernial sac presents on the superomedial aspect of the pubic tubercle, it is of the inguinal type and a hernia which appears on the infcrolateral aspect of the tubercle is of the femoral type.

This important information is dependent upon the correct location of the pubic tubercle which in turn is dependent upon the correct location of the adductor longus tendon.

The subsartorial canal lies on the medial aspect of the middle third of the thigh deep to the sartorius muscle.   Its *lateral boundary* is formed by vastus medialis and its *posteromedial boundary* by adductors longus and magnus. Lying deeply within the canal are the *femoral vessels* and the saphenous nerve. This canal is continuous above with the apex of the femoral triangle and below with the opening in the adductor magnus which leads into the popliteal fossa.

The popliteal fossa at the back of the knee is a diamond-shaped space containing the *popliteal vessels*, some important *lymph nodes* and the terminal branches of the sciatic nerve, viz., the *medial* and *lateral popliteal nerves*.

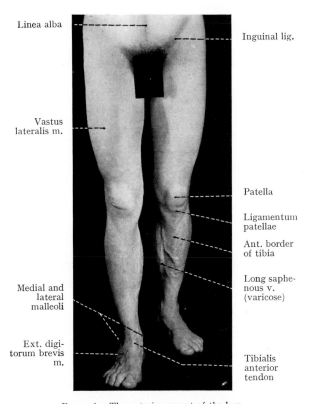

Linea alba

Inguinal lig.

Vastus
lateralis m.

Patella

Ligamentum
patellae

Ant. border
of tibia

Long saphe-
nous v.
(varicose)

Medial and
lateral
malleoli

Ext. digi-
torum brevis
m.

Tibialis
anterior
tendon

FIG. 246.—The anterior aspect of the legs.

The tendons which bound the upper part of this space can be located without difficulty: *laterally* the tendon of biceps can be felt as it passes to the head of the fibula and *medially* the tendons of semimembranosus and semitendinosus. On the medial aspect of the biceps tendon the lateral popliteal nerve can be rolled beneath the examining finger.

The *short saphenous vein* may be seen in the roof of the fossa as it passes to join the popliteal vein. The medial popliteal nerve occupies a central position in the fossa but cannot be palpated since it lies beneath the deep fascia.

The two heads of gastrocnemius can be seen in the lower part of the fossa.

On the lateral aspect of the thigh, extending almost from hip to knee is the *iliotibial tract* of the fascia lata. It will be felt to contract when the leg is extended and abducted.

On the front of the knee, the *patella* and *ligamentum patellae* should be palpated. On the lateral aspect of the upper part of the leg the *head of the fibula* can be felt, and just below this the *lateral popliteal nerve* should be rolled beneath the examining finger as it passes over the bone. The nerve is exposed in this position and is, therefore, liable to injury in this region.

The *adductor tubercle*, surmounting the medial condyle of the femur and the tendon of the hamstring portion of adductor magnus passing into it should be located.

In the leg the medial surface and anterior border of the *tibia*, covered only by skin and fascia and constituting the shin, is easily palpated. The *two*

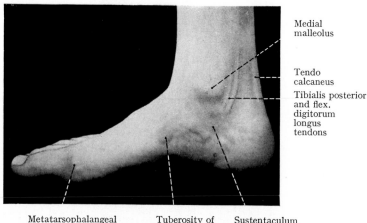

Medial
malleolus

Tendo
calcaneus

Tibialis posterior
and flex.
digitorum
longus
tendons

Metatarsophalangeal   Tuberosity of   Sustentaculum
joint of great toe   navicular bone   tali

FIG. 247.—The medial aspect of the right foot.

heads of the *gastrocnemius* muscle stand out posteriorly when the foot is plantarflexed. The head of the fibula and the lateral popliteal nerve on the lateral aspect of the upper part of the leg have already been mentioned.

In the region of the ankle many structures can be palpated. First, the *medial* and *lateral malleoli*, the former formed by the distal end of the tibia and the latter by the distal end of the fibula. It should be noted that the lateral malleolus extends about 1·5 cm. below the medial malleolus (cf. styloid process of radius and ulna). This is a point of great diagnostic importance in fractures in the region of the ankle joint. (Pott's fracture.)

Behind the medial malleolus are the tendons of *tibialis posterior* and *flexor digitorum longus*, while the *posterior tibial vessels* which run behind the latter tendon can sometimes be felt pulsating midway between the medial malleolus and the heel. The tendon of *flexor hallucis longus* which lies behind all these structures is too deeply situated to be palpated.

On the front of the ankle the tendon of *tibialis anterior* can be seen to stand out when the foot is dorsi-flexed and inverted; the tendon of *extensor hallucis longus* lying lateral to it will come into view when the big toe is extended; next to this are the tendons of *extensor digitorum longus* and *peroneus tertius*. The *anterior tibial vessels* and *nerve* are situated between the tendons of extensor hallucis and extensor digitorum longus, midway between the two malleoli on the front of the ankle.

Behind the lateral malleolus are the tendons of *peroneus brevis* and *peroneus longus* in that order from before back.

The *calcaneum* forming the prominence of the heel is obvious and the tendo-calcaneus can readily be traced passing into it.

The ankle joint is on a plane 1·5 cm. above the tip of the medial malleolus.

On the dorsum of the foot many prominent features are readily verified for the structures here are all subcutaneous.

When the foot is inverted a hard bony swelling is seen and felt just below and 2·5 cm. in front of the lateral malleolus. This is the anterolateral extremity of the *calcaneum* (fig. 249). Medial to this is the *extensor digitorum brevis* muscle which is felt as a rounded soft swelling and medial to the muscle a further bony prominence, the *talus*.

The tendons of extensor digitorum brevis can be determined more readily when the toes are extended. On the lateral aspect of the calcaneum about 2·5 cm. below and 1·5 cm. in front of the distal end of the lateral malleolus is the *peroneal tubercle*, a structure which varies in size in different individuals. Above this tubercle is the tendon of *peroneus brevis* as it passes forwards to the base of the 5th metatarsal bone and below the tubercle is the tendon of *peroneus longus* which is passing to the groove on the plantar surface of the cuboid.

The *base of the 5th metatarsal* bone is especially prominent, and between this bony point and the calcaneum is the *cuboid* bone with the tendon of peroneus longus winding round the middle of its outer border.

On the medial aspect of the foot is the important shelf of bone on which the talus rests, called the *sustentaculum tali*. It lies immediately below the medial malleolus and is in relation with three important tendons, viz., the *tibialis posterior* which lies immediately above it, the *flexor digitorum longus* which is directly in contact with it and the *flexor hallucis longus* which lies directly below it (fig. 110).

The more prominent and no less important *tuberosity* of the *navicular bone* lies on the medial border of the foot in front of the sustentaculum tali. This prominence is formed by the pull of the *tibialis posterior* tendon which is inserted into it.

In front of this prominence is the tendon of *tibialis anterior* passing to the medial cuneiform and to the base of the first metatarsal bone.

The *dorsal interosseous muscles* can be palpated between the metatarsal bones.

A line drawn transversely across the foot immediately behind the tuberosity of the navicular bone indicates the position of the *transverse tarsal joint*.

On the plantar surface of the foot the structures are too well covered to be palpable.

The Femoral Artery can be indicated as follows: with the thigh flexed, abducted and laterally rotated the upper two-thirds of a line from the

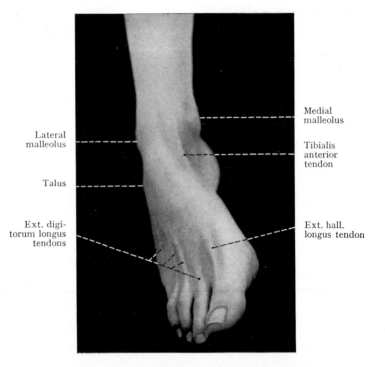

Medial
malleolus

Lateral
malleolus

Tibialis
anterior
tendon

Talus

Ext. digi-
torum longus
tendons

Ext. hall.
longus tendon

Fig. 248.—The dorsum of the foot.

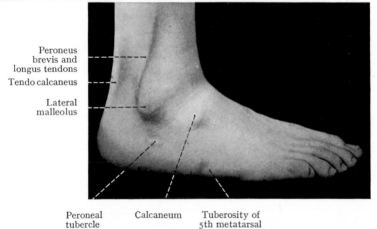

Peroneus
brevis and
longus tendons

Tendo calcaneus

Lateral
malleolus

Peroneal   Calcaneum   Tuberosity of
tubercle   5th metatarsal

Fig. 249.—The lateral aspect of the right foot.

middle of the inguinal ligament to the medial condyle of the femur marks the course of the vessel.

The Popliteal Artery is indicated by a line drawn through the centre of the popliteal fossa. It bifurcates at the lower border of the poplite muscle into anterior and posterior tibial arteries.

The Anterior Tibial Artery is indicated by an oblique line running from a point midway between the head of the fibula and the lateral condyle of the tibia to a point midway between the two malleoli. From here it is continued on to the medial aspect of the dorsum of the foot as the dorsalis pedis artery.

The Posterior Tibial Artery is indicated by a line drawn from the lower border of the popliteus muscle, running obliquely to a point midway between the medial malleolus and the heel, where it divides into medial and lateral plantar arteries.

The superficial veins of the lower extremity originate from a plexus on the dorsum of the foot (fig. 200). From this the *long saphenous vein* ascends in front of the medial malleolus on the inner side of the leg and then passing behind the medial condyle of the femur ascends on the medial aspect of the thigh to end at the saphenous opening where it joins the femoral vein. This vein, as has already been noted, is particularly liable to become varicose. The *short saphenous vein* ascends behind the lateral malleolus and then on the back of the calf of the leg to the popliteal fossa, where it perforates the deep fascia in the roof of that space and joins the popliteal vein.

CHAPTER XI

LEVERS AND LEVERAGE

_____ a device by which force may be applied to greater advantage, and is, therefore, an economiser of power. The mechanical advantage gained by levers is known as leverage.

A lever is a rigid bar which can move at a certain point. The point at which the movement takes place is called the _fulcrum_. The part to be moved is called the _weight_, and the force which performs the work is known as the _power_.

Levers are classified into three groups according to the relative positions of the fulcrum, the weight and the power.

The Three Orders of Levers

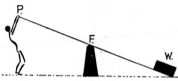

FIG. 250.—First order, See-saw.

In a lever of the first order the fulcrum is between the power and the weight (fig. 250).

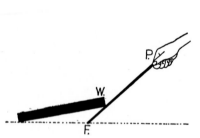
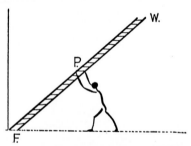

FIG. 251.—Second order, Prising up a weight.   FIG. 252.—Third order, Raising a ladder.

In the second order the weight is between the power and the fulcrum (fig. 251).

In the third order the power is applied between the weight and the fulcrum (fig. 252).

Levers of the Human Body

Mechanical movement in the human body is brought about by means of living leverage. The bones act as levers through which the power of the muscles is used. The joint at which the bony levers meet is the fulcrum and movement takes place as the result of muscle action.

The type of movement and range of movement depend on \
of the joint and the type of muscle acting on it. Where sm. \
required the muscles are short and thick. Where large range is \
the muscles are longer. Muscles act upon the levers of the body, \
shortening (concentric contraction) or in lengthening (eccentric contr.

All three types of levers are found in the human body and it is by ....se
means that the muscles are able to perform the movements of the body.

A lever of the first order. In this the fulcrum, or joint, lies between
the weight to be moved and the power or muscles which move it. This type
of lever is found where stability or poise are required. For example, the
poise of the head on the atlas. Here the fulcrum is the atlanto-occipital
joint, the weight is that part of the head in front of the joint and the power
the post-vertebral muscles attached to the occiput (fig. 253).

A second example may be found in full plantarflexion of the ankle. The
ankle joint is the fulcrum where the movement takes place, situated between

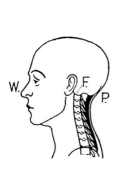

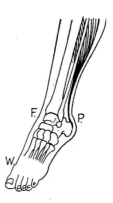

FIG. 253   FIG. 254.

the weight to be moved which is the foot and the power which is supplied
by the calf muscles inserted into the calcaneum (fig. 254).

A lever of the second order. Here the weight is found between the
joint (fulcrum) and the muscle (power). This type is not common in the
human body; its value is that it is designed more for power than for speed.
For example the foot acts as a lever of the second order in walking or in
standing on the toes with heels raised. The heads of the metatarsal bones
on the ground act as the fulcrum. The weight of the body is transmitted
through the tarsus and the calf muscles provide the power (fig. 255).

A second example is flexion of the forearm by brachioradialis. Here
the weight is represented by the forearm, the fulcrum by the elbow joint and
the power is applied at the insertion of brachioradialis at the styloid process
of the radius (fig. 256).

A lever of the third order. This is the most common type of lever
found in the human body, it is designed for speed of action. Here the
power (muscle) is applied to the lever (bone) between the fulcrum (joint)

and the weight to be moved.　A simple example is found in flexion of the forearm by brachialis and biceps.　The elbow joint is the fulcrum, the weight is the forearm and hand and the power is supplied by the chief flexors of the

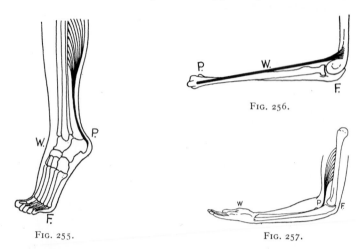

Fig. 256.

Fig. 255.　　　　　　　　　　　　　Fig. 257.

elbow inserted into the bones of the forearm between the fulcrum and the weight (fig. 257).

Because the insertion of the muscles, that is the application of power, is so close to the fulcrum or centre of movement speed is allowed for rather than strength.　If, however, the relative fixation of the attachments of the brachialis are reversed and the muscle works from a fixed forearm, as in the

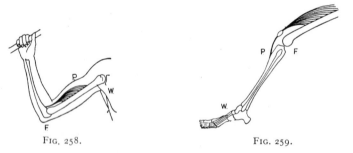

Fig. 258.　　　　　　　　　　　　　Fig. 259.

case of climbing a rope and drawing up the weight of the body towards the hands, the power is greatly increased but the speed of movement reduced. This alteration is due to the extent of the attachment of brachialis on the shaft of the humerus and its distance from the fulcrum.　Note that the type of lever has not changed, the power is still between the weight and the fulcrum, only the distance between the fulcrum and power has been altered (fig. 258).

A second example of a lever of the third order is found in extension of the knee by the quadriceps muscles.　The fulcrum is the knee joint, the weight

is the lower leg and foot and the power is applied at th
the ligamentum patellae (fig. 259).

Some points on the application of power
The more the line of pull of a muscle approaches a right
is the power of leverage, e.g., the power of brachialis is gr

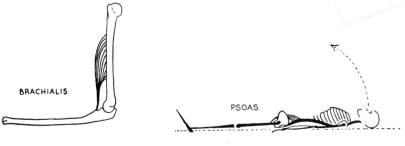

BRACHIALIS.   PSOAS.

FIG. 260.   FIG. 261.

elbow is flexed to a right angle (fig. 260).   Conversely the more parallel the
line of pull of a muscle is to the long axis of the bone or lever upon which it
works, the weaker is its power of leverage, e.g., it is difficult to raise the trunk
from the supine position because psoas is very nearly parallel with its femoral
attachment (fig. 261).

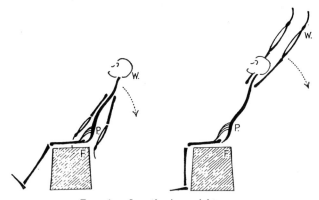

FIG. 262.—Lengthening weight arm.

The part of a lever between the fulcrum and the power is called the *power
arm,* that between the fulcrum and the weight is known as the *weight arm.*
The longer the power arm, the easier the movement and, therefore, less effort
is required to do it.   The longer the weight arm, the more difficult the movement and, therefore, greater effort is needed.   In levers of the second order
the power arm is longer than the weight arm, and because of this mechanical
advantage little force is required to overcome resistance.   In the third order,

ver, the weight arm is longer than the power arm, and because of this mechanical disadvantage greater effort must be exerted to overcome resistance but greater range and rapidity of movement are the result.

In certain movements the weight arm may be lengthened, thus making the movement more difficult, e.g., sitting, trunk falling backward from the hip joints is much more difficult if the arms are stretched above the head than if they are down at the sides (fig. 262).

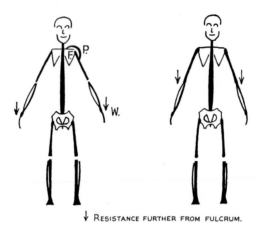

↓ Resistance further from fulcrum.

Fig. 263.

Movements may also be made more difficult by applying resistance to the weight arm, farther and farther away from the moving joint or fulcrum, e.g., arm raising sideways to the horizontal is more difficult if resistance is applied at the hands or wrists than if applied half-way up the arm (fig. 263).

CHAPTER XII

MUSCLES IN ACTION

The three essential physical properties of a muscle are:

(a) Contractility.
(b) Extensibility.
(c) Elasticity.

These three properties not only exist in a muscle at work but are also present in a muscle at rest.

(a) *Contractility.* Skeletal muscles, even when not engaged in performing a movement, are maintained in a state of slight contraction, which is spoken of as *muscle tone*. This *muscle tone* is reflex in character. The muscles are stretched between their attachments and the reflex is initiated by the constant stimulus of this stretch applied to the muscle spindles.

All healthy voluntary muscles show this tone to some degree, but it is greater in the "anti-gravity muscles," i.e., those which maintain the erect posture against the force of gravity, viz. the extensor groups of the lower limbs, the trunk and the head. Tone in these muscles is necessary for the maintenance of balance, for by this means "the body weight is kept within the bony axis" (Lake). Muscle tone may also be described as a state of preparedness of muscle tissue to respond to a call to action, i.e., poor tone produces poor response.

(b) *Extensibility* and (c) *Elasticity*.

A muscle may be compared to a piece of elastic, in that it can be extended by tension and recoils when released. Unlike elastic, it is not, however, uniformly extensible for increasing tension stretches it less and less.

An unexpected finding is that the extensibility of a muscle is actually increased by contraction. That is to say, a given weight stretches a contracted muscle more than it does the same muscle when uncontracted. This is known as *Weber's Paradox* and is an important property, because it reduces the liability of a muscle to be torn from its attachments if contracted suddenly. This property decreases with age.

The muscle is safeguarded still further in this respect by the *lengthening reaction* which depends upon the nervous system. Whenever the tension in a muscle becomes too great, further contraction becomes impossible and it may in fact relax.

The extensibility of a muscle is not to be confused with the *relaxation* of tone in a muscle. As already noted, all muscles at rest are in a state of partial contraction or tonus. During the contraction of any muscle or group of muscles the tone of the opposing group or antagonist is reduced through the automatic action of the nervous system, which brings about an appropriate relaxation. This process is known as *reciprocal inhibition*.

317

Types of Muscle Work

Muscles are described as working in the following ways:

(*a*) Concentrically.
(*b*) Eccentrically.
(*c*) Statically.

(*a*) *Concentric work.* This occurs when the origin and insertion approach each other. Usually the insertion approaches the origin as the latter is the

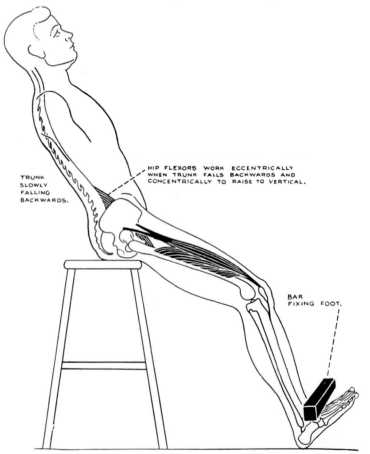

TRUNK SLOWLY FALLING BACKWARDS.

HIP FLEXORS WORK ECCENTRICALLY WHEN TRUNK FALLS BACKWARDS AND CONCENTRICALLY TO RAISE TO VERTICAL.

BAR FIXING FOOT.

Fig. 264.—Trunk falling backwards, illustrating the eccentric work of the hip flexors.

more fixed, but the position may be reversed under some circumstances, e.g., latissimus dorsi adducts the shoulder joint by drawing the arm towards the body, but if the arms are fixed, as in hanging by the arms, latissimus helps to draw the trunk upwards. During concentric work the muscle becomes shorter and thicker in appearance and feels harder.

(*b*) *Eccentric work.* This occurs when a muscle is in action, but the attachments are being drawn farther apart, either by gravity or some outside force (human or mechanical) and the muscle becomes longer and thinner but still feels hard because it is working. In other words it is lengthening by gradually "letting go" to the more powerful outside force, e.g., when sitting with feet fixed and bending the trunk slowly backwards at the hip joints, the hip flexors are lowering the trunk backwards against the force of gravity and are, therefore, lengthening or working eccentrically (fig. 264). (To raise the trunk again to the vertical they would work in shortening or concentrically.)

(*c*) *Static work.* This occurs when a muscle or group of muscles works to hold a given position. No actual movement takes place, although the muscle is definitely in action, e.g., to hold the arm horizontally (as a policeman on point duty), the abductors of the shoulder have to work statically, for gravity is tending to pull the arm to the side.

Static work is considered to be the most tiring of all forms of muscle work. Fatigue products collect, because the circulation is not so rapid as in a more active muscle.

Eccentric work is considered easier muscularly than concentric, and is, therefore, used to re-educate paralysed muscle. It also requires much more concentration, and is useful in making the patient think.

Range of Muscle Work (figs. 265 and 266)

Muscles may work in different ranges (fig. 265).

Full or Whole Range. This is the path traversed by a muscle when it contracts from its greatest possible lengthening, to its greatest possible shortening.

This distance may be divided into inner and outer range, or into thirds.

Outer range is the distance between greatest possible lengthening and the mid-point of full range.

Inner range is the distance between the mid-point of full range and greatest possible shortening.

It is also possible to divide the full range into outer, middle and inner thirds. These divisions are most used when measuring recovery of movement after bone or joint injuries.

Applications of methods of work and range

Stretched muscles are worked concentrically and eccentrically in their inner range in an attempt to shorten them, e.g., weak or stretched abdominal muscles after pregnancy, or visceroptosis, etc.

Shortened muscles are worked eccentrically and concentrically in their outer range in an attempt to increase their habit length, e.g., stretching the hamstrings by bending down slowly to touch the toes with straight knees.

The Group Action of Muscles

By the term the group action of muscles, is meant that harmonious interplay of several groups of muscles which is necessary to bring about a

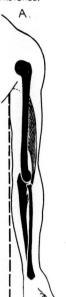

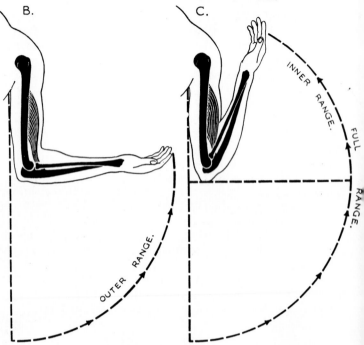

FLEXORS OF ELBOW HAVE
MOVED THE FOREARM THROUGH
THEIR OUTER RANGE.
B.

FLEXORS OF ELBOW HAVE
MOVED THE FOREARM THROUGH
THEIR INNER RANGE.
C.

INNER RANGE.

FULL RANGE.

OUTER RANGE.

FIG. 265.—Range of muscle work.

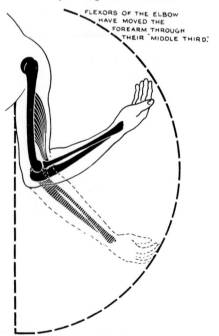

FLEXORS OF THE ELBOW
HAVE MOVED THE
FOREARM THROUGH
THEIR MIDDLE THIRD.

FIG. 266.—Range of muscle work.

perfectly controlled and co-ordinated active movement, no matter how simple or how difficult that movement may be.

The four groups of muscles concerned in this "combined operation" are described as:

   (a) Protagonists
   (b) Antagonists.
   (c) Synergists.
   (d) Fixationists.

The function of these groups has been described fully in a previous chapter (p. 117) and needs no further elaboration.

While constantly bearing in mind the importance of all these groups, when asked to describe the "muscle work involved in holding a certain position, or in performing a certain movement," the student of physiotherapy is primarily concerned with two of these groups, i.e., the prime movers and the fixationists. He is expected to name the joints in which the movement takes place, the axis and plane of movement, the groups of prime movers involved (naming the individual muscles in the group) in the various stages of the movement, how they work (i.e. concentrically, eccentrically) and in what range. When this has been done the fixationists, which work statically to hold the starting position and enable the prime movers to work from a steady attachment, are then tabulated.

When describing the muscles in action in the performance of any movement, whether an everyday movement or an exercise, the power and pull of gravity must always be borne in mind, as this force can entirely alter the muscle work necessary to carry out a movement, e.g., when lying supine, the head is raised (to look towards the toes) by sternomastoid—a flexor; but in extending the head in the standing position the sternomastoid controls the movement by working eccentrically against gravity, which, once the head is off the vertical, is trying to pull it backwards.

Also, lying on the face and arching the back in the lumbar region is performed by sacrospinalis (concentrically in inner range), but standing arching the back in the same region is controlled by the muscles of the anterior abdominal wall working in lengthening (eccentrically, in outer range) (fig. 267).

From this it will be seen that the starting position for a movement must be chosen with just as great care as the actual movement which is to be performed, if the desired effect is to be obtained and the maximum result gained.

As a final example—sitting with the arms swinging sideways and then upwards over the head, and then lowering again, is beneficial for *winged scapulae* as it gives work to serratus anterior, concentrically going up and eccentrically coming down. The same exercise given in the lying position works serratus anterior only while the limb is being elevated, for gravity is now eliminated. Under these circumstances the rhomboids and middle fibres of the trapezius draw the scapulae together as the arms come down and not serratus anterior. Thus sitting is a better starting position than lying for this condition.

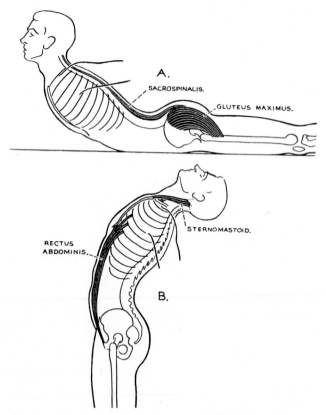

FIG. 267.—Muscle work in arching the back (a) from the horizontal, (b) from the vertical.

Muscle Work involved in Some Commonplace Movements*
The control of the standing position

In standing, the line of gravity falls as nearly as possible through the centre of the supporting surface. That is, the line falls, with slight variations, within the thorax, in front of the lower dorsal vertebrae, and just in front of the axes of the ankle joints.

The erect position, with fixed hip, knee and ankle joints and extended spine is maintained, partly by muscular action and partly by mechanical adjustments, arranged to economise effort.

Posture is determined to a large degree by the variations in the tilt of the pelvis. By pelvic tilt is meant the angle formed between the horizontal and a line drawn from the sacral promontory to the upper border of the symphysis pubis. The normal inclination of the pelvis varies between 60°–65° (fig. 268A). In a slack standing position the pelvic tilt is reduced, possibly to a

---

* A description of the muscle work involved in remedial exercises does not come within the scope of this book.

minimum of 40°–50° (fig. 268c).   In a tense standing position the tilt of the pelvis in increased (fig. 268B).

Muscles maintaining the erect position.   Erect posture is maintained by the balanced interplay of the anterior and posterior muscle groups, but of these the posterior group, including most but not all the extensor muscles, have the most to do.   Because they are continually in action against the pull of gravity they are sometimes termed the "anti-gravity muscles."

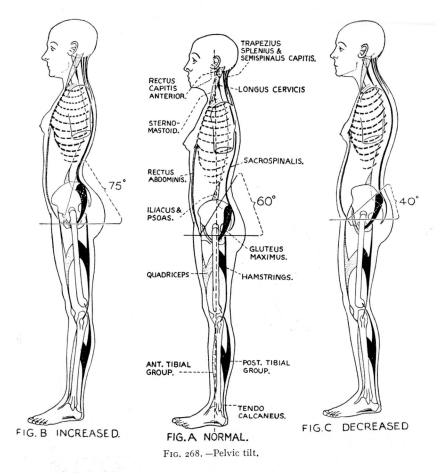

FIG. B INCREASED.   FIG. A NORMAL.   FIG. C DECREASED

Fig. 268. —Pelvic tilt.

Fig. 268A, representing a normal standing position with an average pelvic tilt, shows how and why the various muscle groups are employed.

Commencing with the control of the pelvis on the fixed femoral heads, the pelvis is steadied behind by the hip extensors (gluteus maximus and the hamstrings); in front by the abdominal muscles, iliopsoas and rectus femoris. The spine is held by sacrospinalis and the head and neck by trapezius, splenius and semispinalis capitis.   The poise of the neck and head are controlled by longus cervicis, rectus capitis anterior and sternomastoid—longus cervicis in particular being important in modifying the normal cervical convexity forward.

The knee joint is maintained in extension chiefly by its structure and to a lesser extent by the quadriceps muscles. The ankle joint is stabilised by the anterior and posterior tibial groups and the peronei, which together with the intrinsic muscles of the sole are the main factors in maintaining the arches of the foot.

In a tense standing position or when the pelvic tilt is increased for any reason (e.g., long hamstrings, tight hip flexors, weak abdominal muscles, or over-development of back muscles) certain adjustments and alterations from the normal take place. In this case the pelvic tilt is increased (fig. 268B), the pelvis is tipped up behind and down in front, this may be due to the long habit length of the hamstrings and adaptive shortening of the hip flexors. As will be seen in the diagram, the hip extensors and the anterior abdominal muscles are lengthened and the hip flexors and lumbar extensors are shortened. The pelvis being inclined forwards takes the lumbar spine with it, thus carrying the centre of gravity too far forward. To compensate for this and bring the weight again over the base, the dorsal region and head are carried back, thus increasing the concavity in the lumbar region but maintaining an erect carriage in the upper part of the trunk.

In this type of posture the knees are usually slightly hyper-extended and if the position is forced the quadriceps work to brace the knees back.

In fig. 268C a decrease in the pelvic tilt is shown. The pelvis is pulled down behind, frequently caused by a short habit length of the hamstrings. The iliopsoas in this case is not much stretched as the strain is taken by the iliofemoral ligament and the subject stands with knees slightly bent. The line of gravity falling behind the transverse axis of the hip joints.

Because the pelvis is drawn down behind, the lumbar spine is tilted backwards, thus carrying the centre of gravity too far behind the supporting surface. To counteract this, the head and upper part of trunk are thrust forward, producing an increase in the normal dorsal convexity, a poking head and a general slack posture.

The quadriceps have more work to do as the knees are slightly flexed and are therefore deprived of their mechanical support. The arches of the feet tend to sag owing to the maladjustment of muscles and joints.

Although, normally, habit-length of muscles is responsible for the tilt of the pelvis and thus for general posture, the pelvic tilt may be increased or decreased voluntarily in varying degree in a mobile subject by the necessary adjustments of the muscles concerned.

The muscle work in walking (fig. 269)

The subject is presumed to be standing with the weight equally on both feet: before a step can be taken the weight has to be transferred to one leg, leaving the other free to move (fig. 269A). This is brought about by contraction of the adductor muscles of the supporting leg (say, the left) and is momentary, for as soon as the weight is transferred the abductors of that hip (left) then go into action to prevent the pelvis dropping to the unsup-

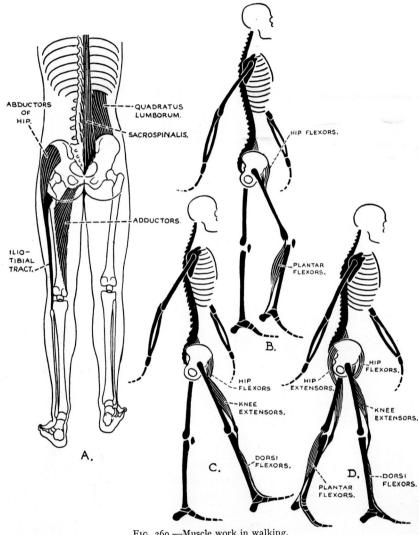

Fig. 269.—Muscle work in walking.

ported side.*   The abductors of the supporting leg are assisted in keeping the pelvis level, by the side flexors of the trunk on the opposite side.†

The weight is now on one leg (left) and the pelvis level, or slightly raised on the side of the moving leg, ready for the first step to be taken.   (The

* Weakness in abductors, allowing this dropping, produces Trendelenburg's sign.
† It has been shown (Sherrington) that this crossed extension reflex also occurs when the feet are not on the ground.

aforementioned muscles worked concentrically to do the movement and then statically to hold it.)   To take a step with the free (right) leg, the hip flexors work concentrically to bring the thigh forward, the knee is bent by its own weight and the ankle slightly plantar flexed (fig. 269B).   The knee is then extended, partly by the contraction of quadriceps, and partly by momentum.   The dorsi-flexors work concentrically to clear the ground and then statically, while the heel is placed on the ground (fig. 269c).   The forefoot is then lowered by the dorsi-flexors working eccentrically and the quadriceps statically to keep the knee straight (fig. 269D).   Simultaneously with the lowering of the heel and the forefoot coming in contact with the ground, the plantar flexors of the supporting leg (left) contract strongly and raise the heel and "push off" so that the weight of the body is now pushed forward over the forward leg (right).   The extensors of the hip and knee of the posterior (left) leg also work.

Once the weight is over the forward (right) leg, the left knee relaxes, the left hip flexors bring the thigh forward and the process is repeated, as already described, but on the other side.

While the moving leg (right) is advancing the pelvis is rotated to the side of the supporting (left) leg.   (It is rotating round the stationary head of the left femur.)   The muscles producing this movement are the medial rotators of the left hip and the lateral rotators of the right hip.

Because of this rotation of the pelvis to the side of the posterior leg, the trunk rotators to the opposite side have to work to keep the body facing forwards, in the line of progress.   In this case the trunk rotators to the right must work, the chief being the right internal and left external oblique abdominal muscles.   (Compare with the exaggerated walk of a mannequin in which the body rotates with the pelvis from side to side.)

The arms swing with the trunk, that is, the trunk is rotated to the right, the right arm swings backwards and the left arm forwards, very little muscle work is required for this, as momentum carries the arms, but if the swing is exaggerated, as in marching, then the respective extensors and flexors of the shoulder joint come into action.   This is really a modification of the walk of the quadruped and is seen in the crawl of children.

In addition to these muscles actually concerned in the act of walking, other groups are involved, which maintain the upright position.   These include the extensors of the hip and knee of the standing leg and the extensors of the spine and head, controlled by the straight abdominal and prevertebral muscles.*

The muscle work in rising from the sitting position

It is impossible to rise to the erect posture from the sitting position if the trunk is at right angles to the thigh and the thigh at right angles to the leg. The first thing to do, therefore, is to move the weight farther forward over the base, or the base farther back under the weight.   Usually both actions are performed to a slight degree.

* Walking has been shown to be a reflex action due to the movement of the centre of gravity.

To move the trunk out of the vertical plane there is slight concentric contraction of the hip flexors, followed at once by eccentric work of the hip extensors as the trunk leans forward.   At the same time the feet are usually tucked under the chair by the contraction of the knee flexors, including gastrocnemius, as the heels are generally raised during this movement. When the weight is sufficiently forward the extensors of both hips and knees go strongly into action, and with concentric contraction in inner range extend both these joints and bring the subject into the upright position.

In addition the extensors of the back, neck and head and the prevertebral muscles work statically.

To sit down again.   This is a reversal of the process, the same muscles which worked concentrically to rise, now work eccentrically in lengthening to allow the subject to sit down gently.

The muscle work in raising the arms from the side to the vertical (fig. 270)

When raising the arm from the side to the horizontal, movement takes place principally at the shoulder joint, although there is slight scapular

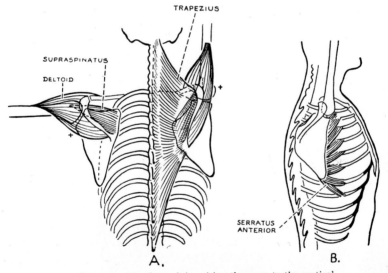

FIG. 270.—Muscle work in raising the arms to the vertical.

movement.   The arm is raised (fig. 270A) by the concentric contraction of the abductors (deltoid and supraspinatus).   These now work statically, except for a slight further contraction of supraspinatus as the head of the humerus sinks lower in the glenoid cavity when the arm is further elevated.

After the horizontal plane has been reached movement is transferred to the joints of the shoulder girdle, viz., the acromioclavicular and sterno-clavicular joints.   There is a gliding movement in the former joint, while the scapula rotates round the chest wall, by the contraction of serratus anterior and by the downward pull of the lower fibres of trapezius, so that the glenoid cavity faces upwards (fig. 270A and B).

There is also a gliding in the sternoclavicular joint as the outer end of the clavicle is elevated. The muscle chiefly responsible for this movement is trapezius (upper fibres).

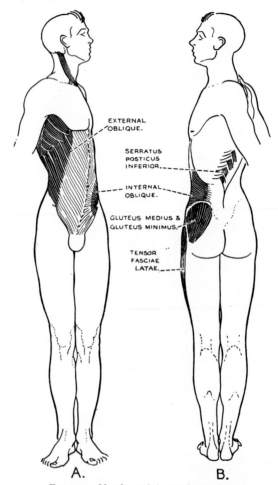

EXTERNAL OBLIQUE.

SERRATUS POSTICUS INFERIOR.

INTERNAL OBLIQUE.

GLUTEUS MEDIUS & GLUTEUS MINIMUS.

TENSOR FASCIAE LATAE.

A.   B.

FIG. 271.—Muscle work in trunk rotation.

It is usual, while performing this movement to rotate the arms, so that at the end of the movement the palms face each other above the head. This is brought about by the lateral rotators of the shoulder joint and the supinators of the forearm and usually takes place just as the arm reaches the horizontal plane.

All these muscles work concentrically as the arms are raised and eccentrically as the arms are lowered.

The anti-gravity muscles (previously named) work statically throughout, to maintain the upright posture. In addition balance is maintained between the flexors and extensors of the wrist and fingers to keep the hand in line with the arm.

Any movement in which the arm is raised above the horizontal, either sideways or forwards, with the elbow straight or bent, e.g., touching the back of the neck or head, or lifting something to the mouth, etc., involves primarily this outward rotation of the scapula.

Muscle work in trunk rotation (fig. 271)

(a) *In standing.* If the body is rotated to one side while the subject is standing, movement takes place in all the joints of the spine, in varying degree, but chiefly in the thoracic region, and also in both hip joints, as the pelvis turns with the trunk.

Muscles working to rotate the trunk to the left. The abdominal muscles and some of the back muscles may be looked upon as forming a spiral round the body (fig. 271A). The muscles concerned in rotating the trunk to the left are the left internal oblique, right external oblique, right serratus posterior superior, right rotatores and right multifidus, left serratus posterior inferior, left internal intercostals and right sternomastoid.

To rotate the pelvis to the left. Movement is performed by the medial rotators of the left hip and lateral rotators of the right hip. Thus in turning from the forward position to the left all the above muscles work concentrically in their inner range and in returning to the starting position the trunk and pelvic rotators to the *right* work concentrically in their outer range.

If the movement is repeated on each side (continuously) as far as possible, both sets of rotators will work concentrically in their full range.

(b) *In sitting.* If rotation is performed in the sitting position, the pelvis is more or less fixed. Thus movement is confined to the spine and the trunk rotators are the muscles brought into action.

Anti-gravity muscle groups work statically to maintain the erect posture.

Muscle work in head rotation (fig. 272)

To turn the head, movement takes place at the cervical joints around a vertical axis on a horizontal plane.

The muscles involved in rotating the head to the left are: Left rectus capitis anterior, left rectus capitis posterior major, left splenius, left longissimus capitis, right sternomastoid, right semispinalis capitis and the right superior oblique capitis.

Muscle work in bending forward with straight knees (fig. 273)

To bend forward with straight knees movement takes place at the intervertebral joints, at both hip joints and both ankles, around a frontal axis in a sagittal plane.

The movement is initiated by a slight concentric contraction of the hip flexors which brings the trunk forward out of the vertical and at the same time the dorsiflexors work eccentrically to allow plantarflexion in the ankle joints, with the result that the hips are pushed backwards, thus maintaining the balance.

The intrinsic muscles of the feet grip the floor statically, then the dorsi-flexors work statically to maintain the plantarflexion in the ankle joints.

The hip extensors and the sacrospinales and their prolongations work eccentrically in outer range to lower the trunk against the pull of gravity.

To regain the erect posture the same muscles work concentrically in the same range.

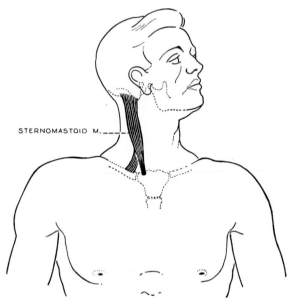

STERNOMASTOID M.

FIG. 272.—Muscle work in head rotation.

The knee extensors work statically throughout to keep the knees straight. If the knees are allowed to bend, then the quadriceps work eccentrically, controlling the amount of flexion and concentrically to straighten them again.

Muscle work in bending the trunk from side to side (fig. 274)

To bend the trunk to the side movement takes place in all the inter-vertebral joints but chiefly in the lumbar region (around a sagittal axis on a frontal plane).

To start the movement, there is slight concentric contraction of the side flexors of one side to bring the trunk out of the vertical position. This is followed at once by side flexors on the opposite side working eccentrically in outer range, against gravity.

To regain the upright position these muscles then work concentrically in the same range. Thus to bend the trunk to the left, once the movement has been initiated, it is the flexors of the right side which work eccentrically to bend and concentrically to raise the trunk.

The side flexors include most of the muscles on one side of the mid-line, the most important being sacrospinalis, rectus abdominis, and quadratus lumborum (fig. 274).

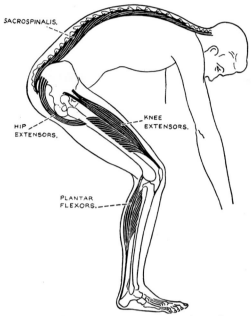

FIG. 273.—Muscle work in bending forward.

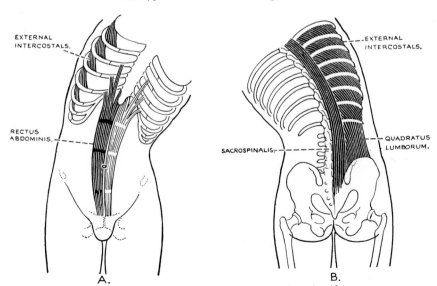

FIG. 274.—Muscle work in bending the trunk to the side.

Note, it is the muscles of the *right* side which are controlling this movement to the left.

PHYSIOLOGY

CHAPTER XIII

THE GENERAL DESIGN OF THE BODY

The Subject of Physiology

The subject of Physiology treats of the function of living things, plant and animal, but in the present connection it is limited to the latter. In all parts of the body, structure and function are extremely closely related. All function is based on an hereditary anatomical structure but it may vary very much according to needs. Thus the strength of a bone and the development of its muscles depend on the extent to which it is used. Actually, however, it is quite remarkable how much a structure which is deficient by virtue of nutrition or heredity, may adapt itself to requirements.

Physiology is part of the subject of Biology and is based on the sciences of Chemistry and Physics, a knowledge of which is essential in order to understand the subject properly. Chemistry indeed bears the same relationship to Physiology as does Anatomy, and most physiological processes are explained in terms of Chemistry and Physics. Such explanations although steadily increasing are, however, far from complete and will not be so until the mystery of life itself is solved. The physiotherapist sees this most clearly, perhaps, in relation to the repair of damaged tissue, for repair depends on the capability of the body to renew itself. In the young this occurs easily, but as the body gets older the tissues become less and less capable of repairing themselves although all known chemical relationships are unchanged. Slowly the vital spark becomes feebler and the body gets older until it is overcome by external forces and returns to the inanimate world whence it came.

All living things have certain activities in common without which life is impossible. They take in oxygen and nourishment from the outside world and having used them they return other substances to their environment. Evidence of their doing so constitutes the signs of life. They reproduce and they grow.

The lowest animals take in substances through their surfaces, but in the higher animals certain areas, which are really inlets from the surface, are specially adapted for this purpose. Thus the lungs are adapted for the intake of oxygen and the giving up of carbon dioxide, and the digestive tract for the intake of nourishment. From these organs the substances are transported by the blood to the areas where they are needed and the waste products are likewise transported to the areas from which they are to be excreted.

By far the greatest amount of nourishment and oxygen supplied is used by the voluntary muscles which from time to time become very active. They constitute about a third of the total weight of the body and with them animals and primitive man not only defend themselves but secure their food and keep themselves alive.

Our voluntary muscles are under the control of the will and messages from the brain reach them by means of the nervous system. The more we study the body the more evident it becomes that it is designed primarily to supply their needs.

Like any other engine, the function of the voluntary muscles is to convert chemical energy into mechanical energy or work. There is a great similarity between the muscles and the engine of a motor car.

The chemical energy is supplied as carbon (C) and hydrogen (H) which unite with oxygen in the muscle to form carbon dioxide (CO_2) and water (H_2O). The tube which carries the supply of the uncombusted mixture is the artery while the products of the combustion are carried away by the veins. The blood in these vessels is specially constituted to perform these functions and is pumped around by the heart. It is not without interest to realise that the essential elements of petrol are also carbon and hydrogen and the exhaust from a petrol engine is similarly carbon dioxide and water. We supply the motor car with petrol while the oxygen of the air is drawn in at the carburettor. In the body the fuel is supplied by the food we eat and the oxygen we breathe. We have already noted that the digestive tract and the lungs are really inlets from the body surface with which they are continuous at the mouth and nose. Many things, notably bacteria, get into the digestive and respiratory tracts normally, which, if they got into the blood stream or the muscles themselves, would cause serious harm. When we come to study the structure of the digestive and respiratory tracts we shall see that they constitute, by virtue of their infoldings, enormous areas upon which the food and air are spread out in intimate contact with the blood and separated from it only by thin layers of cells (e.g., in the lungs, sometimes only by the wall of a capillary blood vessel). From these surfaces absorption into the blood stream takes place for the most part by simple physical processes.

In nature, the food-stuffs exist usually in an insoluble form or are protected by a covering, otherwise they would be washed into the earth. The function of the digestive tract is to break them down into substances which can be readily absorbed into the blood.

The products of combustion, which correspond to the exhaust of a motor car, are likewise transported by the blood from where they are made, to organs which are in more immediate contact with the outside world, namely, the kidneys which produce urine, the skin which produces sweat, and the lungs by which both carbon dioxide and water are eliminated. The faeces (excretions of the bowels) are not products of combustion but substances not needed by the body.

So far we have considered only the fuel and this is by far the most immediate need of an engine and of the body. Fuel for the body is supplied for the most part by the starchy foods such as flour and potatoes and by fats.

A vast number of other substances are also needed to build up and repair the body tissues, but like the running repairs of a motor car they are needed in much less quantity. Actually all human tissue is composed of substances which have been part of the living tissues of plants and animals and this is especially true of protein, the nitrogen-containing substance of which all living tissues are built. In addition to protein, the body takes in minute quantities of other substances such as iron for the blood, calcium for the bones, iodine for the thyroid gland and vitamins for regulative purposes. All these are usually obtained from the bodies of lower animals and from plants, but some of the elements such as iron and calcium may be taken in an inorganic or non-living form.

What has been said for muscle applies to a lesser extent to all the tissues of the body but they do not, with the exception of the heart, use so much fuel. In order to keep alive and to repair itself every tissue has to use a small amount of fuel and to do so it is supplied in the same way as muscle. This repair of the tissues is a constant phenomenon and its slowing down is a characteristic of old age.

This simple view of the design of the body has certain corollaries which are extremely important. In this description such important organs as the heart and lungs are represented as playing a subsidiary part. They are, it is true, essential organs of the body but they act as servants and the amount of work they do depends for the most part on the needs of the muscles. If we take exercise more work is done by the heart and lungs, and as exercise makes us hungry, more work is also done by the digestive tract. When we are in bed we rest all these essential organs and much use is made of this fact in medicine.

For convenience, it is usual to divide the body into systems, such as the muscular, circulatory, respiratory and nervous systems, while the details of the chemical changes which take place are known as metabolism. Each of these will receive consideration in due course.

CHAPTER XIV

THE ACTIVITY OF NERVE AND MUSCLE

When we make a voluntary movement, say of the arm, nerve impulses pass from the brain down the spinal cord to the nerves supplying the muscles concerned. Such activity can be imitated conveniently by stimulating the nerve to a muscle which has been removed from a recently killed animal by a minute electric current. Most studies on the subject have been made on nerve-muscle preparations of frogs which live for several days after removal from the body, provided they are kept moist. All the essential facts obtained in this way have been found to be applicable to the tissues of mammals, including man except that in the latter, changes take place more rapidly than in amphibians.

The motoneurone pool

By cutting the afferent posterior roots and allowing time for degeneration it has been possible to count the number of motor fibres passing to a muscle. A single large nerve-fibre may supply 140–160 muscle fibres, but small nerve fibres may supply only 5–10 muscle fibres. In a muscle there may be several hundreds of such neuromuscular units.

The nerve impulse and the electrical reactions of nerve

When a nerve is stimulated by any means there are set up in its fibres nerve impulses, the nature of which is the same whatever the means of stimulation. Their essential characteristic is that they are self-propagated electric changes. The impulse is therefore sometimes compared with the propagation of the ignition in a train of gunpowder or a burning taper, with, of course, the great difference that the nerve is not destroyed, indeed it very rapidly repairs itself and is ready to carry another impulse. The self-propagation is specially important in regard to afferent nerves carrying impulses into the nervous system, for these impulses would course round the nervous system for ever if they did not arrive at regions where they were blocked.

For the study of the nerve impulse the nerves of the squid (a type of shell fish) have been used, as it is possible to put an electrode inside a large single fibre. It has been found, as in all living cells, that there is a resting potential, that is a difference in electrical potential between its exterior and interior of about 40 millivolts. When a nerve is stimulated by any means it is found that not only is the resting potential lost, but the electric change, or *action potential*, is propagated along the nerve in both directions from the point of stimulation. This may be recorded by amplifying it and connecting it with suitable apparatus such as a cathode-ray oscillograph. The electric change, which is of the order of 80 millivolts is of such short duration (about 0·001 second) that it is commonly known as the *spike*. Since it is greater than the resting potential it is clearly not just a propagated "short" but an additional active process which is believed to be an extremely rapid and selective penetration of sodium ions into the nerve fibre, for if the sodium of the environ-ment is reduced so also is the spike. This spike has an immutable shape and is the same in all nerves, it travels at the same rate as the impulse. When a nerve is anaesthetized the spike disappears. For these reasons the spike is now believed to be the impulse.

Although the nerve impulse is electrical in nature it is not an ordinary electrical current, for if its passage is recorded from two points it is found to be propagated much more slowly than an electric current, viz., at the rate of 27 metres per second in the frog and 120 metres per second in the mammal. The rate of propagation is fastest in the largest, or A fibres and slowest in smallest, or C fibres. Moreover the nerve fibre is not like a wire; it is a living structure which ceases to conduct if cooled and which can be anaesthe-tized. It also requires oxygen and produces carbon dioxide in minute but measurable amounts. It may also be paralysed by pressure, such as may be inflicted by a badly fitting splint, or even a tight bandage. We may readily experience numbness in the side of the hand if the ulnar nerve at the elbow is lain upon.

Humoral transmission

The *neuromuscular junction* is now known to be a region of very special importance, for the electrical change in a nerve is not transmitted directly to the muscle but through the agency of the chemical mediator, *acetylcholine*, which is liberated at the nerve-ending. This substance fires off the highly charged end-plates or sole-plates of the muscle and there is generated a still greater change of electric potential known as *end-plate potential* which, if large enough is propagated along the less excitable muscle and causes it to contract. The most conclusive evidence of the liberation of acetylcholine is the fact that when saline solution is perfused through the blood vessels of a muscle acetylcholine is found in it when the muscle is stimulated through its nerve, and this substance when injected into an artery close to a muscle causes it to contract. In the perfusion experiment it is necessary to add eserine to the perfusion fluid to prevent the destruction of the acetylcholine by cholinesterase, the very active enzyme which normally destroys the acetylcholine immediately it has acted.

Substances which interfere with the action of acetylcholine cause a neuro-muscular block and when this is produced the muscle may be stimulated only by the application of an electric current to it directly, but not through its nerve. Such a substance is curare, the South American arrow poison, and use is now made of this substance to bring about relaxation of muscles during surgical operations. This permits of less anaesthetic and its action is at once antagonised by eserine. A block may also be produced if sufficient acetyl-choline is not made or is not liberated and therefore a neuromuscular block is produced if glucose, necessary for the synthesis of the acetylcholine, is not available or if insufficient calcium is present for the liberation. The physio-logy of the neuromuscular junction is of very special interest because what happens in this region is very like what occurs at synapses in the nervous system generally and is an important factor in many of our movements and possibly in our mental processes. The release of acetylcholine was first discovered in relation to stimulation of the vagus nerve which slows the heart, and its antagonism by atropine has long been known but not wholly understood. It is now known that sympathetic nerves also act by releasing acetylcholine. Some dilate blood vessels but in others the acetylcholine brings about the release of nor-adrenaline which constricts vessels. Acetylcholine is also released by the sympathetic nerves which stimulate the medulla of the adrenal gland and liberate adrenaline.

The electrical reactions of muscle

We have seen that normally when a muscle is stimulated through its nerve a large end-plate potential is set up by the acetylcholine liberated. If the end-plate potential is sufficiently large it spreads over the surface of the muscle and may be picked up by electrodes connected to a galvanometer. It must be clear that this action potential is the cause, not the result, of muscle action, for it precedes the contraction. The action potential appears to be a propagated electrical change very like that in a nerve, and except in very unusual circumstances is always followed by muscle contraction.

Similar action potentials of the heart as taken in electrocardiography, or of the brain in encephalography give information regarding a similar spread of electrical change in those organs. When the nerves to a muscle are degenerated spontaneous discharges of impulses occur at the end-plate and give rise to irregular fibrillations or twitchings of the muscle which are often visible through the skin.

The irritability or excitability of tissues

The contraction of muscle when stimulated is an example of the phenomenon of irritability or excitability which is common to many tissues although it has been mostly studied in muscle and nerve. This excitability depends on the fact that all tissues are normally electrically charged or polarised, that is, the interior of the cell is electro-negative to the outside. This so-called resting potential is very readily observed in a frog's muscle simply by placing one electrode on the cut end of a muscle, another on the outside and connecting them to a sufficiently delicate galvanometer. A difference of 20–40 millivolts may be obtained. This is due to a difference in concentration of ions especially those of potassium inside and outside the cell. There is roughly seven times as much potassium inside as outside, while in the case of sodium the muscle contains only about a seventh of that of the blood or the tissue fluid in which it is bathed. The fact that it is possible to construct a chemical concentration cell capable of producing weak electric currents simply by separating two different concentrations of salts by means of a membrane has long been known.

Studies of the excitability show that an electrical stimulus must not only be of *sufficient strength* to stimulate a nerve or muscle, but it must also be applied for a *sufficient time*. We are familiar with the fact that movements may occur so rapidly that they do not stimulate the retina of the eye. It is for this reason that a modern cinematograph film does not flicker.   In the same way, if an electric current strong enough to light an ordinary 250 volt lamp is made to alternate very rapidly it still may light the lamp but does not stimulate tissues and is quite harmless.   Use is made of this fact in modern physiotherapeutic apparatus such as is used in short-wave therapy which is designed to heat up the interior of the body without causing stimulation of muscle.   The ordinary domestic current of 250 volts alternates relatively slowly (50 cycles per second) and is therefore dangerous.   Fortunately the dry skin offers a resistance of about 50,000 ohms and this reduces its strength, but when the hands and feet are wet, as they are when we are in a bath, contact with faulty electrical apparatus may stimulate the heart muscle causing it to fibrillate.   This may cause death.

These fundamental facts, which are basal to much electrotherapy, are well seen if a strength duration curve for a muscle is constructed (fig. 275).

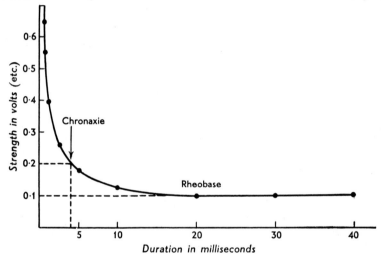

FIG. 275. Note the weaker the stimulus the longer it must act to produce a contraction.
(For explanation see text below.)

The measurement of excitability

This measurement may be made if it is suspected that the nerve to a muscle is injured.   If a simple comparison with a muscle of the opposite side of the body is all that is needed, then it may be measured by finding the *rheobase*, that is the minimum current which when applied to the muscle for an indefinite time will just cause it to contract.   The current may be supplied by an ordinary accumulator or battery and its strength varied by a resistance in the circuit.   Such a current stimulates only at the "make" and "break" and it is found that when the current is made or closed the contraction is greater when the negative pole or cathode is in the muscle, the other pole being at a distance on the body.   The terms cathode closing contraction (CCC), and anode closing contraction (ACC) are used in this connection.

Since the resistance of tissues themselves varies very much it is found, however, to be more accurate to measure the excitability in terms of *chronaxie*, which is the minimum time a current of twice the rheobase must be applied to give a response. There are various devices for producing such accurately timed currents. A heavy pendulum or springs may be used to open and close the circuit, but more commonly use is made of the fact that the time taken for a condenser of a given capacity to discharge depends on the resistance in the circuit. Then by varying the resistance we may vary the time of the stimulus.

The excitability of a nerve is about 10 times greater than that of a muscle and therefore when the nerves to a muscle are injured and degenerate the excitability of the muscle is very much reduced. It will no longer respond to a weak faradic current like a normal muscle, while ACC is now greater than CCC. The muscles also respond sluggishly and often show minute fibrillations. This is known as the *reaction of degeneration*.

Chemical changes in muscle

The outstanding and ultimate chemical change in muscle when it contracts is the burning of the carbon and hydrogen of the carbohydrate glycogen and the production of carbon dioxide and water as in any other engine. A muscle, however, is peculiar in that the combustion may take place a long time in advance of the contraction and the energy is stored in a more readily available form; this is reminiscent of the combustion of petrol used for the charging of the battery of a motor car so that electricity is immediately available for starting. In the case of the muscle the substance stored is adenosine triphosphate (ATP) a substance which by virtue of its two molecules of high energy phosphate liberates much more energy than any other phosphate when split up. If ATP is applied to threads of actomyosin (page 343) it causes them to contract. ATP is made fairly rapidly from ADP (adenosine diphosphate) and from creatine phosphate, both of which have the high energy phosphorus. The making of the latter is a slower and complicated biochemical process, the chemistry of which need not concern us here. A diagrammatic idea of the changes which take place is given in fig. 276.

It will be seen that the first half of the recovery is anaerobic, i.e., it takes place in the absence of oxygen, and that the second half requires oxygen.

This storage of energy as organic compounds of phosphorus makes it possible for a muscle to continue contracting in the absence of oxygen for quite a long time, indeed it can do so until all its creatine phosphate has been converted into creatine. It cannot, however, recover without oxygen for this is necessary to recharge the creatine and adenine with the high energy phosphate. It may therefore accumulate considerable *oxygen debt*. This can be demonstrated readily in man if he takes severe exercise. Although he may take in a large amount of oxygen during the exercise this is not nearly enough to recharge the chemical system. He has to pay off the debt, so to speak, by taking in a large amount of oxygen after the exercise is over. This is indicated by the well-known continued breathlessness after sprinting a hundred yards.

During the oxygen deficiency the body does in fact make a little high energy phosphate as a result of a small anaerobic breakdown of carbohydrate to lactic acid which accumulates in the blood as lactate and is excreted in the urine. This waste of combustible lactate is uneconomical but it makes the body more capable of a physical emergency.

SCHEME OF THE
CHEMISTRY OF MUSCLE CONTRACTION

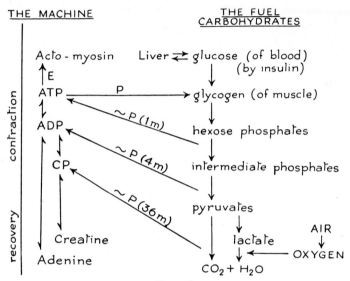

THE MACHINE

THE FUEL
CARBOHYDRATES

FIG. 276.
For explanation see text—"Chemical changes in muscle."

Common electrical apparatus used in stimulating nerves and muscles

These are given in some detail as they are much used in Physiotherapy.

The simplest apparatus used in stimulating nerves is a direct (Galvanic) current supplied to electrodes by wires from an accumulator or battery with a simple key in the circuit. In work on man the resistance of the skin is reduced by moistening it with salt solution and the current is applied through large electrodes to reduce the voltage necessary and the discomfort of the "shock" to the skin. The current stimulates only at the make and break, but the make stimulus is of long duration. It is, however, difficult to adjust the strength of the stimulus to the required strength and therefore an induced or Faradic current is much used. If two coils of wire are placed close to each other, and a current is "made" or "broken" in one of them (the primary), a current is also made or broken in the other (the secondary). If the secondary coil contains many coils of fine wire and the primary fewer coils of stout wire the induced current may be stepped up to a higher voltage than the primary, although the amount of current is less. The reverse occurs if the secondary circuit consists of a few coils of thick wire and use is

23—A.PH.

made of this in the ordinary bell transformer by which it is possible to step down the ordinary domestic current from 250 volts to enable it to activate domestic electric bells. The current in the secondary is of much shorter duration than a primary current depending on the speed with which the current is made or broken, but since the change of current in the domestic mains lasts 1/50 second, the current from a simple bell transformer lasts long enough to stimulate muscle even in the absence of nerves. It is important to emphasize that there is no flow of current in the secondary except when the current in the primary is changed. Mechanical interrupters, similar in principle to that of an ordinary electric bell, are commonly introduced in the primary circuit to produce the faradism much used in electrotherapy to tetanise muscle,

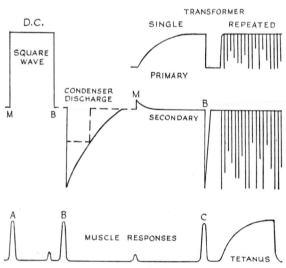

FIG. 277.—Shows the wave-form of different kinds of stimuli and the muscle responses they produce. It is possible to calculate the square wave (dotted line) equivalent of the relatively slow condenser discharge. M = make, B = break, D.C. = direct current. Note that a direct current produces its maximum effect if of sufficient voltage at make. The induced stimulus through a transformer produces a greater response at break because the latter is for physical reasons of greater voltage.

For the production of stimuli of known shorter duration the discharge of a condenser is used and now a large variety of electronic stimulators which give square-wave stimuli of any desired frequency, voltage, amperage and duration are available and are used for routine clinical work. The following simple diagram gives a summary of the main points. It will be noted that although the ordinary transformer with the usual spark interrupter (fig. 278) gives a very irregular current it produces, for reasons described on page 345, a smooth tetanic contraction of the muscle.

The recording and measuring of muscle contraction

When a muscle contracts it shortens and grows thicker, but there is only a minute decrease in volume. It is firmer to the touch. We do not know exactly what causes the muscle to shorten, but X-ray studies suggest that one portion of the protein complex or actomyosin of which the muscle is composed slides into the other. Threads of **actomyosin** still retain their power of contracting to suitable stimuli.

The contraction of muscle may be recorded by attaching one of its ends to a fixed point and the other to a simple balanced lever which writes on a

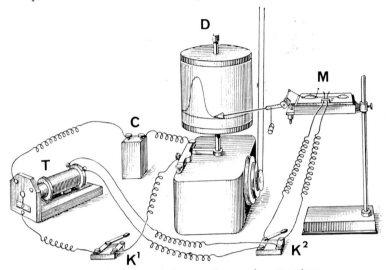

FIG. 278.—Apparatus for recording muscle contractions.
M = muscle.   C = cell.   T = transformer.   D = recording drum.   K¹ and K² = keys.

recording surface, the speed of which is known, as shown in fig. 278. The most generally convenient is a smoked drum but many other varieties are in use. This is known as the isotonic method. Commonly the gastrocnemius muscle from the leg of a recently killed frog with the sciatic nerve attached is used, but we may use any suitable muscle of an anaesthetised animal. In this way we may record the latent period, that is the time between the stimulus and the contraction, how long the contraction is maintained and the relaxation of the contraction, all of which are important as they determine the power of the muscle and are liable to change. We may stimulate the muscle directly or through its nerve. Stimuli of different kinds applied to the muscle or to the nerve will bring about excitation of the preparation. The application of a hot wire or a chemical or a weak electric current from a battery or accumulator may be used but the latter is best as it does not damage the structure.

Wires may be taken directly to the electrode but it is more convenient to stimulate the muscle by means of an induced current through a transformer, because it is easier to vary its strength simply by varying the distance between the primary and secondary coils. A current is induced in the secondary circuit when the current is made or broken by the key in the primary.

The effect of temperature

Cold, at first increases the height of contraction, then diminishes it. Moderate warmth increases the height and diminishes the duration of all stages of the curve, including the latent period. Too great heat induces heat rigor from the coagulation of the muscle proteins.

The effect of strength of stimuli

It can be shown readily that the weakest stimuli are without effect but as the strength is increased the contractions become stronger until a maximal response is produced. This is the maximal stimulus. This phenomenon which may also be observed in human muscle is due to the fact that as the stimulus is increased, more and more muscle fibres are stimulated until all respond. This may be seen microscopically on muscle which has been sprayed with mercury vapour, and it is found that if a fibre stimulated through its nerve contracts at all, it contracts to its full extent. This is known as *the all or none phenomenon*.

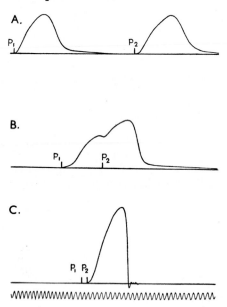

FIG. 279.—Showing the effect of two stimuli P_1 and P_2 at different intervals.

The effect of successive stimuli

If a stimulus which is just sub-threshold is applied it has no effect. If, however, this is followed rapidly by another stimulus there is a summation of stimuli followed by a response because of the accumulation of acetylcholine at the nerve ending. If the stimulus is just above threshold there is a summation of contraction partly because more fibres may be stimulated, as there may not be adequate time for complete relaxation. If several rapid stimuli are applied the responses are fused and a tetanus is produced (fig. 280). This is of special interest since there is now complete evidence that smooth voluntary contractions in man are really tetani produced by irregular showers of stimuli which pass down the nerves.

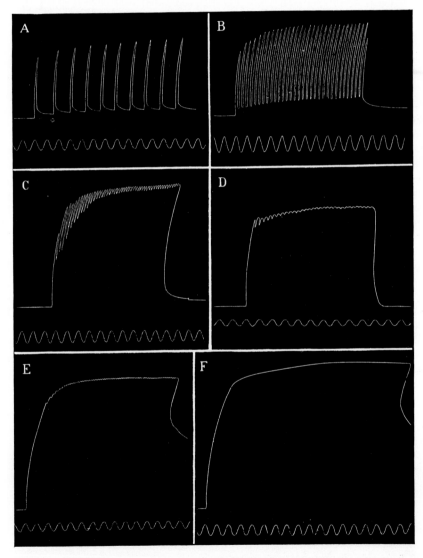

FIG. 280.—Composition of tetanus. These six tracings were obtained on a slowly moving drum from a frog's gastrocnemius, which was excited by a succession of induction shocks. The rate of stimulation was increased from 1 per sec. in A to 30 per sec. in F. In A separate twitches are seen. In B the rate was still insufficient to cause fusion. In both A and B, the staircase effect is well seen. In C and D the rate was insufficient to cause complete tetanus which is nearly achieved in E and completely achieved in F. The time tracing in each case shows half seconds.

An experimental tetanus in which all the fibres contract at one time and which fatigues rapidly differs in this respect from voluntary tetanus in which the muscle is enabled to sustain a contraction by using different fibres in turn. That such fatigue occurs rapidly is of importance in electrotherapy.

Because nerves are more excitable than muscle, the ease with which tetanus can be produced by a galvanic current (the galvanic tetanus ratio) applied to a muscle is reduced if the nerve to a muscle is degenerated and use is sometimes made of this in diagnosis. Different muscles, however, vary very much in this respect, but comparison with the healthy side can often be made.

It must be realised that any stimulus applied to a normal muscle acts on the nerve fibrils in it more easily than in the muscle itself. The slow failure of the muscle to relax in fatigue or oxygen lack causes it to tetanise more easily. These states may also cause the muscle to go into contracture or a state of incomplete relaxation.

The tetanic nature of voluntary contraction was first suspected many years ago when electrodes were inserted into muscle and connected with a telephone and the sound heard. Now that the action potentials can be amplified and recorded by the more modern cathode-ray-oscilloscope showers of action potentials continue to be recorded so long as the voluntary contraction is maintained and their number is in proportion to the tension exerted. If a muscular contraction is maintained fatigue occurs but as it does so the more action potentials occur indicating that more fibres have become "recruited" to the task. If, therefore, we wish to imitate voluntary contraction in therapy we stimulate with short bursts of stimuli. The recording of such potentials is now a diagnostic procedure—electromyography in physical medicine. When the nerve centres in the spinal cord have been damaged, as in poliomyelitis, there is a reduction of the impulses which can be picked up according to the amount of damage present.

The staircase effect (fig. 280A, B and C). After resting, the first few contractions of a muscle, even with the same stimulus, are not maximal but slowly become so. Since increased temperature causes a small increase of contraction the improvement is no doubt partly due to the production of heat and is sometimes known as "the warming up effect," but it is partly due to the liberation of potassium, for if a muscle is being stimulated a short period of tetanus is followed by a marked improvement of the contraction which is temporary and therefore cannot be due to heat only. The warming up effect is commonly made use of by athletes before a race.

The optimal speed of contraction. It can be readily demonstrated that there is an optimal speed of contraction. If muscle contracts too frequently it has not time to recover its stores of immediately available energy; if too slow it does not do the maximum amount of work. Studies of oxygen uptake have demonstrated that each individual has an optimum or most economical rate of walking. In very slow walking, energy is wasted in maintaining contraction between the steps. Therefore we get very tired when we go on a shopping expedition, visit an exhibition or walk with an invalid.

The effect of load and the production of tension. If the lever a muscle is caused to pull is increasingly weighted it can be shown readily that within certain limits the more a muscle is stretched the more tension it can produce although of course a point is reached when it can no longer contract so efficiently. This has been shown to be due to sodium being driven out of the muscle for lowered sodium increases contraction. This increased response to load is a fundamental and most important characteristic of all muscle. Thus in the case of the heart it has been shown that the more its muscle is stretched by incoming blood the better it contracts and within limits the greater its output. Similarly the distention of the intestine by fluid drawn into it by a saline purgative causes it to contract more forcibly.

The power of muscle to produce tension is remarkable. The gastrocnemius of an adult cat can produce a tension of about 50 kg., but as we know in man, the tension produced is greatly increased by use because the fibres hypertrophy. Occasionally a man may tear a tendon or a muscle from a bone, but this is rare because contracting muscle is even more elastic than resting and, as we shall see, the "lengthening reaction" prevents too great tension being developed. It is probably by the emotional loss of this reaction that lunatics may acquire their great strength and as a result they often tear muscle.

The recording of tension. In the recording of muscle contraction by the isotonic method just described it is essentially the shortening which is recorded, but no idea is obtained of the power the muscle can develop. Even if half the muscle were paralysed its shortening would be maximal, although its power would be halved. In accurate work, therefore, the tension which can be produced by a muscle is recorded by the isometric method. In this method, which is most valuable in man, the muscle is made to pull against a stiff spring and shortening is reduced to a minimum. The minute movements of the spring are recorded from a small mirror which is made to reflect a beam of light on a moving photographic film or paper. It is possible to use an electric strain-gauge, the minute movements of which are amplified and recorded from a cathode-ray oscilloscope. Various devices known as dynamometers by which the pull of a limb muscle on the strength of the grasp of the hand can be measured have been devised and are of value in recording clinical improvement after injury. A simple spring balance may also be used—and by this we can study the effect of various bodily states on muscle contraction.

It can be shown that the tension of a muscle depends primarily on the number of its fibres and their size rather than on their length. Some muscles act to greater mechanical advantage than others according to the exact point of insertion in bones relative to the joints they move.

The effects of exercise and training on muscle

It is well recognised that the frequent use of muscle causes it to become more efficient. It would seem that the production of tension is a stimulus to muscle growth or hypertrophy, for there is an increase in both muscle and connective tissue, although exactly how this is brought about is unknown. There is no increase in the number of fibres, but the individual fibres increase in size; there is an increase in the number of blood vessels around them, especially of capillaries while the stores of creatine phosphate, glycogen and oxygen carrying myohaemoglobin is also increased so that the muscle becomes darker in colour. It seems likely too that the "lengthening reaction," p. 456, becomes less effective in reducing the limit of tension which can be produced and it must be emphasised that in training for an athletic event the muscles to be used must be trained.

Sustained activity not involving much tension does not lead to the same increase of bulk. We often see apparently frail individuals who are capable of great endurance. Here it would seem that the mobilisation of energy is an important factor. An increase in connective tissue in more active muscles also occurs and is well seen in the difference between a rump (gluteus) and fillet (psoas) steak, and the difference in tenderness between the legs of hens which have been kept shut up and those allowed to run about.

When a muscle ceases to be used, atrophy sets in and this is of great interest to physiotherapists who seek to arrest it by electrical stimulation. The muscle fibres become smaller and are replaced by fat so that the muscles feel soft and flabby. In the severe forms seen in bedridden patients or after nerve injury the nuclei of the muscle fibres eventually disappear and the muscle consists of little more than fibrous cords, incapable of recovery.

Opinion is divided on the beneficial effects of electrical stimulation as a substitute for voluntary activity in a nerve injury from which recovery may be expected, for although such treatment may maintain muscle size, the movement may delay nerve regeneration. There is no doubt, however, of the benefit of systematic exercise in maintaining the normal efficiency of muscles if the patient is temporarily confined to bed. Convalescence is thereby greatly shortened and after operations patients for this reason are now encouraged to walk as soon as possible.

Local circulatory changes associated with muscle contraction

When a muscle contracts its blood supply is very much increased, partly as a result of the products of combustion and the breakdown of ATP. The vessels in the muscle are opened up by the carbon dioxide, lactic acid and adenine phosphate which is liberated by the contracting muscles and which acts on the thin walls of the capillaries. These substances also draw water into the muscle and should this accumulate in excess, stiffness results. This is specially liable to occur if the blood and lymph circulation is inefficient through lack of exercise in training. This is normally counteracted in part by the fact that contracting muscle massages the blood capillaries and veins in its substance and drives blood back to the heart. Thus massage, movement and heat which open up vessels is the best therapy for such stiffness. Habitually-used muscles develop an increased number of blood vessels.

It is now known that normally the nervous system also plays a part in the opening up of blood vessels during exercise. Sympathetic dilator fibres which have their origin in the higher parts of the brain send down nerve impulses which liberate the very active substance acetylcholine. The dilatation of small vessels is further augmented by the rise of blood pressure in the arteries (see p. 389).

Fatigue

We are all familiar with the fact that excessive use of any particular muscle or set of muscles leads to fatigue. It might be imagined that this is simply due to exhaustion of the muscle but actually the subject is not nearly so simple as it appears at first sight.

If, for example, we study the problem on a nerve-muscle preparation from a frog, it is found that when the muscle can no longer be stimulated through its nerve, it will contract if the electrodes are applied directly to the muscle. On the other hand, if we place a nerve-block, such as a piece of ice, on the nerve and stimulate the nerve for an almost indefinite time, the muscle will at once contract when the block is removed, thus showing that the nerve between the stimulus and the block has not become fatigued. Since fatigue does not depend on the muscle or nerve, it seems justifiable to conclude that the fatigue occurs in the region of the nerve-ending. Possibly there is an exhaustion or upset of the mechanism releasing acetylcholine, but this has not been proved.

Human fatigue, however, appears to be somewhat different. If electrodes are thrust into the adductor pollicis to record its action potential and the ulnar nerve stimulated until the muscle is fatigued, it is found that there is no reduction of the action potential, indicating that there is no neuromuscular block. This severe fatigue must be made in the muscle itself, but there is evidence that impulses pass centrally from the muscles, preventing their being driven to such complete exhaustion.

In addition to fatigue of local muscles there is also a generalised fatigue which would appear to be due to generalised exhaustion and the accumulation of fatigue-products in the body. Such fatigue is prevented by cutting down all unnecessary movements and the movement of large masses of muscle, e.g., those of the back. This variety of fatigue is of interest in industry but it is also of importance in injuries for it has been found that quite small injuries, even a heel blistered by an ill-fitting shoe, may cause fatigue because it calls into use larger amounts of muscle not normally used in walking.

Fatigue is very liable to be produced as the result of work in overheated or humid atmospheres, presumably because the warmth causes a general vasodilatation which tends to interfere with the blood supply to the muscles. On a hot moist day we do not feel as active as on a cool dry day.

The optimum working temperature in factories as judged by the incidence of accidents appears to be from 60–65° F.

The sensation of fatigue occurs when we use muscles to excess. The evidence is clear that chemical products are produced in the fatigued muscles and if these products are sufficiently concentrated they bring about a stimulation of the sensory nerve endings in the muscle, causing pain. This is suggested by the fact that the extent and duration of the pain is greatly increased if the artery to the part is compressed. The nature of the substance or substances concerned are not known and the term P. (*pain-substance*) has been suggested, but it would seem that *lactic acid* is almost certainly concerned for this substance accumulates in fatigued muscle, especially when the circulation is deficient.   There is also evidence that an extract of fatigued muscle or a solution of lactic acid produces fatigue and it is known that fatigue in the body as a whole depends upon the total amount of muscle used.   In factories is has been shown that fatigue is more liable to occur in overheated rooms.

Of recent years great emphasis has been placed on the importance of the psychological states in relation to fatigue; indeed we are all familiar with the fact that we get more tired when we do things we do not wish to do or at which

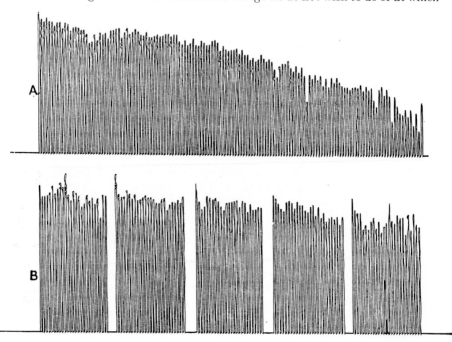

FIG. 281.—A, shows fatigue of an ordinary voluntary muscle of a finger, doing work on an ergograph at the rate of 48 contractions per minute.   In B, the subject worked for the same length of time—three minutes—but took four rest periods of five seconds each.   In A, the amount of work done was 1·80 kilogramme-metres.   In B, the amount of work done was 2·23 kilogramme-metres (Whittles).

we are not very successful.   It must be realised that all sensation is fundamentally a mental phenomenon (see Sensation) and the acuteness of the sensation of fatigue must therefore be greatly influenced by mental states.

Rest pauses

It can be readily shown experimentally that if we wish to get the maximum amount of work from a muscle in a given time it must not be over-fatigued but rested from time to time.   It can indeed be shown that almost all activities are benefited by properly spaced rest pauses.   Too much rest leads to a reduction of output, but too much work is just as effective in so doing.

During the war of 1914–18 detailed studies of this problem were made and the output of factories greatly increased when the workers had more leisure. So-called time and motion studies have, however, not been generally popular, since workers imagine they lead to exploitation.

Muscle Tone

If we place a hand over one of our muscles we feel it to be firmly elastic. It is not fully relaxed even when it is not being voluntarily contracted. It is said to be in a state of tone, but this is reduced if the opposing muscle is contracted.

A muscle may become flabby from disuse or from damage to its nerve supply; indeed, we know that muscle tone depends upon the integrity of the reflex arc (p. 452).

Since the muscles are constantly maintained in a state of tone they can no doubt respond more quickly as there is no slack to be taken up. The tone merges imperceptibly into that slight muscular contraction which it is so essential to avoid when muscles are to be massaged.

This subject is dealt with further in relation to the nervous system, upon which muscle tone depends.

Muscle Cramps

Intense contractions producing very severe pain occur from time to time in normal persons, especially after excessive use. They are not completely understood but they appear to be associated with excessive loss of salts (see sodium) from the body such as occurs after sweating or diarrhoea. Loss of calcium may also produce cramps in lactating women.

CHAPTER XV

THE BLOOD AND ITS CIRCULATION

The blood transports various substances to different parts of the body. It is composed of red and white blood cells and blood platelets suspended in the blood plasma which forms 55 per cent of its volume.

The Red Blood Cells (erythrocytes) are so called because they contain a red iron pigment called *haemoglobin*, the substance chiefly responsible for the carriage of oxygen and carbon dioxide. When fresh, blood pigment is soluble and can be washed easily out of linen; when dry it changes its character, becomes insoluble *methaemoglobin* and is difficult to remove. Red blood cells live only a few months but are constantly renewed.

The White Blood Cells are of two types—granular and non-granular. The granulocytes have a lobular nucleus and stain with neutral, acid, or alkaline dyes. Neutrophils form over 70 per cent. of the white cells and ingest bacteria, the acidophils, called eosinophils, form only about 2 per cent. and are increased in allergy (hypersensitivity to a foreign protein). The non-granular cells are the lymphocytes.

The colour of pus is largely due to the leucocytes, some of which may be living, but many have been killed by the toxins produced by bacteria.

The Platelets which initiate or hasten blood clotting are present normally at the rate of 300,000 per cubic millimetre of blood. They also contain a highly specialised protein which apparently plays a part in the retraction of the clot. They live only a few hours and are removed by the reticulo-endothelial system.

For further details of the cells of the blood see the section on Histology, page 13.

Blood Formation and the Origin of the Blood cells. We have already observed that in post-natal life all the cells of the blood with the exception of the lymphocytes are derived from the red bone marrow. In the foetus, the liver and spleen are concerned with their manufacture, but these organs do not function in this way after birth. Red bone marrow occupies the marrow cavity of all the bones in the body throughout childhood, but afterwards it is replaced by yellow bone marrow (fat) except in the flat bones such as the ribs and sternum, the vertebrae, pelvis and skull bones in which the red marrow persists throughout life. If, however, a patient suffers from frequent haemorrhages, the yellow marrow of the long bones becomes transformed into red marrow and again forms blood cells.

It is now clear that vitamins C, B_{12} and folic acid of the diet are important in blood formation. Some factor—*the intrinsic factor of Castle*--probably protein in nature is responsible for the absorption of vitamin B_{12}, and in its absence pernicious anaemia occurs when immature cells are seen in the blood. The vitamin responsible for the full development of the red cells is stored in the liver from which it can be extracted. It has recently been isolated in crystalline form and is used in the treatment of pernicious anaemia.

The **Reticulo-endothelial system** consists of a series of phagocytic cells which are widely distributed throughout the body. Some are present in the form of the wandering cells of the connective tissue and the mononuclear cells of the blood and spleen. Others are fixed in position such as the Küpffer cells of the liver which line the hepatic blood sinuses and have the property of taking up particulate matter such as Indian ink by which they may be stained or the haemoglobin liberated from the disintegration of red cells. The reticulo-endothelial system liberates the iron content of haemoglobin and this is stored in the liver, spleen and bone marrow. The iron-free blood pigment is called *bilirubin* and this is liberated into the blood, altered slightly by the liver and is excreted in the bile. Some of the bilirubin is oxidised into the green pigment *biliverdin*. These pigments give the bile its characteristic greenish colour and eventually they give the dark colour to the faeces. The green colour of a bruise is due to a similar change in the blood pigment which has escaped from the injured blood vessels.

Other reticulo-endothelial cells are to be found in the alveoli of the lungs where they are active in removing carbon particles which have been carried in with the inspired air.

Further reticulo-endothelial cells are to be found especially in the lymph nodes which become black after an injection of Indian ink (Gilding's experiment).

The **Blood Plasma** or fluid of the blood is composed of 90 per cent. water. The remainder is protein or albuminous substances like white of egg, and salts, especially sodium chloride (common salt) which is present to the extent of 0·69 per cent. This is an important figure and must always be remembered, as *normal saline* (salt solution of this strength) is sometimes used as a blood substitute after severe haemorrhage, for keeping exposed abdominal organs moist and for washing the bowel. It also contains minute but essential quantities of calcium and potassium phosphates and bicarbonates without which no organ can function properly.

The blood plasma is faintly *alkaline* in reaction, having a pH of 7·4.* It may become appreciably more alkaline but only very slightly less so. It never becomes acid since an acid blood is incompatible with life. There exist in the body a large number of chemical mechanisms to maintain its reaction constant.

The plasma proteins consist of *serum albumin, serum globulin* and *fibrinogen*. Their molecules are too large to filter freely through the capillary walls into the tissue fluid except in injury or disease and remaining in the blood plasma they exert an osmotic pressure which tends to return the tissue fluid into the blood stream. Fibrinogen forms the fibrin in a blood clot and plasma from which the fibrin has been precipitated by clotting is called *serum*. The presence of these proteins in the blood increases its viscosity and, therefore, raises the blood pressure slightly. The plasma proteins may be increased in disease, and it is believed that they are the source of the antibodies which help to fight infection. They also assist in maintaining the normal reaction

* A solution exactly neutral has a pH value of 7. Higher values indicate alkalinity, lower values acidity.

of the blood which is slightly alkaline. After injury, those plasma proteins which may escape into the tissues form an important medium into which new blood vessels grow and in which fibrous tissue is formed as part of the process of repair.

Besides the proteins and salts which are present in the plasma there are various substances which can be extracted from the blood. They comprise nutritious substances such as glucose and fats, substances necessary for the repair of effete cells such as amino-acids, substances which activate certain tissues such as hormones, as well as waste products such as carbon dioxide, urea and uric acid.

The Haemoglobin content of the Blood. Haemoglobin is the iron-containing pigment found in the red cells and is responsible for the red colour of the blood. It is of the greatest importance in the carriage of oxygen and indirectly of carbon dioxide.

A deficiency in haemoglobin may be due to a variety of causes, the commonest being haemorrhage following childbirth or excessive menstruation. In this simple anaemia each red cell may be deficient in iron and the mucous membranes such as those of the conjunctiva or lips become pale. It is treated by giving iron. In pernicious anaemia on the other hand there are too few red cells but each has an abnormally large amount of haemoglobin. In both varieties, however, the total haemoglobin of the blood is low. On the other hand ascent to high altitude or in some congenital heart conditions (blue babies) there is compensatory increase in normal red blood cells and the haemoglobin content of a given amount of blood may be high. In such cases the bone marrow in which the red cells are made becomes very active as it does after haemorrhage.

The haemoglobin content is expressed as a percentage of an average blood which is capable of carrying 20 ml. of oxygen per 100 c.c. of blood (i.e., blood which contains 15 per cent. haemoglobin). Such blood is said to contain "100 per cent." haemoglobin and is a measure of the oxygen carrying capacity of the blood. If the number of red cells in the blood is also counted and their haemoglobin content estimated it is possible by means of a *haemoglobinometer* to determine the *colour index* of the blood. Thus if there are 5,000,000 red cells per c.mm. of blood and their haemoglobin content is 100 per cent. then the colour index is said to be 1. If on the other hand each cell contained only half the normal amount of haemoglobin then the colour index would be 0·5.

The Salt content of the Blood is maintained at a fairly constant level of concentration for on this depends the normal functioning of many organs and tissues of the body, notably the heart. The most important salts are sodium, potassium, calcium, iron, magnesium and phosphorus but there are minute amounts of many others the importance of which is just becoming known, such as fluorine for the teeth and cobalt for vitamin B_{12}.

Blood volume, etc. This is found by injecting into the blood stream an easily recognisable substance such as Evans Blue which mixes rapidly yet remains in the circulation long enough to be estimated. After a short period a sample of blood is withdrawn, an anticoagulant added, the blood cells centrifuged off and the degree of dilution of the blue determined by reference to standard dilution in a colorimeter. In man it is found that the blood volume is about 70–100 ml. per kilo or 1/11th of the body weight or about 6 litres in the average adult. Of this about 600 ml. can be removed with safety.

The total water in the body is estimated on the same principle by injecting D_2O (heavy water) which distributes itself throughout the whole body while the *extracellular* water may be obtained by injecting a substance such as inulin which will pass through the capillaries but not enter cells. Subtraction gives the *intracellular* water.

Blood Groups

In patients who have suffered a severe haemorrhage a transfusion of blood from a normal healthy individual has been found most efficacious. It is known, however, that the blood of different people is not necessarily compatible. Precautions, therefore, have to be taken in order to prevent the mixing of incompatible blood, which would have most serious results. The red blood cells of the donor are tested against the plasma of the recipient to make sure that no agglutination (clumping together of the cells) will occur. According to the behaviour of these cells when tested in this way, people are divided into four blood groups usually called AB, A, B, and O. It has been found that cells in group O are not agglutinated by any type of plasma. People whose cells are in this group are therefore known as "universal donors."

Blood Clotting

Blood plasma has the peculiar property of clotting when it comes in contact with the juices of damaged tissues or blood platelets, both of which contain the enzyme *thrombokinase*. This substance, which is not normally in contact with the blood plasma, initiates the clotting process. *Prothrombin* and *calcium*, which are normal constituents of the plasma, in the presence of thrombokinase are necessary for the first stage of clotting by converting prothrombin into *thrombin*. The latter substance then combines with *fibrinogen* which is one of the plasma proteins, converting it into *fibrin*. Fibrin consists of masses of web-like threads which entangle the red blood corpuscles in a jellified clot. For the production of the essential prothrombin by the liver, vitamin K is essential.

If the calcium is put out of action, e.g., by adding sodium citrate, the blood does not clot and use is made of this in blood transfusions. Various other substances, such as leech extract and heparin, may also be used to prevent clotting.

All these facts of blood clotting are based on strict experimental evidence, but there is considerable controversy as to how the blood is kept from clotting in the body. Some hold that a very active anticoagulant *heparin* or *anti prothrombin* which is produced by mast cells and may be extracted from the liver and especially from the lungs, is normally present in the circulation and is rendered inactive by the thrombokinase.

The clotting of blood may be hastened by increasing the surface wetted by applying cotton wool which soaks up the blood. Heat also reduces the time required for clotting, thus the local application of *hot* water is of great value in the arrest of haemorrhage.

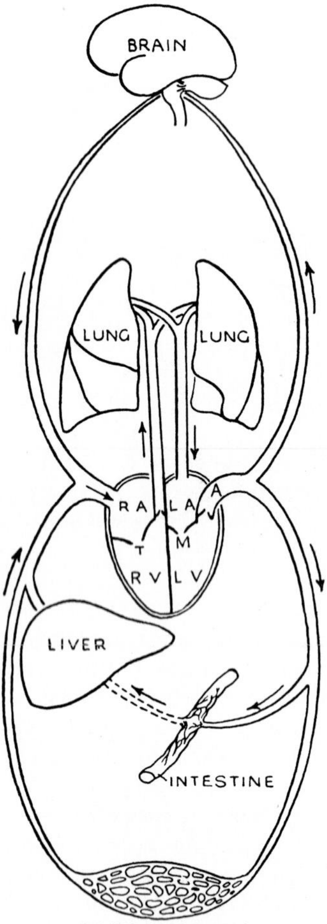

Clotting is facilitated if the flow of blood is slowed or arrested. Fortunately, the nature of the injury commonly causes the severed blood vessels to contract. Further contraction may be produced by the use of astringents such as alum or dilute ferric chloride, or by other substances which act on the vessel walls, e.g., adrenaline or ephedrine. Contraction of the vessels may also be brought about by the application of cold to *another* part of the body. Thus bleeding from the nose may be benefited by the application of cold to the back of the neck.

Commonly, pressure applied to the bleeding point by causing stasis (standing) of the blood at the site of the injury is also of advantage as it gives time for a clot to form at the openings of the severed vessels. When arterial bleeding is severe or where large areas are involved, the pressure is best applied to the main artery supplying the part at the pressure point, in which case the vessel is compressed against the underlying bone.

Substitutes for Blood are considered on p. 378.

THE CIRCULATION OF THE BLOOD

Arteries pass to all parts of the body supplying the tissue cells with blood in which oxygen and nourishment is carried. The tissue cells are constantly removing these substances from the blood and giving up carbon dioxide and waste products which are then returned to the heart by *veins*.

FIG. 282.—A scheme of the circulation.

RA, right atrium; LA, left atrium RV, right ventricle; LV, left ventricle T, tricuspid valve; M, mitral valve; A, aorta.

The actual transfer of substances from the blood to the tissues takes place in the thin walled *capillaries*, which link the arteries with the veins. The capillaries can be observed only with the aid of a microscope and it is seen that in them the blood cells move in a steady stream and in single file. On the arterial side of the capillaries are the very muscular *arterioles* which play such an important part in controlling the blood pressure and the blood flow; on the venous side are the *venules*.

The Heart is the central pump which is responsible for the circulation of the blood.   It is a hollow muscular organ, composed of cardiac muscle which has the special property of rhythmic contraction and relaxation known as "beating."   The heart is constantly receiving blood from the veins and pumping it round the body via the arteries.

The circulation of the blood is, however, complicated by the necessity for the blood to be purified in the lungs (reloaded with oxygen and relieved of carbon dioxide) before it can be of use to the body.   The heart is so designed that it sends oxygenated blood to all parts of the body except the lungs; and the so-called deoxygenated blood to the lungs only; the circulation is, therefore, a double one.   The two parts of the circulation are the *pulmonary* and *systemic*.   The right chambers of the heart receive venous blood and send it to the lungs; the left chambers receive arterial blood from the lungs and send it round the body.

It will be seen (fig. 282) that venous blood arriving at the heart from the body passes into the *right atrium*; before it can again be sent to the body it

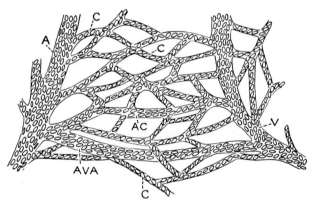

Fig. 283.—A capillary network.

A, arteriole; C, capillary; AC, arterial capillary; AVA, arterio-venous anastomosis; V, venule.

must go to the *right ventricle*, then to the *lungs* by the pulmonary artery, whence it is returned to the *left atrium* of the heart by the pulmonary veins; from the left atrium it passes to the *left ventricle* and from here it passes into the general circulation via the aorta.

The cardiac cycle

The series of changes which the heart undergoes constitute the *cardiac cycle* and the student should not confuse this with the course of the circulation.   These changes consist of a series of contractions and relaxations, contraction being known as *systole* and relaxation as *diastole*.

The contraction of the two atria takes place simultaneously and is known as *atrial systole*, this is followed by the simultaneous contraction of the two ventricles and is known as *ventricular systole*.   After each systole the atria and ventricles relax and go into diastole in the same order, thus we speak of *atrial diastole* and *ventricular diastole*.   The atrial diastole commences before ventricular systole is completed and is followed by ventricular diastole. The cycle commences again with atrial systole.

The average heart contracts 72 times per minute, each cycle will occupy therefore 0·8 of a second. This may be accounted for approximately as follows:

atrial systole 0·05 sec. + atrial diastole 0·75 sec. = 0·8 sec.
ventricular systole 0·3 sec. + ventricular diastole 0·5 sec. = 0·8 sec.

If the speed of the heart is quickened, the time occupied by each cycle is diminished, but the diminution affects chiefly the diastole. The filling of the heart and the phases of the cycle will now be studied in more detail, and

EVENTS OF THE CARDIAC CYCLE

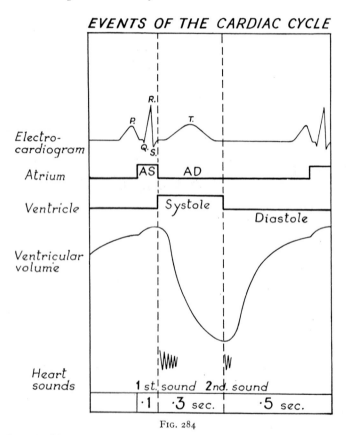

FIG. 284

The student should note:

1. That the electrical change precedes the contraction.
2. That atrial contraction is very short.
3. That the filling of the ventricle is most rapid in the first third of diastole.
4. That for a fraction of a second the ventricle although contracting does not diminish in size because the pressure inside it is not sufficient to open the aortic valve.

The volume of the ventricle is taken by placing it in an air-tight chamber (cardiometer) connected with a rapidly moving photographic recorder.

For an explanation of the electro-cardiogram see p. 361.

in this connection it must be noted that the atria are much smaller than the ventricles.

Atrial diastole. During this stage the blood from the veins is flowing into the atria, for although the pressure in the veins is low it is greater than that in the empty atria. As the atria fill, their walls expand. When the pressure in the atria exceeds that in the ventricles i.e. at the beginning of ventricular diastole, the atrioventricular valves open and the blood passes into the ventricles.

Atrial systole. The atria now fill a second time and then contract and empty their contents into the ventricles which are already full. Contraction commences at the junction of the large veins with the right atrium and is propagated towards the atrio-ventricular opening and by this means regurgitation into the veins is prevented.

Ventricular diastole. During the latter part of atrial diastole and the whole of atrial systole, the ventricles are relaxed and are then filled with blood. The ventricles dilate under the pressure of the venous blood.

Ventricular systole. The contraction of the ventricles is more prolonged than the contraction of the atria. When it occurs the atrioventricular valves close, thus preventing regurgitation into the atria and when the pressure in the ventricles exceeds that in the large arteries which emerge from them, the semilunar valves open and the blood is pumped into the aorta from the left ventricle and into the pulmonary artery from the right ventricle. During rest the ventricles do not empty completely but during exercise they do.

It should be emphasised that the ventricles are filled by the pressure of blood in the veins and that the blood ejected from the atria during atrial systole causes slight additional distension of the ventricles. The atria are not therefore essential for ventricular filling but are important accessory factors. In a certain type of heart disease known as auricular fibrillation the atria do not contract rhythmically and so the filling of the ventricles depends solely on the venous pressure. It is important to realise that the main filling of the ventricles takes place in the first third of ventricular diastole. The cusps of the atrioventricular valves are lifted up by the pressure of blood in the ventricles and their margins interdigitate, being held taut in this position by the chordae tendineae which are themselves tightened by the simultaneous contraction of the papillary muscles to which they are attached. This arrangement also prevents the cusps from being ballooned into the atria during ventricular systole.

The first result of ventricular systole is, as we have said, the closure of the atrioventricular valves and in this way intraventricular pressure rises. When the heart has emptied itself, the ventricles relax and the semilunar valves close because of eddies set up behind them by the outrushing blood.

Heart Sounds. When a stethoscope or even the ear is placed over the region of the heart two sounds can be heard in quick succession followed by a pause. The heart sounds are often compared to the syllables lubb-dupp. The *first sound* is due to the muscular contraction of the heart and the closure of the atrioventricular valves and coincides with the impact of the heart against the chest wall. It lasts during the greater part of ventricular systole and it just precedes the pulse at the wrist. The *second sound* is due to the closure of the aortic and pulmonary valves and is shorter and sharper. It marks the end of ventricular systole and it follows the radial pulse. The impact of the apex of the heart against the chest wall is called *the apex beat* and this is normally felt in the fifth intercostal space, three and a half inches from the mid-line. It is due to ventricular systole causing a rise of pressure in the aorta so that the vessel tends to straighten and this presses the heart firmly against the chest wall.

The Properties of Cardiac muscle

When considering the properties of cardiac muscle, it is important to bear in mind that its unique feature is that it is a syncytium. This factor accounts for most of its properties which may be seen if a strip of cardiac muscle is attached to a lever and stimulated. They are as follows:

A fundamental property of cardiac muscle is that it exhibits the phenomenon of *rhythmicity*. The isolated heart which is not under the control of the central nervous system can be made to contract both spontaneously and rhythmically. That this property is inherent in heart muscle is shown by the fact that a single muscle cell which has been grown outside the body in tissue culture exhibits the same phenomenon.

Cardiac muscle exhibits the "*all or none*" *law*, which means that a stimulus strong enough to produce a contraction produces a maximum contraction. Thus the amount of contraction does not vary with the strength of the stimulus for if the muscle contracts at all it does so to the limit of its capacity.

Heart muscle also exhibits the *staircase phenomenon*. Like muscle generally, heart muscle requires to be "warmed up" before it can become fully effective, a factor which is dependent not only on an increase of temperature but also to the beneficial effect of the metabolites produced. To demonstrate this, a heart is stopped and then stimulated artificially a number of times with the same strength of stimulus. It will be observed that the first few contractions increase in size and when recorded on a drum it produces a staircase effect.

Heart muscle exhibits a *refractory period*, which means that after the application of a stimulus, a second stimulus will not cause a further contraction until after the initial contraction is completed and it is for this reason that heart muscle cannot normally be tetanised. If the heart is stimulated during systole it therefore has no effect, but if the stimulus is applied during diastole an *extra systole* is produced. If the normal stimulus from the atrium reaches the ventricle during this extra systole, it produces no effect and the heart appears to have missed a beat and this is known as the *compensatory pause*. This refractory period gives the heart an intermittent rest and makes it possible for the organ to continue to contract throughout our lives.

Like all other muscles, that of the heart has the very important power of contracting more forcibly when stretched. This confers on the heart its power of expelling blood according to the amount it contains (see Starling's Law of the Heart).

The origin and conduction of the cardiac impulse

An individual heart cell has the power of inherent rhythmicity, even when removed from the body. This appears to be due to a build up of potassium inside the cell and the extrusion of sodium. In this way the cell becomes charged and when the difference of potential is large enough there is an electrical discharge and the cell contracts.

In the mammalian heart this rhythmicity is developed in a group of specialised cells in the right atrium near the entrance of the great veins. This is known as *the sino-auricular node or pace-maker.*

From the pace-maker the impulse spreads out fan-wise over the atria and causes them to contract. It then passes to a similar neuro-muscular area known as *atrio-ventricular nodes* where starts a specialised bundle of conducting tissues called the *atrio-ventricularbundle of His*. This conducts the impulse to the Purkinje tissue which lies just under the endothelial lining of the heart and is distributed especially to the papillary muscles. This tissue conducts the impulse five times more rapidly than ordinary cardiac muscle and ensures that the impulses reach all parts of the ventricles almost simultaneously, while the early contraction of the papillary muscles supports the atrio-ventricular valves as soon as the ventricles contract.

The Electrocardiogram

The electrical changes are recorded in man by attaching electrodes to the hands or feet or by placing them on the chest. The impulse of the pacemaker is known as the P wave, Q is associated with the contraction of the papillary muscles and the complex RST is associated with the contraction of the ventricles (fig. 284). The electrocardiogram is an important aid in diagnosing heart disease. The T wave may be reversed in coronary thrombosis.

The nourishment of the heart and of tissues generally

The heart is, as we have seen, composed of cells linked together into a muscular mass which beats as a whole.

All large masses of cells must therefore have an efficient blood supply to carry oxygen and nourishment and to provide for excretion. In the case of the frog, they manage to seep through from the blood in the interior of the heart, but in higher animals a separate series of blood-vessels called the *coronary vessels* supply the organs.

By passing blood or other nutrient fluid into these vessels it is possible to keep even the heart of a mammal alive for several days after removal from the body. In this way the optimum conditions and the composition of the nutrient fluids essential for the normal contraction of the heart have been ascertained. It has been found, for example, that the mammalian heart beats well on the artificial nutrient solution known as *Ringer-Locke fluid* containing sodium chloride 0·9 per cent. together with traces of calcium chloride which is essential for its contraction, and potassium chloride which is needed for its dilatation. The fluid must also be made slightly alkaline with sodium bicarbonate, warmed to body temperature and supplied at sufficient pressure to force it through the coronary vessels. Normally this pressure is supplied by the blood pressure.   If it is desired to keep the heart beating for more than a very few hours some form of fuel must be provided and the whole procedure carried out under aseptic conditions.

Most of the tissues of the body can be kept alive if the same principles are applied and so may most plants.   An apple-tree planted in minute glass beads will not only live but bear fruit if it is supplied with such a solution together with nitrogenous material from which it can build up its body substance of protein.

The body possesses a large number of mechanisms which keep the composition of the tissue fluid almost constant (see p. 374 et seq).

Most hearts eventually stop at death because of oxygen deficiency from failure of respiration or from a decreased pressure in the coronary arteries. More rarely they fail from weakness of the muscle from other causes such as the poisoning which occurs in the severe infections and incompetency of the valves.

The pulse

The pulse is defined as the response of the arterial wall to the changes in lateral pressure caused by the heart.   At each beat of the heart a pulse wave is set up in the blood in the same way as a wave is set up in a pond if a stone be thrown into it.   It travels at the rate of about 7 metres per second to the more distant vessels and is, therefore, felt in the carotid arteries appreciably before it is felt in the radial artery at the wrist.

It is at the wrist that the pulse is most conveniently taken and from it information can be obtained regarding the following points:

Its *rate*, in the absence of rare diseases, usually indicates the rate of the heart and may vary from 50 to 80 beats per minute in the normal adult. An increase usually indicates an infection but is normal in mental excitement and physical exercise.

Its *rhythm* and regular beat indicate the regularity with which the contractions of the left ventricle are taking place.

Its *force* and *fullness* indicate the force of the heart and give some idea of the amount of blood which is being pumped out per beat.

Its tension, i.e., the force necessary to obliterate it.

The *condition of the vessel wall* (e.g., thickening or otherwise) should also be noted.

Graphic records of the pulse may be taken with a suitable apparatus (the sphygmograph) but this is becoming obsolete since it is difficult to use and more accurate methods are now available for studying the limited facts obtained.

Frequency of the heart.   This is indicated normally by the frequency of the pulse and varies very much even in health.   The average heart rate in the resting adult is about 72 per minute but it increases in the erect posture, in mental excitement, in exercise and in raised body temperature (fever).   It is highest in the late afternoon when body temperature tends to increase. Individuals in good physical training have a very slow heart as have individuals with deficient thyroid activity.   Abnormally high resting rates are found in thyroid excess and in some varieties of heart failure. At birth the pulse rate varies between 120/140. In animals other than man it may be stated generally that the smaller the animal the more rapid the heart rate since the metabolic rate in small animals is much greater than that in large ones.

The arterial blood pressure

The blood is circulated through the body at a considerable pressure which is maintained by the combined action of the heart and blood vessels. This blood pressure as we have just seen is necessary for the maintenance of the activity of the heart itself.

At each beat of the heart more blood is forced into the arteries than escapes into the capillaries during the contraction. The arteries which are elastic are thereby distended. When, therefore, the heart is filling, the blood pressure does not have time to fall to zero but is maintained to some extent by the recoil of the arteries. This produces the *diastolic pressure* which is about 80 millimetres of mercury in a normal young adult. The pressure during the contraction of the heart is known as the *systolic pressure* and is about 110–120 millimetres of mercury in the resting subject. The difference between the diastolic and systolic pressures is known as the *pulse pressure* and is normally about 40 mm. of mercury.

In man the systolic pressure is taken by applying an inflatable bag to the arm and ascertaining the pressure which is just sufficient to obliterate the pulse. This may be felt at the wrist or heard at the bend of the elbow. The apparatus is shown in fig. 285, and students should be familiar with its use.

The arterial blood pressure is maintained by three factors:
  (i) the output of the heart;
  (ii) the peripheral resistance to the blood flow put up by the smaller vessels;
  (iii) the elasticity of the vessel walls.
The part played by the viscosity of the blood is small.

The output of the heart depends on the strength of the contraction of the cardiac muscle. This depends on the amount of blood reaching the heart. Thus the blood pressure falls if the heart muscle fails or if there is a reduction in blood volume such as occurs after severe haemorrhage.

A fall of blood pressure will also occur if the smaller blood vessels, especially the arterioles, which normally resist the flow of blood, are opened up. This occurs in the common faint when the brain fails to keep the peripheral blood vessels in their normal state of tonic contraction. A rise of blood pressure on the other hand is produced by vasoconstriction. It occurs normally and temporarily in emotion and exercise when there is an increased output of the heart in combination with a constriction of the blood vessels, especially of the skin and splanchnic area.

In advanced age the arterioles become less elastic and the blood pressure tends to rise, but the whole picture of high blood pressure in apparently healthy people is not fully understood.

Many of the facts can be appreciated by simple experiments with the well-known wartime "stirrup pump," the extent of the stroke being considered comparable to the filling of the heart, the nozzle, to the resistance, and the distance the water is thrown by the jet, to the blood pressure.

The special importance of high blood pressure is that the heart has much more work to do in forcing the blood into the aorta and may fail in so doing. Also this raised pressure may cause some of the more fragile vessels, especially those of the brain, to burst resulting in a cerebral haemorrhage and sudden death.

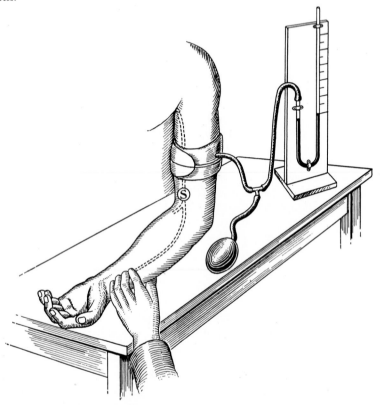

Fig. 285.—Apparatus for recording the blood pressure (Sphygmomanometer). The subject's hand is best supported by a table to promote relaxation of muscles. The stethoscope is applied at S. The pressure on the arm cuff is raised by rhythmically compressing the bulb and is shown on the manometer.

The Venous blood pressure.

The pressure of the blood in the veins is very low compared with that in the arteries. Indeed in the veins of the head and neck it is negative when the subject is in the erect posture. The blood in the veins of the lower limbs as would be expected is much higher in persons whose occupation prevents them from sitting, the veins may become distended and the valves within them cease to be patent. This is the explanation of varicose veins. In heart failure there is a marked increase in venous pressure (see also the effects of gravity on the circulation, p. 371).

THE CONTROL OF THE CIRCULATION AND BLOOD VESSELS

The circulation of the blood is so controlled that it can increase the amount of blood to those parts of the body which are most active. The whole mechanism is subordinated to the needs of the voluntary muscles. It can also compensate for a considerable loss of blood and adapt itself to changes in the posture of the body. The changes during activity are brought about in two ways: by raising the blood pressure, and by opening up the blood vessels in the active part at the same time. The latter process is facilitated and increased by massage but is normally due to chemical and nervous mechanisms.

The control of the blood vessels

Chemical mechanisms.   When a muscle contracts a number of chemical substances are produced which are very active dilators of capillaries. The most important are carbon dioxide, lactic acid and possibly histamine. It should be noted that these substances are produced outside the capillaries, but as these vessels have very thin walls they penetrate easily and are carried away by the blood into the general circulation to be destroyed or excreted. The fact that these substances are dilators can be seen under the microscope if they are applied in very dilute solution to capillaries. They can also be seen to open up the blood vessels in the limb of an animal if they are added to the blood passed through the limb even when it has been removed from the body.

Some idea of this dilatation is also obtained by simply tying a piece of string round a finger for a few minutes. When the circulation through the finger is thus stopped the chemical substances produced by the tissues accumulate, for all living tissues are constantly producing such substances in very minute quantities even when they are not specially active. When the ligature is removed from the finger it will be seen to flush because of the greater amount of blood which is present in the dilated capillaries of the skin. This is known as *reactive hyperaemia*. This simple method of temporarily increasing the blood flow through a part has been used in surgery (Bier's method) to hasten repair but is not very popular because it demands more co-operation by the patient than is usually possible. It should be emphasised that the constriction must not be applied too long since it cuts down the oxygen supply to the part.

When a muscle contracts the heat produced also brings about the relaxation of the muscular walls of the blood vessels. This is the basis of many methods of producing heat artificially in the tissues, e.g., by short-wave therapy, infra-red rays and by the direct application of heat. A hot-water bottle is a most effective means of producing a vasodilatation.

Nervous mechanisms.   The blood vessels are also under nervous control. This is of two kinds, vasodilator and vasoconstrictor, of which the latter is probably the more important in most parts of the body. Vasodilator and vasoconstrictor fibres are incorporated in the sympathetic nervous system (p. 225). *Vasoconstrictor fibres* arise in the medulla of the brain, pass down the spinal cord and eventually pass out in the anterior nerve roots to the sympathetic chain where there is usually a relay and are distributed with the ordinary motor nerves so ending as plexuses around the vessels.　These fibres conduct impulses which keep the blood vessels in a state of partial contraction or tone.　This we know because there is a dilatation of blood vessels if the appropriate nerve supply to any part of the body is cut.　Thus if the nerve supply to a limb is cut there is at once a flushing of the skin of the part. This operation which has often been done in man to relieve spasm of vessels also shows that the vasoconstrictor nerves exercise a tonic control over the blood vessels, i.e., are constantly sending out nerve impulses which keep the blood vessels partially constricted.　The vasoconstrictor nerves act by liberating an adrenaline-like substance probably nor-adrenaline at their nerve endings.

The practical importance of the vasoconstrictor nerves is that they reduce the capacity of the circulation when blood is lost or by varying the peripheral resistance bring about a redistribution of the blood when it is needed in any specially active organs such as the muscles in exercise.　They are chiefly responsible for the raised blood pressure during mental excitement and exercise, which is considered in a separate section.　They are of the greatest importance in the maintenance of the blood pressure in response to change of position and haemorrhage.

All the vasoconstrictor nerves are under the control of a *vasoconstrictor centre* in the medulla and if this is put out of action a fall of the blood pressure at once occurs.　This may occur if there is over-ventilation of the lungs. because carbon dioxide is essential for its action, and this is the great disadvantage of breathing exercises which are not accompanied by muscular exercise.　The vasoconstrictor centre may fail for psychological reasons, producing the ordinary faint.

It is now known that there is a separate sympathetic vasodilator system. The *vasodilator fibres* have the same course as the vasoconstrictor fibres. They originate in the cerebral cortex and appear to be especially concerned with dilatation of the active muscles in exercise.

There is good evidence that the stimulation of posterior spinal roots or sensory nerves bring about vasodilatation—possibly by releasing histamine or acetylcholine at their endings.　Such stimulation is responsible for several important reactions.　If the skin of an area is irritated it becomes red as the result of what is known as an *axon reflex*　It is known that nerves are involved in this reaction because it is very markedly reduced if the nerves have been cut and allowed to degenerate.　This was observed in patients in whom the 5th nerve had been cut for neuralgia.　The importance of this observation lies in the fact that it explains the action of counter-irritants, such as mustard and of turpentine, the common ingredients of liniments, while researches have shown that there may be a dilatation not only of the skin vessels but of those of the underlying tissues.　The flushing of the part with blood is beneficial to healing.　In this connection it may be noted that the blood flow through the superficial tissues of the body at rest, especially in the limbs, is insufficient to keep them at normal body temperature. They may be several degrees lower.

A peculiar characteristic of the vasodilator fibres is that they react to electrical stimulation differently from the vasoconstrictor nerves. Thus if the sciatic nerve, which contains both constrictor and dilator nerves, is stimulated with a faradic current alternating at over 50 times per second, vasoconstriction is produced, but if galvanic stimuli at the rate of 1–5 per second or mechanical stimulation such as tapping is used there is vasodilatation. Why different kinds of electric currents have such reverse effects has not been satisfactorily explained, at least the evidence is very contradictory.

There are two chief possibilities: the different nerves may have different excitabilities or the different stimuli may produce amounts of some substance or mixture of substances (e.g., acetylcholine and adrenaline) which act differently according to their concentration. It is unfortunate that we should have so little information on these points upon which so much electrotherapy is based. The important fact, however, is that the faradic current produces a tetanus if applied to the leg and thus liberates more chemical substances than the galvanic current. Surges or bursts of faradic current applied directly to the muscle causing it to contract are on the whole most effective in producing maximal dilatation, but normal exercise, when possible, is more effective than either, because it involves also a psychic factor which raises the blood pressure at the same time. In some circumstances normal exercise is impossible because of pain or excessive fatigue while in other cases it cannot be carried out because of nerve injury.

The output of the heart

The efficiency of the heart may be gauged by measuring its output, but unfortunately there is no easy way of doing this in man. The most accurate method is to pass a tube down a large vein to the right atrium to obtain a sample of the mixed venous blood. Then the oxygen content of this is compared with a sample of blood taken from an artery. If at the same time we find the amount of oxygen taken up by the lungs per minute and from the samples we know the amount taken up by each c.c. of blood we can easily calculate the number of c.c. of blood which must have passed through the lungs in the same time.

At rest this is about 4 to 5 litres* but in exercise this may be increased enormously—in the average individual to about 15 litres or 3 gallons per minute. In athletes it has been calculated that it reaches 30 litres or 6 gallons per minute, a most remarkable performance for such a small organ.

The heart increases its output in three ways, by contracting more forcibly and thereby emptying itself more completely, by increasing its output per beat and by increasing its rate. The increased force and rate are brought about by the sympathetic, which is still further augmented by the effect of

*1 litre = 1·75 pints

increased filling of the heart; indeed until comparatively recently this was considered to be the chief factor in promoting an increased output.

Any increase in the volume of the blood returning to the heart causes a stretching of its muscular walls, and since heart muscle responds in a similar manner to muscle generally, it follows that the greater the filling the more forcibly will the heart contract. This is known as *Starling's law of the heart*. It will of course be realised that in whatever way the heart increases its output it can only do so if at the same time it receives more blood, such as happens in exercise.

The control of the heart

The rate of the heart is governed by a neuro-muscular area known as the *sino-atrial node* or *pace-maker* in the atrium near the entrance of the great veins. It is also extremely sensitive to changes in temperature; indeed it was by applying a warmed glass rod to different parts of the heart that this sensitive area was discovered. An acceleration of the heart in a resting person is commonly associated with raised body temperature.

The heart rate is controlled by the sympathetic which accelerates and the parasympathetic which retards its action. Both sets of nerves act on the pace-maker like governors and are constantly active. But for the action of the vagus (parasympathetic), the heart would beat very much faster during rest. Normally these nerves do not, as might appear at first sight, act in opposition. They should be regarded as collaborators, for when sympathetic activity is increased that of the parasympathetic is decreased. This occurs in states of mental excitement and physical activity. It can be shown that most of the increased heart rate in exercise is really due to the mental state, although increased venous pressure in the right atrium causes the heart to accelerate. This is known as *Bainbridge's reflex* or the right atrial reflex, by which impulses are sent up the vagi to the medulla depressing the cardio-inhibitory centre and stimulating the cardio-accelerator centre so that the heart rate increases.

The range of the change in the heart rate during exercise is an important factor in determining the efficiency of the circulation. Individuals in good physical training have slower hearts than sedentary persons. Long-distance runners and especially swimmers may have very slow hearts; rates less than 40 per minute have been reported. The injection of atropine shows that the slowing is due to increased action of the vagus nerves. These facts are important as they emphasise that a heart rate of 72 may be fast for a subject in training. They will be referred to again in relation to exercise (see After-effects of Exercise).

This vagus activity and slowing of the heart depends on the increased development of what are known as the *depressor reflexes*. At each beat of the heart, nerve impulses pass up the glossopharyngeal and aortic depressor nerves (which run in the vagus) to the vagal nucleus in the medulla, from the carotid sinus at the bifurcation of the carotid arteries, from the arch of the aorta and from the left side of the heart. These impulses continually stimulate the vagal nucleus which in turn sends down the vagus nerve impulses having a continuous restraining influence on the heart. At the same time the impulses inhibit the sympathetic centre. These depressor reflexes have a twofold action. During rest they restrain the heart, and thus give it a greater range of activity during exercise. Also by inhibiting the activity of the vasomotor centre, they keep the blood vessels and blood depots dilated, and in this way make available a large amount of blood for the active muscles.

In exercise the depressor reflexes are themselves inhibited chiefly by impulses from the cerebrum with the result that the blood vessels and blood depots constrict, throwing more blood into the active circulation and increasing the venous return to the heart while at the same time the vagus restraint of the heart is reduced and the heart beats faster.

At rest the depressor reflexes are also responsible for maintaining the blood pressure at a constant level. In this way the capillary pressure is kept constant and filtration through the capillary walls does not vary, but anything which tends to raise the blood pressure (except emotion and exercise) slows the heart. The action of the depressor reflexes keeps a large volume of blood especially in the skin and splanchnic area which is immediately available for exercise. Rest in bed causes these reflexes to fall into disuse with the resultant fall in blood volume.

There is good evidence for suggesting that on these depressor reflexes depend many of the beneficial effects of exercise generally, for the vagus controls digestion and many other activities.

The efficiency of the circulation

On the capability of the circulation to carry out its functions man's capacity for work depends and the efficiency of the circulation is, therefore, of considerable importance in convalescence from disease or injury. As has just been said the circulation may, like the neuromuscular system generally, become inefficient from lack of movement which may result from confinement to bed or as a result of disease or therapeutics involving the heart itself or the control of the circulation. Many of the fevers cause impairment in this way and a valuable therapeutic agent such as emetine, used for the treatment of tropical amoebic dysentery may do likewise, temporarily.

Many attempts have been made to arrive at some standard by which the efficiency of the circulation may be measured, since failure of the circulation, especially of the heart, is a common concomitant of disease and limits capability for physical work. The difficulty is that muscular capability varies very much, and what may be strenuous exercise to one subject may be negligible to another. All such tests attempt to ascertain the tolerance of the heart to effort.

The effort tolerance test consists of stepping on and off a stool 18½ in. high 5 times in 15 seconds and recording the time taken for the pulse to return to normal. This mild exercise causes a moderate rise in the heart rate but there is a rapid return to normal.

If the heart does not return to normal in one minute (i.e. does not get rid of the increased venous pressure) it is probably inefficient. In all such tests it is essential that the subject should be at physical and mental rest before commencing the test.

The forty-millimetre test.   In the Royal Air Force the 40-mm. test is used. In this test the subject after a deep breath blows (with his nose clipped) into a mercury manometer and maintains its level at 40 mm.   A fit subject should maintain this pressure for 52 seconds and show no change in blood-pressure or heart rate until he reaches "breaking point."   The test is purely arbitrary and is somewhat difficult to analyse, as it involves respiratory acid-base and mental as well as circulatory considerations.

The response to posture may also be taken as an indication of circulatory efficiency.   The more efficient the circulation the less is the increase of the heart rate when a recumbent subject assumes the erect posture.   In efficient persons the heart rate does not increase on standing nor should there be any fall of arterial pressure, indeed there is commonly a rise of 5–10 mm. of mercury.   The test has been elaborated by Crampton in America who devised a scale by which an efficiency index was arrived at.

Turner has elaborated the test still further and in arriving at an index takes into consideration the reclining pulse rate, the pulse pressure, the diastolic pressure, and the effect of prolonged *quiet* standing (15 minutes).

The oxygen consumption test.   This test has not been much used, but it would seem that it is probably the best test in fit persons—in whom the oxygen-uptake should reach 2,000 c.c. per minute in exercise, but may actually reach 5,000 c.c.   It is a combined test for the haemo-respiratory system.

All such tests may be supplemented by noting the effect of a moderate exercise on respiration and the sensations of the subject generally.

The relation of the circulation to the needs of a tissue.

The control of the circulation which has just been described makes possible, as we have seen, an increased supply of blood and of oxygen to an active part, and this relationship between activity and blood supply is essential to the health of any organ or part of the body.   If this fails pain is produced and the tissue may die.   Thus a patient who lies too long in one position may develop areas of dead skin, bed sores or even gangrene, as the result of a diminished blood supply.   This reduction of the blood supply to a part may be caused by injury, compression or disease.   Compression may result from too tight bandaging or splinting of a limb.   Fortunately the discomfort which such procedure produces acts as a warning, but in stoical patients or patients who are anaesthetised or who have sensory nerves "destroyed" by the injury, the danger of producing permanent damage in this way is very real and can only be avoided by care in observing, when possible, the colour and temperature of the part.   When splinting a limb it is always as well to test the pulse to the part as a final precautionary measure.   It is quite remarkable, however, the extent to which a limb may recover from blockage or damage even to its main artery, provided the vessels are healthy and no attempt is made at too early a stage to use or stimulate the muscles.   Anastomatic vessels rapidly open up which by-pass the block and supply the limb with a normal amount of blood.   Thus the subscapular artery may take the place of the axillary (collateral circulation).

When a muscle is deprived of blood and continues to work it becomes very painful as the result of the accumulation of chemical substances or P-(pain) substance which stimulate the nerve endings. The intense pain of angina pectoris is produced in this way. This occurs when the coronary arteries of the heart become occluded by an embolism (clot) or by spasm of their walls. Cramp in the limbs is similarly produced and may be imitated by exercising the hand while the circulation is occluded in the upper arm.

The Return of Blood to the Heart. It should be realised that in man, except when he is lying down, the blood from the lower half of the body is returned to the heart against gravity. Many factors are concerned with this phenomenon. In the first place the arterial pressure behind the venous stream is an important factor, but this is insufficient to return the blood from the lower limbs in the erect posture. The return of the blood is also greatly facilitated by muscular contraction by which the capillaries and veins are compressed. The dilatation of the capillaries due to nervous impulses and metabolites permits a more rapid flow of blood from the arteries to the veins between the contractions.

In standing the pressure in the veins on the dorsum of the foot is between 80/90 mm. Hg and it has been estimated by Lewis that the taking of a few steps reduces the pressure by nearly half. Thus standing tends to produce a stagnation of blood in the lower extremities and prolonged standing is an accessory factor in the production of varicose veins and swelling of the feet.

The return of the blood to the heart is greatly facilitated by respiration and so the diaphragm has been termed the *respiratory pump*. The pressure in the chest is normally negative. At inspiration this negative pressure is increased as is the positive pressure in the abdomen. The negative pressure in the thorax tends to suck the blood into it and the positive pressure in the abdomen drives the blood out of that cavity and into the thorax. The reverse does not occur during expiration because the blood is trapped in the lungs by the pulmonary valve. In expiration extra blood is driven into the left side of the heart and so to the aorta. The action of the respiratory pump is greatly increased with increased respiration during exercise. The valves in the veins of the limbs are an accessory factor in facilitating the return of blood to the heart for they prevent regurgitation.

The effect of gravity on the circulation

The liability of patients to faint or feel giddy when they assume the erect posture is well known and is of special importance to physiotherapists, as this is especially liable to occur when patients have been exposed to heat of various kinds or after illness. The cause of this is fundamentally mechanical.

The blood vessels are a system of tubes and if any such system is held erect blood tends to accumulate in the dependent parts. This is particularly well seen in the snake and the eel or even a tame rabbit. If they are held erect for a few minutes they rapidly become unconscious and may even die. If this is done in anaesthetised animals it is seen that their hearts do not fill adequately in the erect position and the blood pressure falls. This does not normally occur in man because the fall of blood pressure at once causes the vasoconstrictor centre in the brain to bring about constriction of the blood vessels throughout the body but especially those of the abdominal organs and the skin. At the same time there is an increased heart rate and an increased respiration which sucks more blood into the chest at inspiration where it is trapped in the lungs by the pulmonary valves. In a healthy person the compensation is commonly so good that the blood pressure may be actually higher in the erect posture than when prone. If, however, the patient's skin vessels are dilated by the application of heat, then the normal compensation is interfered with. It is liable to occur also in those who have been confined to bed for some time and whose vasomotor systems have become inefficient through disuse after surgical operations or after infections, notably influenza which poisons the system. These facts emphasise the importance of prescribing suitable exercise for convalescent patients, for this sluggish response of the vasomotor centre is in part responsible for the sense of fatigue and weakness experienced after illness.

Haemorrhage and its natural arrest

When a blood vessel is opened the body loses blood in greater or less amount according to the size of the vessel, unless steps are taken to prevent it. There are, however, many reactions designed to prevent excessive loss of blood which would of course be fatal. First, the mechanical damage to the blood vessel causes it to contract, its lumen is diminished while at the same time it retracts and shortens. In a matter of a few minutes the blood begins to clot (see p. 355) and the opening in the blood vessel is blocked. Vasomotor reactions occur in response to the fall in blood pressure, for the vasomotor centre is activated and this sends out impulses to the blood vessels all over the body causing them to contract. This is particularly noticeable in the skin which thereby becomes pale. At the same time the sympathetic is stimulated and the heart rate increases causing the blood to be pumped round more rapidly. There is an increased respiration which further facilitates the return of blood to the heart.

A greatly increased heart rate associated with intense pallor is therefore a most important sign in the diagnosis of internal haemorrhage.

After moderate haemorrhage the blood, or more especially the circulating blood volume rapidly returns to normal. At least a pint of blood is held in reserve in the blood depots (*q.v.*) and this is squeezed by the contracting vessels and spleen into the general circulation. As a result of the fall of blood pressure in the capillaries, fluid is transferred from the tissue spaces to the blood vessels—a reverse process to the formation of tissue fluid and lymph—while at the same time the bone-marrow accelerates the manufacture of red blood corpuscles and the liver adds the proteins, especially fibrinogen.

The blood depots

Certain organs of the body contain more blood than they need for their own activity, and are known as the blood depots. Of these the most important are the skin, the intestines and the spleen, although other organs, such as the liver, the lungs and even the large veins probably store blood. The spleen of man which has no muscular capsule is, however, not so important as a store as it is in lower animals.

The advantage of this store is that blood is available for emergencies. The commonest "emergency" is physical exercise when the needs of the muscles are increased. Under these circumstances the blood depots contract and send their store into the general circulation. This also occurs in conditions of mental stress, in haemorrhage and in infections. It is this which makes the sick or frightened person pale, and the withdrawal of the warm blood from the skin makes him feel cold. Pallor of the skin associated with a very rapid pulse is a valuable indication of haemorrhage.

The Control of the Blood Depots, including the Spleen. It now seems probable that the blood depots are controlled by the depressor reflexes from the carotid sinus and the arch of the aorta. When blood from these depots is needed, e.g., after a hæmorrhage or during muscular activity, these reflexes are reduced resulting in a vasoconstriction so that extra blood is thrown into the circulation and there is an increased flow to the heart.

Other functions of the Spleen. The spleen is not essential to life and the organ is sometimes removed without the patient being any the worse apparently. Its most important function is that it is a storehouse for blood, but like all lymphoid tissue it plays a part in the formation of lymphocytes. It is particularly rich in reticulo-endothelial cells and so assists in the destruction of effete red cells and because of this property it contains a relatively large quantity of lipides—cholesterol and lecithin—and of iron which is stored in the organ. Because it is engaged in the destruction of red cells it is also concerned with the liver and other organs in the manufacture of bile pigments. The spleen is also said to participate in nitrogenous metabolism especially in the formation of uric acid.

Fainting. This occurs when for some reason the brain does not get sufficient oxygen. This may occur in severe haemorrhage or when a large amount of blood accumulates in the blood vessels. Sometimes several factors are concerned, thus menstruating women are especially liable to faint in a hot room especially if they are anaemic, i.e., if the red blood cells are deficient in oxygen-carrying power. The blood accumulates in the lower limbs during prolonged standing or in the skin during excessive heat. Convalescents after a long period in bed may faint for similar reasons. In this case the vasomotor centre has suffered from disuse, but sometimes as after influenza the centre may have been poisoned. Psychological fainting is less easy to understand but we know that the dilatation of the vessels occurs in the muscles while those of the skin constrict, indeed the pallor of the skin may be seen before the subject becomes unconscious.

Stretching of the spine, which is now practised by physiotherapists, may lead to temporary faintness or fainting when the subject resumes the erect posture. This would seem to be produced by an inhibition of the vasomotor centre by impulses from the stretched parts.

CHAPTER XVI

THE LYMPH

In addition to the veins, there is a completely separate set of vessels which carry fluid from the tissues. These are the lymphatics which carry the lymph. In order to understand the formation of lymph it is necessary to know a few facts of physical chemistry.

Processes governing the passage of substances through the membranes of the body

All cells, as we have seen, are surrounded by an exceedingly delicate membrane, and in the body there are many instances of structures which are simply very thin cells fastened together at their edge, e.g., the walls of very minute blood vessels, the pleura and the peritoneum.

Diffusion. The simplest animal consisting of a single cell, such as the amoeba which lives in water, absorbs its food and oxygen and excretes through the simple membrane which covers it, by the process of diffusion. This is the process by which all substances in a gaseous or liquid state tend, by virtue of the movement of their molecules, to pass from areas where they are most concentrated to where they are less so. We are familiar with the process in the spread and dissipation of scents and smoke. Similarly a drop of ink in a glass of water will gradually colour all the water.

By this process oxygen passes from the air in the lungs through the walls of the blood vessels into the blood and the carbon dioxide passes out. This process also plays an important part in the absorption of foodstuffs from the alimentary canal into the blood.

Filtration. We are familiar with the fact that pressures tend to equalise. For this reason air leaks out of a punctured tyre or water from a cracked glass. The creation of a blood pressure in the blood vessels has certain similar consequences, for the fluid of the blood tends to leak through the walls of the thinner blood vessels, as it would through a tube of any slightly pervious material. Moreover the volume of the leakage must depend on the hydrostatic pressure inside and the permeability of the tube. This process is constantly going on from the blood vessels all over the body and by it all the body fluids are formed from the blood, e.g., the tears, saliva, urine, cerebrospinal fluid, lymph, etc. It is responsible also for the filling of joints with fluid after injury.

It must, however, be emphasised that it is only water and the salts of the blood dissolved in it which are filtered off in this way, but there may be added in certain organs, substances produced by cells through which the fluid passes. Substances which exist in the blood whose molecules are too large cannot as it were pass through the sieve of the membrane and are retained in the blood. The proteins of the blood, therefore, do not normally pass through to any extent, unless the walls of the blood capillaries have been damaged.

374

Osmosis. Compared with gases, the process of diffusion in watery solutions is very slow, because most substances attract water. Thus the sugar which we put in our tea although it may dissolve would remain at the bottom of the cup were the tea not stirred. This would occur still more if the sugar and tea were separated by a membrane although the sugar would diffuse through eventually. There are, however, substances which would not pass through the membrane at all but would attract water in the same way; these are *the colloids* and all proteins are of this nature. They mix freely with water like egg-white but are not really soluble. They cannot pass through animal membranes because their molecules are too large and, therefore, are separated by the membrane. The power of attracting water in this way is known as osmosis and this is a most important property of substances in the body. Thus the protein of the blood attracts water from the tissues and thereby counteracts filtration and, to take a further example, if blood corpuscles are put in distilled water the protein they contain attracts water until their envelopes burst.

Osmosis is also made use of therapeutically in the well-known application of strong solutions (e.g., of Epsom salts) to inflamed parts and is probably also important in relation to poultices. They attract water and are, therefore, said to have a "drawing" effect on the local poisons formed by bacteria and local tissue damage, and as a result the local defences have more chance of overcoming the infecting bacteria and so a boil or carbuncle is "brought to a head." In the case of the poultice the drawing effect is still further increased by the heat which also dilates the local vessels. The injection of an antibiotic such as penicillin which prevents the bacteria from growing is now, however, much more rapidly effective.

The factors which control the formation of tissue fluid, viz., hydrostatic pressure on the one hand and an osmotic pressure on the other, also in the same way control the production of other body fluids, e.g., the formation of the urine, sweat, digestive secretions and the cerebrospinal fluid.

The fluid of joints is also lymph to which a minute quantity of lubricant, mucous-like substances, have been added. The lymph indeed is the typical body fluid which is the basis of many other fluids known by other names as has been indicated in relation to filtration (p. 374).

The *lymph* is a clear fluid formed from tissue fluid which is derived mostly from the blood, having seeped through the capillary walls. Tissue fluid together with other substances especially water which are added in the tissues constitutes lymph (fig. 286). Normally only the water of the blood, together with the salts dissolved in it, can filter through the capillary walls, the blood corpuscles and blood proteins being left behind, but if the capillaries are injured or widely dilated, some of the protein also passes. The tissue fluid is constantly being formed by filtration through the arterial ends of the capillaries, for the pressure in these vessels is higher than in the tissue spaces. Under normal circumstances it is as rapidly removed through the venous end of the capillaries where the blood pressure is lower and by lymphatics which carry it to the central lymphatic channels, notably the thoracic duct. Throughout the body there are, however, in addition, frequent communications by which the lymph may pass from the lymphatics to the veins.

It is of special interest to physiotherapists to understand exactly what causes the fluid to return through the wall at the venous end of the capillaries.

The proteins of the blood plasma, by virtue of their osmotic pressure, exert what might be described as a "sucking" action on the fluid in the tissues, but normally this is more than counterbalanced by the blood pressure in the arterial end of the capillary and so filtration, not absorption, results. At the venous end of the capillary the blood pressure is lower and thus its filtering effect is overcome by the osmotic suction of the plasma proteins. In injury there is commonly a swelling of the injured part, partly from the extravasation of blood from ruptured vessels and partly as a result of the accumulation of tissue fluid in the region. This accumulation takes place because the injury damages the capillary walls which dilate and become more permeable. Not only is filtration increased but proteins leak into the

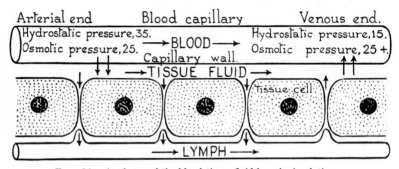

FIG. 286.—A scheme of the blood-tissue fluid-lymph circulation.

tissue spaces and thus further hinder reabsorption. Bacteria produce a similar local reaction.

This protein may eventually coagulate and become the seat of the formation of strands of fibrous tissue which later may prevent the return of the normal movement of muscles and especially of joints. The breakdown of such strands (adhesions) or the prevention of their formation is the aim of many remedial exercises after injury.

This "sucking" action of the proteins is also of importance in haemorrhage, for when the capillary pressure falls from loss of blood, filtration ceases while the proteins of the blood plasma continue to exert their action and draw water from the tissues into the blood stream and thus assist in making up the blood volume.

The function of the lymph is to carry away the products of chemical change from the tissues, e.g., carbon dioxide, lactic acid and water. The more active the tissues the more these products are produced. In such circumstances the flow of lymph is greatly increased because the increased blood pressure increases filtration from the capillaries and the products of chemical change attract more water from the blood by osmosis. The lymph flow is greatly increased in exercise because the capillary pressure rises with the blood pressure.

Lymph also carries away bacteria which become trapped in the lymph nodes. These, in turn, may become inflamed and painful. Thus after vaccination in the arm the axillary nodes become painful and similarly in tonsillitis those lying behind the angle of the jaw.

In the intestine the lymph has the additional function of carrying away some of the fat which is absorbed from the digestive tract. The fat is added to the lymph in the form of minute droplets so that after a fatty meal the lymph channels from the small intestine are full of a milk-like fluid called *chyle*. These lymph channels join together and eventually empty into the *receptaculum (cisterna) chyli* whence the chyle is carried by the *thoracic duct* to the blood stream.

A depletion of fluid in the tissue-spaces is known as *dehydration*, a condition which may be produced by insufficient intake or excessive loss of water such as occurs in vomiting, diarrhoea and excessive sweating.

Factors affecting the flow of Lymph

Since the lymph stream has no pump behind it, as has the blood stream in the form of the heart, its propulsion throughout the body is due to outside agencies. The lymph leaves the tissue spaces under pressure and this initiates the flow. It is believed also that the lymph vessels contract and thus propel the lymph, the valves inside the lymph vessels would successfully prevent regurgitation, but the propulsion of lymph is due chiefly to respiratory movements and to muscle action generally. Thus the lymph flow is greatly increased during exercise and is retarded during rest.

Accumulation of Tissue Fluid

Tissue fluid may accumulate in various parts of the body and produce swelling, oedema or dropsy which is characterised by the fact that it may be driven out readily by pressure with the finger on the skin and subcutaneous tissues which are therefore said to "pit on pressure." Several conditions cause it:

1. Increased capillary pressure produces an accumulation of tissue fluid. A mild degree of oedema occurs normally in the feet in prolonged standing, especially if there is little muscular movement and the feet are warm. A more severe variety (dropsy) is seen in cardiac failure when the venous pressure rises. Blockage of a vein produces a similar state limited to the area drained by the vein.

2. Obstruction of the lymphatics, especially a block of the nodes, may also cause swelling of a part. Such a block may be caused by the inflammatory state of the nodes such as occurs occasionally after vaccination in the arm, but an enormous swelling (elephantiasis), especially of the legs, is seen in filariasis when the blockage is due to minute worms. It may also be seen after surgical excision of the lymph nodes in cancer of breast.

3. Increased permeability of the capillary walls produces a swelling of the tissues when the vessels dilate or are damaged; the latter occurs in burns,

frostbite or chilblains. It occurs also in inflammation and this is seen in pleurisy when the cavity of the chest may fill with a very coagulable fluid.

4. Unaccustomed exercise may, by producing metabolites, cause muscles or the feet to swell. This causes the stiffness which occurs after much exercise and is benefited by massage or more exercise.

5. The taking of large quantities of salt which is not rapidly excreted also causes water retention and likewise extracts of adrenal cortex which produce salt retention.

6. Oedema may also be produced by decreased osmotic pressure of the plasma. This occurs as a result of inflammation of the kidneys or when there is abnormal loss of plasma proteins. A low plasma protein also occurs in starvation.

Blood Substitutes

We are now in a position to consider blood substitutes. When blood is lost from the body it is best replaced by blood, and this may be achieved by direct transfusion from person to person. Usually, however, it is more convenient to withdraw blood from the donor, add citrate* to prevent clotting, and inject or store it until required. It cannot, however, be stored in-. definitely, for after about a month the older blood corpuscles die and break up (haemolyse) and are no longer efficient as oxygen carriers. In practice it is found that plasma is more convenient, largely because it may be concentrated or dried and is, therefore, more portable. It has also the advantage that blood groups (q.v.) can be ignored. It has, however, the disadvantage of having little oxygen-carrying power and is, therefore, very inferior to blood in cases of very severe haemorrhage for oxygen-lack eventually brings about death.

When blood or plasma is not available or when the body suffers from dehydration without loss of blood cells as in diarrhoea, vomiting or severe sweating, salt solution, such as that referred to on p. 361, may be used of approximately the same concentration as blood, or a 0·69 per cent. solution (a teaspoonful to the pint) of common salt.

The disadvantage of salt solution compared with plasma or blood is the absence of protein to retain the fluid in the blood vessels. This has been circumvented by adding to the saline harmless carbohydrates which attract water. Gum acacia 9 per cent. has been used but is now replaced by dextran, which is, however, very expensive. All artificial fluids must be sterilised by boiling before injection. All such fluids are usually injected or allowed to flow by drip into the median basilic (antecubital) vein of the arm, care being taken to avoid the entrance of air into the vessel. It should be emphasised that the administration of fluid is not free from risk. Too much may lead to a high venous pressure and cardiac failure.

*See blood coagulation.

CHAPTER XVII

RESPIRATION

All living things require a supply of oxygen or they die. Many of the lower animals with very thin skin, e.g., the frog, can take in oxygen through the body surfaces, but the higher animals are dependent upon the lungs for their oxygen supply. The oxygen, we have seen, is used to burn the carbon (C) of the foodstuffs and to convert it into carbon dioxide (CO_2) while hydrogen (H) is converted into water (H_2O).

The trachea is kept patent by a series of incomplete cartilaginous rings, some of which can be felt in the neck. It divides into two main bronchi in the upper part of the chest and these subdivide into smaller bronchi and these into bronchioles.

The *bronchioles* open into the air sacs of the lungs called the *alveoli*. In the bronchioles the cartilages seen in the bronchi are replaced by rings of thin muscle fibres. These minute tubes control the intake and exit of air to and from the lung alveoli. They contract at the beginning of expiration or on coughing and thus offer some resistance to the exit of air, a fact which is of considerable importance in that this causes stretching of the lung and the barrel-shaped chests of those with chronic coughs. The bronchioles become constricted if they are inflamed as in bronchitis and this is responsible for the sense of tightness of the chest which may then be experienced. They constrict excessively in asthma for various reasons of which excessive sensitivity to certain dusts and mental states are by far the most important. Breathing exercises designed to empty the chest completely are found most valuable in asthmatics and chronic bronchitics (see p. 387).

All the large tubes are lined by columnar ciliated epithelium. The cilia carry foreign particles and mucus up the respiratory tract where they can be expectorated.

Mucus is a slimy substance which is secreted by glands lying under the surface membrane lining the various large tubes of the body. It acts both as a protective and lubricant. It is present in the fluid secreted by the nose, mouth, stomach and especially the large intestine. When these parts are inflamed or irritated the secretion of mucus may be enormously increased. An over-secretion of nasal mucus is manifested in the common cold.

Gaseous Exchange in the Lungs and Tissues

In the section on Anatomy we have seen that the capacity of the thoracic cavity is increased by the raising of the ribs and the descent of the diaphragm. Since there is no other patent opening in the thorax except the trachea and the blood vessels, air (and blood) is sucked into it during inspiration. The lungs themselves are quite passive as is well seen if an opening be made into the chest wall (pneumothorax). Students should see a model in which these facts are easily demonstrated.

The structure of the lung is peculiarly adapted to its function. In the alveoli the air comes into almost immediate contact with the blood—in some places, indeed, the same cells act as a wall to both an air alveolus and a blood capillary.

All gases are made up of vast numbers of minute particles or molecules which are invisible and which are in constant movement in every direction. This gives the gas the power of diffusion, a process which tends to make gases mix and to pass through thin membranes from a high to a lower concentration.

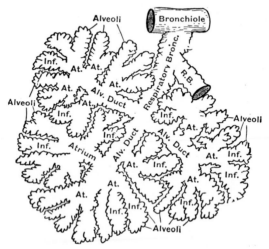

FIG. 287.—Diagram to show the general arrangement in a piece of lung. (McDowall, modified from Miller.)

The capillary walls in the lungs and tissues are so thin that gases can diffuse through them almost as rapidly as if they were not present.

The *atmospheric air contains* the following gases:

20·96 per cent. oxygen (O_2).

0·04 per cent. or practically no carbon dioxide (CO_2).

79 per cent. nitrogen (N).

The air to which the blood is exposed in the lungs is, as might be expected, richer in carbon dioxide which is constantly being added, but poorer in oxygen, which is constantly being withdrawn.

The *alveolar gas** can be obtained by asking a subject to breathe out through a piece of tubing of about 2·5 cm diameter. It is the last portion of air expired. In normal persons at rest it contains:

13 per cent. oxygen.

About 5·5 per cent. carbon dioxide.

82 per cent. nitrogen.

* This term has now replaced alveolar air.

It should be understood that these figures vary in different circumstances. This concentration is normally kept almost constant by quiet respiration, but it is evident that we can, by voluntarily increasing respiration, make the concentration of the gases in the alveoli almost like that of the outside air.

In the blood, although the same principle of diffusion applies, there is present in the red blood corpuscles the special red-coloured iron-containing pigment *haemoglobin*, which has the power of taking up more oxygen than an ordinary fluid—100 ml.* of water if shaken with pure oxygen can take up only 4 ml. of the oxygen while blood can take up about 20 ml. The oxygen in the alveoli is in a higher concentration than in the blood and, therefore, diffuses into the latter. From the lung alveoli it is carried by the blood to the tissues where the opposite state of affairs is present. There, oxygen is being used by the tissue cells and the concentration is less than in the blood. Oxygen, therefore, passes from the blood into the tissue cells by a similar process of diffusion.

A similar principle applies to the carriage of carbon dioxide by the blood from the tissues to the lungs. The concentration is highest in the tissues and it therefore passes readily into the blood and consequently, via the lungs, into the expired air just as soda water, which has been saturated with CO_2 in the factory, gives off this gas when the water is exposed to air.

Since the diffusion of gases depends on their concentration, the amount of carbon dioxide which leaves the blood in the lungs depends on the concentration of the carbon dioxide in the alveoli. Thus in excessive breathing exercises too much carbon dioxide may be lost from the blood.

The whole process of gaseous exchange is still further facilitated by a number of delicate chemical processes of which the most important is a competition by oxygen and carbon dioxide for the haemoglobin of the blood. Thus in the tissues the balance is in favour of the carbon dioxide, and the more the latter gas is produced the more oxygen is driven off. Actually this competition is indirect for the carbon dioxide is mainly carried by the plasma but to make room for it some of the chlorine of the sodium chloride leaves the plasma and enters the red cells.

The actual exchange of gases which takes place in the lung at rest is quite small as is indicated by the following table:

	100 ml. Venous Blood contain	100 ml. Arterial Blood contain
Oxygen	13·5 ml.	18·5 ml.
Carbon dioxide . .	56·0 ml.	52·0 ml.

It will be seen that only 5 ml. of oxygen are taken up by each 100 c.c. of blood passing through the lungs. During exercise, however, much more oxygen is used by the tissues and the venous blood therefore contains less oxygen and a correspondingly greater amount of carbon dioxide. It will also be noted that even the arterial blood contains a relatively large amount of carbon dioxide. It is this carbon dioxide in the arterial blood going to

* The term millilitre (ml.) has now replaced cubic centimetre (c.c.) in respiratory physiology.

the brain which is responsible for stimulating the parts of the brain controlling the respiratory and vasomotor centres. So-called "breathing exercises" do not produce a beneficial effect unless most carefully done, i.e., extremely slowly. If done at the normal rate of breathing, the deeper respiration of the breathing exercise brings about a washing-out of the carbon dioxide from the blood which, as we have already noted, is so essential for the proper action of the mechanism which controls the blood vessels. Breathing exercises may produce fainting.

When the blood is saturated with oxygen it is bright red, but when it loses its oxygen it becomes more purple in colour. The colour of blood from a vein is, therefore, darker than that from an artery.

THE CONTROL OF RESPIRATION

Respiration is controlled by the chemical composition of the blood and by nervous impulses.

Chemical Control. There exist in the lower part of the brain, especially the medulla, areas which together are termed the *respiratory centres*. These are exquisitely sensitive to changes in the concentration of carbon dioxide in the blood, indeed it has been found that a 0·2% rise in the alveolar carbon dioxide is sufficient to double the pulmonary ventilation during rest. It can be shown that a certain amount of carbon dioxide in the arterial blood is, however, necessary for the normal activity of the respiratory centres. This may readily be shown in man. If we voluntarily overbreathe and thus renew rapidly the alveolar air so that it becomes almost like atmospheric air, an excessive amount of carbon dioxide leaves the blood and passes through the lungs. In these circumstances less goes to the brain, and the normal stimulus to the respiratory centre is reduced. Respiration ceases until carbon dioxide again accumulates in the blood. We cannot, however, hold our breath for a long time, because of the accumulation of carbon dioxide in the alveolar air and consequently in the blood supplying the brain, and because of the lack of oxygen which also occurs. We have already seen that the concentration of the gases in the blood depends on the concentration of the gases in the alveolar air.

Oxygen lack alone may cause an increase in respiration. This can be proved by causing an individual to rebreathe his own expired air at the same time preventing an accumulation of carbon dioxide by passing the air through soda lime. It must, however, be emphasised that the increase is slight compared with the effect of increased carbon dioxide. Were it not for the fact that oxygen lack stimulates respiration, respiration would cease at high altitudes where for example the partial pressure of alveolar carbon dioxide may be as low as 28 mm. Hg instead of the normal 40 mm. at sea level.

In addition to the respiratory centre, there are *chemoreceptors* in the carotid body at the bifurcation of the carotid artery and the aortic body at the arch of the aorta, which are sensitive to the concentrations of carbon dioxide and oxygen in the arterial blood. Any increase of carbon dioxide or fall of the oxygen content in the blood acts on the nerve-endings of these special bodies and from them messages are transmitted to the respiratory centres in the brain. It can be shown that oxygen-lack acts solely through these chemoreceptors otherwise it depresses the brain.

Nervous Control. The respiratory centres are also stimulated by sensory nerves, especially from the skin; indeed, the first breath that many of us took possibly resulted from an energetic stimulation of the skin by the relatively colder air of the outside world comparable to the deep breathing which results from plunging into cold water.

In addition to stimulation by the ordinary sensory nerves, the action of the vagus nerves limits the depth of respiration. At each inspiration, when the lung is stretched, impulses pass up the vagus nerves to the respiratory centre and expiration follows. This is known as the *Hering-Breuer reflex* and its importance lies in the fact that in inflammation of the lungs (pneumonia) this reflex becomes unduly exaggerated and breathing which is normally from 15 to 25 per minute, becomes so very rapid and shallow that it may be insufficient to change the air in the alveoli. If we breathe rapidly but shallowly, like a dog or sheep on a hot day, we can readily appreciate that deeper respiration becomes a necessity.

From the above it will be evident that the adequate oxygenation of the body depends on the following factors:

(i) The circulation of the blood.
(ii) The adequacy of the lungs as an aerating area.
(iii) The patency of the trachea and bronchi..
(iv) The adequacy of the blood as a carrier of gases.
(v) The adequacy of the respiratory movements.
(vi) The power of the tissues to use oxygen.

Breathlessness occurs whenever there is an accumulation of carbon dioxide in the blood provided the respiratory centre is active. Typically this occurs in exercise. At first the additional carbon dioxide produced by the burning of carbon gets through the lungs into the arterial blood. This stimulates the respiratory centres which in turn send down messages to cause the subject to breathe more deeply and rapidly until the respiratory movements are adapted to the needs of the body.

Breathlessness, while the subject is at rest, also occurs in many diseases of the lungs and heart which interfere with the aeration of the blood. It is always a serious symptom.

General blueness of the skin or *cyanosis* is produced by the same causes as breathlessness but it may be localised when there is a slowing of the blood through an area of skin. This is seen if we obstruct the flow of blood through a finger by tying a ligature around it. The blood already in the finger loses its oxygen to the tissues and becomes blue. In cold weather, when the arterioles in the skin close down to conserve body temperature, local stagnation of blood may cause blueness of the extremities (e.g., the hands, feet and ears).

Ventilation of the lungs

At each breath about 500 ml. of air enters and leaves the lungs; this is known as the *tidal* volume. We can take in about 1,600 ml. more air now known as *the inspiratory reserve volume* and also at the end of a normal expiration expire another 1,600 ml. known as the *expiratory reserve volume*. The maximum expiration after the maximum inspiration, i.e., the *vital capacity* is from 4,000 to 6,000 ml. in most persons. The actual amount may be measured by means of a spirometer which is really an inverted bell suspended in water and it is found that individuals differ very much. A vital capacity of 10,000 ml. is not unusual. This is by far the most important chest measurement which can be made for it indicates the amount of lung surface available and the amount of oxygen which can be taken in per breath. It is a much more valuable index than the circumference of the chest but is roughly parallel to the chest expansion during inspiration. There is in addition a quantity of air always in the lungs even after the deepest possible expiration. In the adult this *residual capacity* may amount to 1,600 ml. but it is increased in exercise. It is this residual air which makes the lungs float in water and is an important indication, in medico-legal work, that an infant has breathed.

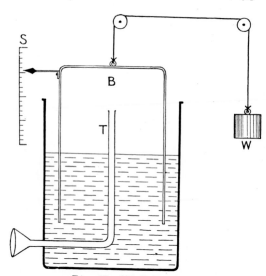

FIG. 288.—The Spirometer.
B. Bell.   W. Weight.   S. Scale.   T. Tube.

An increase of the residual capacity is of special interest to physiotherapists because they are frequently called upon to treat it. It occurs notably in asthma and in emphysema. Emphysema is caused by an over-distension of the lungs and results in the alveolar partitions becoming destroyed. It is often the result of frequent coughing over a period of years and produces the typical barrel-shaped cheat. There is not only a faulty aeration of the blood but a resistance to the pulmonary blood flow and this results in a failure of the right ventricle of the heart from which the patient dies (see p. 387).

The important datum in relation to ventilation is that from 250 to 300 c.c. of oxygen are required per minute by the body at rest. Adequate ventilation of closed spaces is based on this figure. It has been found by experiment that closed spaces, such as sealed air-raid shelters, may be occupied safely until the oxygen has fallen to 14 per cent. with the carbon dioxide accumulating to 6 per cent. It can, therefore, be calculated that a sealed room of 250 cu. ft. can be safely occupied by one person for twenty hours.

The frequency of respiration. The average adult breathes from 15/18 times per minute, but those who take in large amounts of air per breath, breathe correspondingly slower. Normally an increased frequency occurs in exercise, but it also occurs when the body temperature is raised, sometimes from nervous causes, and whenever there is inadequate aeration of the blood in the lungs.

Forced expiratory volume. It is now realised that the speed with which a subject can expire is of considerable importance, as a reduction of this may be a prelude to the more dangerous emphysema. The forced expiratory volume is the proportion of the vital capacity which can be expired in the first second of expiration. It is reduced in asthma.

Asphyxia

This term is applied to the accumulation of carbon dioxide and lack of oxygen in the body. It occurs when there is interference with pulmonary ventilation as in immersion under water, strangling, severe bronchitis or an impairment of the movements of the chest. The latter condition is not infrequent in babies who have been overlain. The movements of the chest and diaphragm may also fail in poliomyelitis or in damage to the spinal cord. Asphyxia may occur also in poisoning by narcotics or anaesthetics which paralyse the respiratory centre.

The typical sign of asphyxia is blueness of the skin and mucous membranes because the oxygen of the blood becomes used up and haemoglobin is much darker in colour than oxyhaemoglobin.

Except when the asphyxia is due to depression of the nervous system, the accumulation of carbon dioxide causes a marked stimulation of the respiratory and vasomotor centres with the result that breathing is very much increased and there is a large increase of arterial and more especially of venous pressures so that the veins of the skin stand out and are easily seen. If the asphyxia is severe, consciousness is lost and convulsions commonly occur. The heart at first beats faster but very rapidly fails because of the oxygen want. It is therefore essential to begin artificial respiration as soon as possible. While the heart is beating there is hope of survival.

A slow type of asphyxia of the tissues occurs when the blood pressure falls or the circulation is slowed. The tissue metabolites accumulate, the capillaries open up and act like a sponge to soak up the blood. There is a reduced return of blood to the heart and a corresponding reduced output, and so a vicious circle is produced. This may occur rapidly or slowly in untreated haemorrhage, but is the common end result of cardiac or respiratory failure. It is the lack of oxygen to the tissues which does harm rather than the accumulation of carbon dioxide which can be excreted by the kidneys.

Anoxia

In this state there is lack of oxygen but no accumulation of carbon dioxide. It occurs typically at high altitudes where the air is thin, that is its molecules

are widely separated.   In anoxia the stimulative effects are less and unconsciousness ensues rapidly.   If any gas other than oxygen is breathed
unconsciousness is produced in about two minutes.   Anoxia, or more
correctly hypoxia (reduced oxygen), is produced if for any reason the blood
is unable to carry sufficient oxygen.   This occurs in haemorrhage, in
anaemia and in coal-gas poisoning when the carbon monoxide of the gas is
taken up instead of oxygen by the red blood cells.   It is also produced in
heart failure.   The ultimate effect of both anoxia and asphyxia is due to
the uptake of sodium by the cells of the respiratory centre which thereby lose
their electrical potential and so become unexcitable.   Death occurs very
rapidly if the anoxia is severe.

Artificial Respiration

A most satisfactory method is that of *Schafer*, which consists in laying
the patient on the face and kneeling beside him with the hands on the loins
and compressing the abdomen rhythmically at the rate of normal breathing.
This forces up the diaphragm and drives air out of the chest.   The diaphragm
recoils when the pressure is released and air is sucked in.

The *Neilsen* method is now in considerable vogue.   In this method the
patient is also placed face down and the ribs are raised by pulling up the
arms.   Expiration is assisted by compression of the back.

Mouth to mouth breathing, "the kiss of life" may also be used when there is
no obstruction to the air passages.   In this method, the operator simply
blows intermittently into the mouth while holding the subject's nose.   It is,
however, not a very hygienic procedure and there is always the danger that
fluid and foreign bodies may be blown into the lungs.

In the *rocking method of Eve* the patient is placed on a stretcher or plank
and rocked through a central axis.   The method so overloads the heart that
it has been generally abandoned, except for newly born children when it can
be readily carried out in the nurse's arms.   In all types of asphyxia the right
side of the heart is engorged with blood and the venous pressure is very high
because of the stimulation of the vasomotor centre and the failure of the heart.

Anaesthetists commonly carry out artificial respiration by driving air or
oxygen mechanically into the lungs through a tube inserted into the trachea.

In all methods of artificial respiration the criterion of efficiency is whether
or not the lungs are ventilated adequately but not excessively.   Excessive
ventilation by washing out carbon dioxide prevents normal breathing
restarting.   It must be remembered that any type is better than none and
must be begun as soon as possible as failure of respiration leads to heart
failure, in a few minutes.

If the patient is on an operating table the ribs may be elevated by fully
extending the arms above the head (inducing inspiration) and then compressing the chest with the flexed forearms (inducing expiration).   This is
known as *Silvester's* method of artificial respiration.   Pulling the tongue
forward rhythmically is also beneficial.

In the so-called *iron lung*, the patient is placed in an air-tight chamber
with the exception of the head, and the volume of the chest is altered by

inflating and deflating the chamber. It is used especially when the origins of the phrenic and intercostal nerves have been affected by anterior poliomyelitis.

The Effects of Respiratory Movements on the Circulation

At each inspiratory movement, the pressure inside the chest falls about 25 millimetres of mercury, and at each expiration the pressure rises, although it never becomes positive.

At each inspiration blood is sucked into the lungs via the pulmonary veins. It cannot escape backwards and so at each expiration it is driven into the arteries. Moreover, at each expiration the resistance to the blood flow through the lungs rises, thus the blood pressure shows a normal rise and fall with respiratory movement, which is increased when there is obstruction to the nasal passages as in tonsils and adenoids. If we expire violently against resistance as with the glottis closed, so little blood passes through the lungs that the arterial blood pressure falls violently (Valsalva's experiment). A lesser degree of this occurs in coughing when the systolic pressure in the pulmonary artery may rise from its normal 30 mm. of mercury to over 400 mm. This throws considerable strain on the right side of the heart, a fact which must be remembered in the conduct of expiratory breathing exercises.

Breathing Exercises

Breathing exercises commonly come under the control of physiotherapists and are of considerable value. Many children are born with poorly developed chests and so have a poor vital capacity. They have a poor tidal volume and readily become breathless on exercise. The subject may have to be taught to use the diaphragm or the chest if either is deficient. In asthma and emphysema the patient has difficulty in expiring because of an excessive contraction of the bronchial muscle at the commencement of expiration. An accumulation of residual gas adds to the distress. In such cases the patient is encouraged to empty his chest as far as possible at each expiration. A valuable illustrated system of expiratory exercises is published by the Asthma Research Council. It must be understood that in cases of cardiac failure, expiratory exercises may, by raising the pulmonary resistance, put a strain on the right side of the heart.

In all breathing exercises the primary object is to assist and facilitate normal respiration but if deep breathing is taught care must be taken that it is not too fast, otherwise an excessive amount of carbon dioxide may be washed out of the blood and the subject therefore may become giddy or exhibit muscular spasm or even faint. It must be remembered that respiration is best stimulated by physical exercise, as in running, and this should be encouraged in the young whenever possible.

The Effect of Atmospheric Pressure on Respiratory Processes

The atmospheric pressure as measured by a barometer varies at different altitudes. At sea-level it is 760 mm. Hg or approximately 15 pounds per square inch, although we do not notice this pressure since it is diffused. Below sea-level it is greater, above it is less. This is because the molecules of the atmospheric gases are more tightly packed together at the lower than at the higher altitude. Their concentration relative to each other remains the same.

Although the composition of the air remains the same whatever the altitude, a breath of a given depth will take in much less oxygen at the top of Mount Everest than at sea-level.*

High atmospheric pressures occur in diving bells or caissons which are lowered under the water in the building of bridges. To keep the water out air is pumped in under pressure. All the gases in such air are more concentrated than at sea-level, and not only more oxygen is taken up by the blood but also nitrogen. While a man remains in this atmosphere no ill effects occur but when he comes up to sea-level, the extra nitrogen which has been absorbed by the body as a whole, begins to bubble off, especially in the nervous tissues, and produces paralysis and cramp, popularly known as "bends." The condition is prevented by slow decompression. The extra oxygen which has been absorbed is used by the tissues.

Low atmospheric pressures. At high altitudes, such as are attained in the ascent of mountains or in aircraft, the opposite state of affairs occurs. Since the molecules of oxygen are more dispersed fewer are taken in per breath. The oxygen is still less concentrated in the alveoli of the lungs and therefore less of it diffuses into the blood and each 100 c.c. of blood cannot take up its normal 18–19 c.c. of oxygen.

To some extent the concentration of oxygen in the alveoli is increased by deep and rapid breathing, but in addition there are adaptations of the circulation. The blood is pumped round more rapidly so that each 100 c.c. makes, as it were, a double journey; also more blood corpuscles appear in the circulation as a result of stimulation of the bone marrow.

In modern aircraft which commonly fly at over 20,000 ft. air is pumped into an airtight cabin and so the atmospheric pressure is maintained at that of 8,000 ft. In practice it is found that at this height an individual can by slightly deeper and more rapid breathing keep his alveolar gas at a normal concentration with no apparent discomfort. It is not considered safe for mountaineers to go beyond 20,000 ft. without having oxygen available, although with training 28,000 ft. has been attained. With a supply of oxygen a man can apparently go to any height as in a space ship.

---

* The actual concentration of oxygen is sometimes expressed as the partial pressure of the atmospheric pressure. At sea-level the atmospheric pressure is 760 mm. of mercury. Of this, 20·96 per cent., i.e., about one-fifth, is due to oxygen. Thus the partial pressure of oxygen is 150 mm. of mercury. On the top of Mount Everest the atmospheric pressure is about 250 mm. of mercury, but one-fifth only of this is oxygen. The extent to which the blood will take up oxygen is then described as proportionate to its partial pressure.

CHAPTER XVIII

THE EFFECTS OF EXERCISE AND MASSAGE

We have seen that the body generally is designed to supply oxygen and nourishment to the voluntary muscles and that the majority of the organs in the body are subservient to the needs of the muscles. Physical activity brings into increased action directly or indirectly most of the body and it is for this reason that moderate exercise is most health giving, for disused organs tend to degenerate and become incapable of maximum use. Unaccustomed exercise on the other hand throws a strain on the organs. It is convenient to consider the effect of exercise in relation to the various systems concerned.

Effect of Exercise on Respiration   *Running*

We can appreciate the effect on this system if we take the exercise of running as an example. During the exercise, carbon dioxide and lactic acid are produced while additional oxygen is used.

The venous blood returning to the lungs contains more carbon dioxide and less oxygen than at rest. If respiration remains as at rest the ventilation in the lungs is insufficient to allow of adequate gaseous interchange in the lungs and imperfectly aerated blood gets through to the arteries. When this occurs the arterial blood supply to the brain is affected and as a result the respiratory centre is stimulated and the movements of the respiratory muscles are increased in both rate and depth, the Hering-Breuer reflex (*vide* Respiration) being temporarily in abeyance. Exercise is the only physiological method of increasing respiratory activity and increasing the capacity of the lungs and chest. The disadvantage of breathing exercises has already been discussed (p. 387).

Actually before the exercise begins respiration may be stimulated merely by anticipation and some stimulative impulses pass to the brain from the active muscles.

Effect of Exercise on the Circulation

In exercise the rate of circulation may be increased threefold in the normal person and much more in the trained athlete. This is achieved by a rise of blood pressure and a dilatation of the blood vessels in the active muscles.

The dilatation of the peripheral vessels has been referred to already. The capillaries are dilated by the chemical substances produced in the active tissues and the larger vessels by impulses which pass out by the sympathetic vasodilator nerves and by nervous reflexes which reduce the normal tonic activity of the vasomotor centre.

The rise of blood pressure in exercise is produced by the shutting down of vessels in the less active parts of the body, together with an increased output

26—A.PH. 389

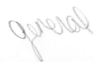
General

of the heart which is really due indirectly to the closing down of vessels. The generalised constriction of vessels and of the spleen greatly reduces their capacity and in addition to raising the peripheral resistance causes blood to be squeezed into the veins and thus the venous pressure rises. This is still further augmented by the pumping action of the muscles, for when a muscle contracts, it compresses the dilated vessels within it, as one might compress a sponge, and thus drives its blood still more rapidly into the veins. The return of the blood to the heart is further increased by the so-called respiratory pump. As we have seen at each inspiration the negative pressure in

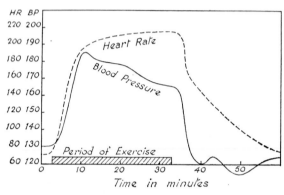

FIG. 289.—Effect of moderate exercise on heart rate and blood pressure. (After Bowen.)

the thorax rises and the pressure in the abdomen is increased. This forces blood from the abdomen into the thorax, but the reverse does not occur at expiration for the blood which is taken into the chest is trapped in the lungs by the valves in the pulmonary artery at its exit from the right ventricle.

As has been said (p. 367), the heart increases its output by increasing its rate and output per beat. Students should take their pulses before and after varying degrees of exercise.

The actual cause of the constriction of the vessels and of the increased heart rate is primarily *psychic*, i.e., it is due to the same cause as that which causes the exercise to be performed. Work performed with a grudge is not accompanied by a rise of pressure. Mental excitement alone is sufficient to bring about these changes, the higher centres apparently sending impulses down the sympathetic nervous system to the organs concerned. Emotional factors alone may raise the blood pressure by as much as 60 mm. of mercury, a fact which must be taken into consideration when the blood pressure of an apprehensive patient is being taken. -

Adrenaline and nor-adrenaline are secreted from the suprarenal glands and the action of these hormones are selective for they force the blood from the blood depots, e.g., the skin, spleen and intestine, and send it into the vessels supplying the active muscles which are dilated by this and other substances. Adrenaline also further accelerates the heart and raises the blood pressure.

The Limiting Factor in Physical Exercise

Provided nutrition is adequate, exercise is limited by the physique of the individual and by his training. In the average healthy person the limitation is set by the power of the circulation and of respiration to adapt themselves to requirements. In most of us the limit is set by our power to ventilate adequately, but a well-trained athlete with a vital capacity of over 10,000 c.c. may not experience breathlessness.

Effect of Exercise on the Alimentary Canal and on Metabolism

All severe exercise or mental excitement reduces the activity of the alimentary canal. Glandular secretion ceases, the normal movements are inhibited and the blood vessels are constricted. Food is therefore best digested when the subject is in a state of mental and physical rest.

At the same time the glucose of the blood passes into the muscles to be converted into glycogen and burnt to carbon dioxide and water, but the blood sugar does not normally fall because of this, for the liver stores glycogen which is converted into glucose and is poured into the blood as required. This breakdown of liver glycogen occurs as a result of the activities of enzyme systems by the action of the sympathetic and adrenaline. Before a very strenuous exercise it is, therefore, an advantage to take a large quantity of glucose and this is sometimes done before athletic competitions, although the taking of any starchy food a little earlier has exactly the same effect for starch is converted into glucose in the body with surprising rapidity and is much cheaper.

The After-effects of Exercise

When the exercise is over and the mental excitement involved is at an end, the sympathetic activity is reduced leaving the parasympathetic in preponderance. This is well seen in the circulation. As has been said, in those who habitually take large amounts of exercise the resting heart rate is slow. Immediately after the exercise the blood pressure also may fall appreciably below normal. This may be readily demonstrated and is due to the vessels in the recently active muscles remaining open while the constriction in other parts has passed off. If there has been fatigue, such as after a long march or a strenuous game, the fall of blood pressure may be prolonged as shown by the effects of long forced marches. Even small amounts of exercise in healthy persons result in a delayed slowing of the heart. Students may demonstrate this on themselves. Training also increases the vital capacity and the tidal volume at rest.

The after-effects of exercise on the other systems has not been accurately studied but by analogy and from general experience it is probable that parasympathetic activity is increased also in relation to the alimentary canal. Alimentary movements, digestion and appetite improve as the result of exercise, provided it is not so strenuous as to induce excessive fatigue which has the opposite effect.

Strictly speaking it is not, however, certain how far some of the beneficial effects of exercise are due to the circumstances attendant upon the exercise, e.g., relaxation from confined mental work, the effects of breathing cool air and the general stimulation of the skin.

The Effect of Massage, etc.

There seems to be little doubt that one of the benefits of massage is its effect on the circulation of the area treated. By improving the circulation of blood and lymph it facilitates the removal of deleterious substances formed in excess during disease or injury or liberated by movement.

Superficial light massage can be expected only to affect the skin circulation, the actual vessels affected being the skin capillaries, superficial veins and lymphatics. The two former, however, hold so much blood that massage in the direction of their flow must materially increase the return of blood to the heart and produce an effect rather like exercise without the more exhausting effects of fatigue. Since the superficial veins draw blood from the muscles as well as the skin, the drainage of the part generally is facilitated. Massage of the lymphatics increases the flow of lymph and the removal of tissue fluid, the accumulation of which causes pain and stiffness. In injury this fluid contains an abnormally large amount of protein and if allowed to remain stationary may be converted into fibrous tissue and cause permanent stiffness of the part.

Deeper massage hastens the circulation through the muscles and through the soft tissues as each compression tends to drive the blood towards the veins where the pressure is least. It similarly facilitates the dispersal of accumulated lymph or blood in the deeper parts.

It cannot, however, be over-emphasised that movements, preferably active, are the best stimulants to the circulation. In the limbs the circulation can be much improved by raising the part and it is doubtful if adequate use has been made of this fact therapeutically.

Mere rubbing of the skin is also presumably valuable as it sends a vast number of impulses into the nervous system. It seems most likely that this is the chief cause of the sense of well-being which undoubtedly follows massage. Other forms of skin stimulation, such as sea bathing and rough towelling, have the same effect. The effects of mechanical and chemical irritation of the skin are dealt with separately (p. 436).

"Hacking" may be effective also in this way, but it is possible that such mechanical stimulation brings about local vasodilatation by stimulating nerves. This is suggested by the fact that slow galvanic stimuli (1–5 per second) applied to a mixed nerve brings about vasodilatation. Experimental evidence on this point is, however, desirable.

It now seems probable that mechanical stimulation may have a direct dilator effect on the blood vessels. The application of heat and cold alternately and of counter-irritants such as liniments dilate the skin vessels by local irritation and also bring into operation reflex nervous reactions which dilate the larger vessels, not only of the skin, but also of the underlying structures. They also mobilise the leucocytes of the blood which are the scavengers of bacteria.

Electric currents act in a variety of ways, according to their type and may be summarised thus:—

Slow galvanic currents only stimulate the muscle at the make and break but if not too slow may stimulate the vasodilator nerves. They do not stimulate when flowing.

Fast faradic currents cause tetanic contraction of muscle and vaso-constriction, but this is followed by vasodilatation because of the action of the chemical substances produced.

Very rapid alternating currents (short wave high frequency) are used to produce heat in the tissues (see page 339).

Reactive hyperaemia has been used to promote the circulation through a limb. This consists simply in bandaging a limb for a short time to allow the products of metabolism to accumulate and dilate the vessels. When the bandage is removed the circulation is greatly increased as seen by the flushing of the skin. It is doubtful if this method is used as much as it deserves to be.

The Effect of Artificial Movements

Passive movement probably produces increased blood circulation in the joints only, but firm massage of the muscles also increases the blood flow through them. An important result of such passive movements is that they break down adhesions or prevent their formation but the psychological factor which raises the blood pressure is absent. They can never be so effective as active movements in promoting an increased blood flow through the part. Short bursts of faradic stimulation simulate most closely voluntary activity, which is tetanic in nature (see p. 346), and use is made of this in physiotherapy.

CHAPTER XIX

DIET

The chief functions of the diet are:

1. Energy producing.
2. Body building.
3. The regulation of the body functions by the vitamins and hormones.

It has to provide carbon and hydrogen which may be burnt as fuel and converted into physical work and heat as we have seen in relation to muscle contraction. These necessities may be derived from carbohydrates, fats and proteins. It also has to provide for the growth and repair of the body which is built largely of protein and for this purpose proteins only will suffice. The protein taken into the body in excess of what is needed for repair is partly burnt as fuel and partly excreted.

The Energy requirements of the body or Metabolic Rate

The amount of fuel needed, as in any engine, depends on the amount of work that is required to be done and is usually expressed as large calories. A calorie is the amount of heat required to raise 1 c.c. of water 1° Centigrade and a large Calorie* 1,000 times this amount. The therm of the gas company is a similar kind of unit.

The amount of fuel burnt by a man may be measured directly by placing him in a special chamber (calorimeter) in which the heat he gives off may be measured.

The direct method of measurement is now obsolete and use is made of the indirect method in which the amount of oxygen used is measured and the amount of heat produced calculated. In the Benedict method the subject breathes to and from a spirometer (see p. 384) filled with oxygen, the carbon dioxide he produces being taken up by soda lime. The descent of the spirometer indicates the amount of oxygen used. For measuring the usage in more active pursuits an impermeable Douglas bag is strapped on the back and the expired air collected by having a special valved mouthpiece. A measurement of the amount expired and an analysis by which the composition of this air is compared with normal air, indicates the amount of oxygen used. Since one litre of oxygen produces on the average 5 large Calories, the number of litres used multiplied by 5 gives the number of calories produced. This method shows that the major factor determining the metabolic rate is the amount of physical exercise taken and the figures obtained indicate the calorie requirements of the body and are the basis of all rationing.

During rest in bed an average individual uses calories at the rate of 1,600 large Calories per day. This is known as the *Basal Metabolic Rate* (B.M.R.) or *basal metabolism*. A sedentary occupation increases this to

---

* This is sometimes known as the Kilocalorie and is written with a large "C."

about 2,500 Calories, but an active physical life needs about 4,000. Very heavy manual work may need Calories at the rate of 10,000 per day. Since long thin subjects have a larger surface area than those who are short and fat they lose more heat through the skin and therefore waste calories in keeping themselves warm. For comparison of one subject with another the metabolism is given in terms of square metres of body surface calculated from specially constructed body height and weight tables. A normal person uses about 40 calories per square metre per hour. The metabolic rate is controlled by the thyroid gland (see page 445). Young persons, especially females, have a slightly higher metabolic rate than adults, but in old age the rate falls. It is increased in cold weather and by proteins.

The Calorific Value of Foods

In order to adapt a diet to requirements it is necessary to know how much heat any given diet will produce.

This may be done as in the case of the man, by putting the food in a special chamber known as the *bomb calorimeter* in which it is burnt on a miniature electric fire, or by the more modern methods the amount of oxygen used in burning the fuel is found and the heat produced calculated. By such means it has been found that:

1 gramme of carbohydrate produces about 4 calories of heat.

1 gramme of fat produces about 9 calories of heat.

1 gramme of protein (in the body) produces about 4 calories of heat.

It has in this way been found that all carbohydrates, whether starch or sugar, produce almost exactly the same amount of heat and that protein (meat) does the same. This is a point of great practical importance as these substances vary very much in price.

Fat becomes essential only when it is necessary to supply very large amounts of energy for severe physical work. It also supplies some of the essential vitamins (A and D), but these can be supplied in other ways.

Diet for Growth and Repair

All the tissues of the body are composed of the nitrogen-containing substance, protein, details of which are given later.

This protein structure is like the structure of a motor car, constantly subjected to wear and tear and requiring repair. Sometimes in injury or disease the wear and tear is excessive. The growing body, up to the age of 25, also requires more protein than the adult with which to make new structure and this applies indirectly to the pregnant female and convalescents after an exhausting illness, injury or surgical operation. For such individuals the supply of an adequate amount of protein is especially important.

Protein is, however, the most expensive part of our diet and its assimilation throws more strain on the liver and kidneys than do carbohydrates and fat. Much discussion has, therefore, taken place regarding the term "essential protein."

If a man is starved the amount of nitrogen in the urine gives an idea of the wear and tear of the protein structure of the body and attempts have been made to reduce the amount of protein in the diet to this amount. The subjects of such experiments invariably feel very cold. Moreover nature does not deal in minima and the child at birth is normally provided with as much as ten times the minimum amount of protein.

Another point to be remembered is that protein is not only required for growth and repair, but that the hormones of the ductless glands are also manufactured from it, e.g., thyroxine by the thyroid and adrenaline by the suprarenals, which are so important for the control of the body functions. The presence of protein is also necessary for the proper absorption of calcium from the alimentary canal.

It has been found, too, that all proteins are not equal in their growth-promoting qualities. Those from meat, fish, eggs and milk are very much more efficient in this respect than the proteins of vegetables. The former are, therefore, known as first-class proteins of which a small amount is considered most desirable if not essential in human diets. It would seem that this difference in proteins depends on their chemical structure. They are built up of amino-acids, some of which, it has been found, are essential for growth. They also increase the metabolic rate.

Protein is contained to a small extent in all plants but especially in the legumin or pea family of which peas and beans are the common representatives. Even wheat contains as much as 12 per cent. of protein and rice 8 per cent. Vegetable proteins are deficient in the growth-promoting amino-acids. It has been found, too, that the plant proteins are very difficult to digest and that large amounts are wasted. At the same time it must be remembered that very many animals live successfully on a purely vegetable diet. This subject is discussed further in relation to the metabolism of proteins.

On the whole, therefore, it can be said that while plant protein can replace animal protein to a large extent it should not be allowed to do so altogether, especially in the young or convalescent in whom a full supply of amino-acids is most desirable, but at the same time it is evident that many persons eat expensive protein much in excess of their real requirements and that purely for the supply of energy or fuel, carbohydrate or fats are equally efficient.

For the adequate use of these materials for growth, the activity of the hypophysis and thyroid gland are necessary; without these the child fails to grow in spite of an adequate diet. By far the commonest cause of failure to grow amongst poor children is an inadequate supply of calories. This is the chief reason why milk is so valuable to such children, and also because it contains the growth-promoting vitamins and salts.

Vitamins

It has been shown that artificially prepared foods, although they may contain most of the elements necessary as fuel and for tissue repair, do not maintain the body in perfect health, and young animals do not grow if fed on them exclusively. For this, certain substances, present in fresh foods and known as vitamins, are necessary. Many have now been recognised, and it has been shown by biochemists that the vitamins are really chemical substances which the higher animals cannot make in sufficient quantity for their needs. It must be realised that a generous mixed diet containing meat, milk and vegetables contains abundant vitamins. They are the regulators of the body but their actions are supplemented by the hormones produced by the ductless glands. The following are the chief vitamins:—

Vitamins A and D. These are present in animal fats and in green plants. We take them in fresh salads and in milk and butter provided the cows have been properly fed. They are present in fish-liver oils because the large fishes feed on smaller ones which eat the green growth of the sea. The two vitamins may be separated by chemical means.

If deprived of vitamin A, young animals do not grow and are prone to conjunctival infection, but there is no evidence that infection in humans is reduced by its administration. Vitamin A deficiency causes night blindness for the vitamin is specially concerned with the formation of visual purple. A deficiency also leads to a gross over-growth of the bones, especially of the spinal column, which may press on the spinal cord and cause paralysis. If deprived of vitamin D, the animals do not absorb sufficient calcium from the alimentary canal and develop rickets. The bones and teeth, being deficient in calcium (chalk), become abnormally soft. The bones of the skeleton bend easily and the teeth are liable to decay and there are other signs of calcium deficiency. It has now been clearly shown that normally the ultra-violet light of the sun enables this vitamin to be produced in plants and animals exposed to it by activating a precursor substance, *ergosterol*, in the skin. The recognition of these facts has caused the virtual disappearance of this deforming and disabling disease in the last twenty-five years.

Vitamin B. This vitamin is contained in seeds, but may be lost if the seeds are unduly milled and the darker part removed. Normally we take it in nuts, whole meal, bran, yeast and eggs—but many artificial foods prepared from these are undoubtedly deficient.

Vitamin B is not really a single substance but a group of substances several of which have now been identified chemically as thiamine, nicotinic acid, riboflavin, nor is this list complete.

Their absence leads to inflammation of the nerves (neuritis) which gives rise to a great variety of pains, inflammation of the eyes, dryness and itching of the skin, many digestive complaints, stunted growth and anaemia.

A good supply of these vitamins is obtained from yeast or preparations made therefrom. Vitamin B is that most likely to be deficient on a modern artificial diet in which white bread replaces brown. Fortunately it is also made by bacteria in the large intestine so long as there is no abnormal use of purgatives or intestinal antiseptics. Vitamin B^{12} is of special importance in the formation of red blood cells and failure to absorb it leads to pernicious anaemia.

Vitamin C. This is present in certain vegetables and fresh fruit, especially black currants, lemons, oranges, rose-hips, kale and potatoes.

In its absence scurvy occurs, in which there is great muscle weakness, a tendency for the bones to break and a tendency to bleeding from the gums and in the skin generally. The vitamin has been shown to be *ascorbic acid*. It appears to be specially concerned in the growth of fibrous tissue and is of importance in the healing of wounds. If a person is deficient in this vitamin, as indicated by its absence in the urine, the scar over a simple healed cut may be torn open easily. This vitamin is stored in the cortex of the supra-renal gland.

Vitamin P. This vitamin would also appear to be present in citrus fruits (lemon peel), but is not ascorbic acid, for such fruits have been shown to prevent a tendency to haemorrhage and oedema when ascorbic acid will not. It acts by decreasing capillary permeability and is called *citrin*.

Vitamin E. Rats fed on synthetic diets do not breed unless given a supply of vegetable fat, usually available from the germ of cereals. Vitamin E is fat soluble but is not present in animal fats. Its absence prevents the proper development of both the male and female reproductive elements, but its action in man is disputed.

Vitamin K. This vitamin is stored in the liver and found in green foods, eggs and meat. In its absence prothrombin is not formed in sufficient amount and the blood does not clot properly. Bile is necessary for its absorption.

The effect of cooking on vitamins. Most vitamins are destroyed by prolonged heating, so that the foods which contain them are best eaten fresh. If they must be cooked, then this should be reduced to a minimum and the use of alkalies such as sodium bicarbonate (baking powder) which is commonly used to preserve the green colour of vegetables is to be avoided. Even the mashing and cutting up of vegetables into small pieces tends to cause a destruction of vitamins. Vitamin B is relatively resistant.

The Weight of the Body

The weight of the body depends on its size and structure but can be made to vary enormously with the number of calories taken and the amount of physical work done.

If calories in excess of requirement are taken they are stored largely in the form of fat; if insufficient are taken, the body becomes thin. It is possible then to put on weight by eating more or by taking less physical exercise and to lose weight by the reverse. These facts depend on simple physical laws from which normal persons cannot escape. There are a few rare individuals who store fat abnormally as a result of disease of the hypophysis.

Individuals vary, however, in their metabolic rates and in the extent to which protein stimulates their metabolism, for protein in addition to its other qualities appears to fan the body fires somewhat. Thus if a person wishes to lose weight the taking of protein instead of carbohydrate or fat is advantageous. It seems probable, too, that many individuals are fuel wasters and do not absorb, because of bad digestions, all the nourishment they swallow. This failure to absorb into the blood things taken by the mouth is seen in the case of certain inorganic substances, e.g., iron, iodine or calcium, an insufficiency of which may cause anaemia, goitre or rickets respectively.

It can easily be demonstrated by regular weighing, that if a diet consisting solely of vegetable products (apart from legumins and cereals) is taken (e.g., oranges) weight is rapidly lost, for, since the cellulose of vegetables is not digested by man, in reality little or no nourishment is taken. It should be emphasised, too, that if exercise is taken to reduce weight it should be adequate to produce slight breathlessness and should not be compensated by taking additional quantities of food.

The laziest method of getting thin is to take extract of thyroid which stimulates the resting metabolism, but this is not free from danger because of its effect on the heart (see Thyroid gland).

It should be realised, however, that since the body is composed of over 75 per cent. water the amount of water retained materially affects body weight. The taking of salt therefore by causing water retention tends to increase weight and gross increases of several stones occur as the result of the injection of cortisone for rheumatic and other states, since this causes marked salt retention.

The Chemistry of Living Things and of Food

All living things are made up of chemical elements like the things of the inanimate world. These are carbon, hydrogen, oxygen, iron, phosphorus, calcium, sodium, potassium and many others.

The food of animals comes from the animal and plant kingdoms, and is similarly composed.

It is convenient to divide the chemical substances concerned into three main groups, carbohydrates, fats and proteins, but in addition there are other important substances needed such as vitamins, salts and water. These, however, are commonly present in plants and animals.

Carbohydrates

These are substances like starch and sugar, and are composed solely of carbon, hydrogen and oxygen, the latter two being in the proportion as they are in water $2:1$.

The great source of starch in nature is the cereals such as wheat, oats, rice and potatoes, but it is present in small amounts in meat.

Sugar is commonly available as the commercial sugar made from sugar cane and from sugar beet. Sugar of a slightly different kind is also available from fruit (fructose) and from milk (lactose).

At this stage it should be emphasised that starches and sugars are not nearly so dissimilar as their taste might lead us to suppose; indeed, when digested they all very quickly become the same substance, glucose. It is important to understand that all the carbohydrates must be converted into glucose before they can be utilised in the body. Fortunately this conversion is a process which the body can do very easily.   The chemical formula of the substances indicates their essential chemical similarity.

$$(C_6H_{10}O_5)^n \qquad C_{12}H_{22}O_{11} \qquad C_{12}H_{22}O_{11} \qquad C_6H_{12}O_6$$
$$\text{Starch.} \qquad\quad \text{Cane sugar.} \qquad\quad \text{Milk sugar.} \qquad\quad \text{Glucose.}$$

A variety of starch known as *glycogen* occurs in the animal body.   It is stored especially in the muscles and the liver and can be very rapidly converted into glucose by body ferments.

Fats

Fat may be described as concentrated carbohydrate, but the concentration completely alters its physical characteristics, the chief of which are its greasiness and its insolubility in water and solubility in such substances as ether and chloroform.

Its essential chemical nature is indicated by the formula of a typical fat, tristearin $C_{57}H_{110}O_6$.   Unlike the carbohydrate, the fat molecule contains little oxygen.   A given weight of fat, however, contains very much more carbon and hydrogen than a corresponding amount of starch and, therefore, when burnt it gives off more than double the amount of heat.   Fat, therefore, is the fuel to be consumed where there is difficulty in maintaining body temperature.

Fat, however, is not burnt so easily as carbohydrate.   We cannot set fat alight easily but it burns readily if it is put into a coal fire, which vaporises it.   In the body also, fat is liable to be incompletely burnt.

Fats are the natural solvents and therefore carriers of the important vitamins A and D which are intimately concerned with growth, especially of the bones, and with the deposition of chalk within them.

Fat is available in nature for the most part from the fat of animals which have the power of making it from carbohydrates.   It is stored whenever the carbon and hydrogen intake is in excess of immediate needs.   Fats are composed of different fatty acids linked together and the fats of different animals vary in that they have different proportions of fatty acids.   When mutton fat is eaten it is broken down by digestion into its component fatty acids and then rebuilt into human fat.

An important source of fat is milk which is really an emulsion of fat suspended in water.   When examined under the microscope milk may be seen to consist of vast numbers of minute globules of fat.   When concentrated the globules form cream or butter.

In the plant world the most important source of fat is seeds, nuts and various vegetable oils, e.g., linseed and cotton-seed oils, and these are used in the making of margarine and other animal foods.   Olive and corn oils are also extensively used for cooking.

The disadvantage of fats is that they are not very digestible and they tend to slow the digestion of other substances, especially in children in whom fat dyspepsia is very common.   Thus fatty foods are less easily digested than others.   Modern milk from artificially fed cows may contain from two to three times as much fat as human milk.   Thus it is that many children thrive much better on skimmed milk than on whole milk.

Proteins

Protein, as has been observed already, is the essential substance of which living tissue is made. It is the body builder.

In addition to carbon and hydrogen protein contains nitrogen, sulphur and commonly phosphorus.

A protein is composed of amino-acids linked together and the proteins of the different animals and plants vary by being composed of different amino-acids into which they are broken up by the digestive juices. It appears that certain of these amino-acids, known as the *essential amino-acids*, are more important than others and that all animals do not have the power of making them. The carnivorous animals and man do not appear to have the power, for example, of making the amino-acid lysine, which is necessary for growth.

The proteins are utilised in the body for repairing the body tissue in the adult and for building it in the young. If more than necessary is taken into the body, the amino-acids needed for repair are first used and of the remainder, the carbon and hydrogen are used as fuel and burnt or stored, while the rest of the molecule is excreted in. the urine. The nitrogen is excreted as urea, uric acid, ammonium salts and creatinine; the sulphur as sulphates and the phosphorus as phosphates.

In nature the proteins exist in the cellular parts of animals and plants. Typical proteins are the white of egg and meat. Milk contains the important protein caseinogen. Many substances of plant origin also contain protein, e.g., wheat and potatoes, in small quantities but leguminous plants such as peas and beans which have a special power of taking up nitrogen from the air contain larger amounts. Rice may contain as much as 8 per cent. of protein. The importance of these facts is discussed further in relation to metabolism.

The Minerals of the Diet

Sodium. All the cells of the body are bathed in tissue fluid which is a dilute solution of salts of sodium, potassium, and calcium of which sodium chloride (common salt) predominates to the extent of about 0·9 per cent. (see Ringer Locke fluid). It has been suggested that when our remote ancestors left the sea they brought sea water with them in their blood vessels. The cells of the body have a special mechanism known as the sodium pump which keeps the sodium in the cells relatively low in amount, about $\frac{1}{7} - \frac{1}{12}$ of that in the surrounding fluid. This difference in concentration between the inside and outside of the cells assists in the maintenance of the excitability of cells. A heart perfused with fluid without sodium chloride will not beat.

The maintenance of the sodium chloride content of the body is essential to life, as is well seen if excessive amounts of this salt are lost. This occurs in excessive sweating in hot atmospheres and in diarrhoea and vomiting; indeed, salt loss is the common cause of death in cholera and dysentery. Less severe sodium loss shows itself in cramps of muscle, tremor and sometimes unconsciousness. Fortunately if recognised early the condition is easily and rapidly treated by taking additional salt in the food. The taking of excessive salt may, however, lead to the accumulation of water in the body, especially in the feet and legs.

Potassium has long been known to be necessary for the relaxation of the heart, but now it is recognised that it is essential for maintaining the electrical potential of cells generally and for their excitability. This element indeed preponderates in all cells.

After injury or surgical operations, there is a general breakdown of body proteins with a loss of protein and potassium, and this is probably responsible for weakness in convalescence which may be out of all proportion to the injury, a fact which emphasises the desirability of giving diets rich in cells (i.e. proteins) rather than starch.

Iron. There may be, however, deficiencies in the diet in some localities of other essential elements and these are commonly the ingredients of various tonics. Of these *iron*, of which haemoglobin of the red blood corpuscles is made, is the most important. Women who lose blood at the menstrual periods and at childbirth are specially liable to suffer from a deficiency in this element and from the anaemia which results. Normally we get iron in meat, eggs and vegetables, especially spinach. Milk contains very little, and children kept too long on a milk diet tend to look pale from the attendant anaemia. Loss of potassium may accompany severe sodium loss or may occur independently, especially after severe injury or surgical operations, when for some unexplained reason there is great tissue breakdown. The loss produces great muscle weakness. Fortunately it is contained in all the cells we eat, but it tends to be boiled out in some kinds of cooking.

Calcium is a very important mineral constituent of the diet, indeed it is the specific duty of a group of ductless glands (the parathyroids) to keep its concentration at a constant level in the blood stream. They do so by calling on the store of calcium in the bones when necessary. Calcium is one of the chief inorganic constituents of bones and is chiefly responsible for their hardness. Calcium deficiency in children occurs if the vitamin D content of the diet is deficient or if they do not receive sufficient sunlight. It gives rise to a softening of the bones, whereby they easily bend and become misshapen, the condition being known as rickets. It has been estimated that growing children utilise in this way about one gram of calcium daily. A further manifestation of calcium deficiency is seen in chilblains, for a lack of calcium causes an increased permeability of the walls of blood vessels whereby more fluid escapes into the tissues, giving rise to the irritating and often painful swelling which is associated with this condition. Calcium is deficient in the soft Moorland waters with which some of our large towns are supplied but some authorities, e.g., Birmingham, add it at the waterworks.

Calcium deficiency is specially liable to occur in a mother after childbirth, because of the loss of calcium in the milk. Softening of the bones and even deaths occurred before it was realised that the condition could be prevented by giving calcium. When the lungs are over ventilated the available (ionised) calcium of the blood falls and a hyperexcitability of the nervous system occurs resulting in muscular spasms (tetany). This is a danger if breathing exercises are too vigorous.

Calcium is necessary for a great variety of bodily functions, indeed its presence is essential for the normal activity of all organs and especially for the contraction of all muscles and for proper neuromuscular transmission throughout the body including the heart. It is especially necessary in nursing mothers in order to maintain the calcium content of the milk. Calcium is essential for the clotting of blood and of milk.

Calcium is found in hard water, meat, cereals, certain vegetables and in milk. Cheese made from milk is especially rich in calcium. Vitamin D is essential for the proper absorption of calcium from the small intestines and it is lack of this vitamin rather than a lack of calcium which is usually the cause of a deficiency of calcium in the blood. Lack of calcium may also occur during lactation.

Iodine is necessary for the normal activity of the thyroid gland.

Phosphorus is necessary for the formation of bone but it is specially important in the utilisation of glucose and the provision of energy. We have already noted that energy for immediate use is stored in the form of adenine triphosphate (A.T.P.). Fortunately phosphorus is present in most foods and the daily requirements are so small that we excrete it in the urine. We probably use the same phosphorus over and over again.

Fluorine is necessary for the enamel of the teeth and is sometimes added to public water supplies.

Magnesium is required in minute quantities for the action of many enzymes.

Some Common Foods

Milk

Milk is produced by the mammary glands of lactating mammals. During pregnancy the glands under the influence of the anterior lobe of the hypophysis and the corpus luteum of the ovary develop enormously and a great increase of glandular tissue occurs. The breasts become harder and more distinctly lobulated while the veins on the surface become more prominent. The nipple and the areola surrounding it become dark in colour. Eventually milk may be squeezed out of the 15 to 20 ducts which converge at the nipple. Into each of the main ducts a number of smaller ducts from the lobules open. These ducts dilate and act as reservoirs. In late pregnancy secretions of the placenta of the foetus inhibit the glands until the child is born.

Once lactation has begun its continuance depends on the sucking activity of the child which stimulates the hypophysis to secrete the hormone lactogen.

Milk has the following composition per cent.:

	Woman	Cow
Protein (caseinogen and lactalbumen) .	1·7	3·5
Fat	3·4–4·5	3·7–8·0
Sugar (lactose)	6·2	4·9
Salts	0·2	0·7

It must be understood, however, that the milk of all varieties of cows is not identical or that of the same cow at different times of the year. After calving, the fat content of cow's milk may rise to 8 per cent. and the administration of such milk to infants causes indigestion.   Human milk may also vary from time to time.

The first milk after the birth of the child, known as *colostrum*, is richer in proteins and salts but poorer in fat.   It is also more yellow.

From the point of view of nutrition the caseinogen of milk is the more important protein.   Lactalbumin is present in small quantities only, but occasionally children become hypersensitive to the lactalbumin of cow's milk and develop eczema.   In such circumstances the milk has to be treated to remove the lactalbumin which is precipitated by boiling after adding dilute acid.

As indicated by the comparison of human and cow's milk the latter may be adapted for infant use by diluting it with its own volume or more of water and adding a small amount of sugar.

The butter-fat of milk is in the form of a very fine emulsion, the globules of which may be seen under the microscope and it is these which make it white.   It is more digestible than other fats.   In the fat, the valuable vitamins A and some D are dissolved, but these vary with the animal's diet. In winter when cows get little fresh grass, the vitamins may be deficient. Lactose, the sugar of milk, is less sweet than cane sugar and is commonly used as a medium in the making of medicinal tablets.

The salts of milk are especially phosphorus and the chlorides of calcium, magnesium, potassium and sodium.   Iron is deficient and hence children fed largely on milk tend to become anaemic.   An infant, however, is born with a store of iron derived from the blood of its mother.

The clotting of milk occurs when rennin, the ferment produced by the wall of the stomach, comes into contact with it.   The clot is really an insoluble salt of calcium and casein which has been formed from the soluble protein caseinogen.   This clot, which is known as junket or curd, is the first stage in the making of cheese which is essentially compressed curd suitably flavoured.   The fluid which escapes from the jelly when it shrinks is known as whey.

It should be noted that this clotting normally occurs in the stomach and some children find the clot or curd difficult to digest.   Its digestibility is improved by diluting with soda water or by the addition of sodium citrate. The latter reduces the action of calcium which is essential for the clotting of milk as it is for the clotting of blood.

The souring of milk.   If milk is exposed to the air it sours as a result of the production of acid by the lactic acid bacillus.   The acid causes acid curdling, like rennin.

The sterilisation of milk.   The souring of milk may be prevented by destroying the bacteria by boiling and keeping it protected from the air. This simple experiment was performed by Lister to prove the existence of bacteria and the value of such treatment in milk preservation.

Many kinds of bacteria can live and grow very freely in milk.   The bacteria of diphtheria, scarlet fever, typhoid and tuberculosis may be carried in milk, the latter organism being derived usually from the cow, the others from those who handle the milk. The prevalence of bovine tuberculosis which spreads in this way has led to special preventive care being taken. At one time it was found that in some districts as much as 70 per cent. of the herds were infected with the tubercle bacillus and tuberculosis of bones was very common.

Ideally, milk should be taken from tuberculin tested (T.T.) cows under hygienic conditions into sterilised cans and kept cooled till consumed. This is compulsory in Britain and tuberculosis is becoming rare.

When milk is sterilised, i.e., its bacteria killed by boiling, the fat emulsion is made coarser (use is made of this in the making of Devonshire cream), the lactalbumin is coagulated and the caseinogen is less digestible. Its vitamins may also be destroyed.

A partial sterilisation known as pasteurisation in which the milk is kept for half an hour at 145° F. and rapidly cooled has been found to kill most disease-causing organisms including the tubercle bacillus. It is, however, a laborious and expensive process.

The advantages and disadvantages of milk in the diet. There can be little doubt that to under-nourished children a ration of milk is of enormous advantage because of the additional calories and vitamins supplied. Children otherwise well fed do not necessarily benefit in the same way and in them the disadvantages become apparent. Fat dyspepsia may lead to faulty nutrition including dental decay (see fat). Some children appear to have an inherent difficulty in digesting milk and it should not be forgotten that milk is not a normal diet of animals after they are weaned and rennin disappears from the stomach of the adult. Fortunately the vitamins present in milk are as easily obtained from green foods and sunlight.

Derivatives of Milk

Cream is the lighter fat portion of the milk which rises to the surface if the milk stands. It rises more rapidly if the milk is warmed (Devonshire cream). It may also be separated mechanically by a separator.

Cheese is essentially the caseinogen of milk, precipitated as casein by rennin with a certain amount of fat. Depending on whether or not the cream has been previously removed the product is flavoured or coloured and otherwise treated according to the special variety of cheese made.

The Cereals

Cereals form much the largest part of the diet of civilised man. The chief are wheat, oats, rice, maize, rye and barley. In Britain flour made from wheat may be looked upon as the staple article of diet. The cereals consist for the most part of starch, but there is an appreciable amount of protein (5 per cent. to 10 per cent. in most cereals).

The stickiness of wet flour is due to the proteins, especially the gluten, it contains. These hold together the various foodstuffs prepared from wheat and oats and its absence accounts for the difficulty of making bread with maize or barley.

Unfortunately it has become usual to separate the starch from the seeds

27—A.PH.

by milling in order to obtain a white flour which keeps better* and makes the articles baked from it more agreeable in appearance. With the removal of the covering from the seed the valuable bran and the germ in the embryo are lost. These not only contain vitamins B and E but are important in giving bulk to the diet and acting as a stimulant to the secretion of mucus by the large colon. Bran is therefore often added to the diet of both man and animals to prevent constipation. The covering of the seed also contains the protein, salts and small quantities of fat. Brown bread is better than white in this respect, but wholemeal bread is to be preferred. It should, however, be pointed out that these articles are not desirable for those suffering from irritative conditions of the intestinal tract.

Cooking greatly improves the digestibility of cereals; indeed, badly cooked starch may escape ordinary digestion and subsequently ferment and be responsible for the formation of gas in the lower parts of the bowel. This is particularly true of some of the starch contained in the coarser vegetables and of starch added to thicken soups or gravies. The digestion of uncooked starch by animals is assisted by the digestive enzymes present in the seed in its wild state.

The starch granules are burst by adequate boiling or baking. Baking, like toasting, converts the starch granules into soluble starch and the slightly sweet dextrins which are really the first stage in digestion. In the making of bread, yeast is added to cause fermentation with the formation of carbon dioxide and alcohol. Practically all the latter is lost in the baking but the gas gives to the bread its lightness and sponginess which facilitates the access of the digestive juices. In baking articles such as cakes, a baking powder consisting largely of sodium bicarbonate and acid is added to the flour and when wetted the bicarbonate and acid react together to give off the gas.

Oatmeal is coarser than wheat-flour because it is more difficult to remove the seed covering by milling. It has, however, more protein, fat and salts but unfortunately it also contains a considerable quantity of phytin which interferes with the absorption of calcium and tends to cause rickets and bad teeth. Oatmeal porridge should, therefore, be accompanied by large quantities of milk to antagonise the phytin, which contains phosphorus.

Rice is also very rich in starch but also contains protein.

Various Starch products. *Cornflour* is almost pure starch made from maize. *Macaroni and vermicelli* are preparations of wheat flour forced through tubes and dried. *Arrowroot* is prepared from the roots of maranta, a West Indian plant. Its starch is specially digestible because of its association with digestive enzymes. It will digest itself if kept wet and warm. *Sago* is prepared from the pith of the sago palm. *Tapioca* is prepared from the roots of cassava, a tropical plant. *Semolina* is a granular preparation of wheat flour.

Various other proprietary foods are chiefly composed of starch in association with enzymes which may be sufficient to partly digest the starch if the

* Since most of our wheat comes from North America this is an important economic fact.

preparation is added to water and kept warm.

Eggs contain all the elements necessary for the formation of a young animal. The white consists of a richly protein fluid in a network of firmer material. The yolk contains the important phospho-protein, vitellin, cholesterol and fatty substances. Eggs are most nourishing and very readily digestible but they are much less so when cooked. They are also an important source of the vitamins A, B and D.

Meats are composed of muscle with an admixture of fibre and collagen (gristle) according to cut. It is composed of about 75 per cent. water and 25 per cent. protein. Its flavour is due to the different mixtures of salts and extractives regarding which little is known. There is no reason to believe that the nutritive value of meat is in any way reduced by freezing although in some way the flavour is affected, while the cheaper cuts are just as nutritious as the more expensive. On hanging, meat tends to become more tender because of the acid substances formed in it which facilitate the conversion of collagen to gelatine. Steak is commonly made more tender by mechanical rupture of its fibrous parts by beating or cutting with minute knives. On the whole the more tender the meat the more readily it is digested because the digestive juices penetrate more easily between its fibres. It is of interest to remark that animals which bolt their food, such as dogs, digest minced meat less effectively than meat in large pieces, since the latter remains in the stomach longer.

Cooking precipitates the proteins and causes a marked loss of water. Boiling tends to dissolve out the extractives and the flavour of the meat but otherwise there is little difference between this and roasting. It is important to remark that these meat extracts are much more important than is generally recognised. They not only create an interest in the food and thus stimulate digestion but they also have a beneficial effect on the secretion of the gastric juice. The protein value of cooked meat varies from 20 to 30 per cent. Different meats vary appreciably in their fat content, a fact which materially affects their digestibility by invalids who have difficulty in digesting fats. Roast pork and roast duck have over 23 per cent. Stewed steak and roast chicken have under 10 per cent. Boiled chicken, on the other hand, has a slightly higher fat content.

Fish is generally less fatty and more readily digested than meat but some fish, e.g., herring, mackerel and salmon, contain much fat.

When, however, fish is fried about 12 per cent. fat may be added to it, hence the desirability of steaming or boiling fish for invalids. High-speed cooking in deep fat does not allow so much fat to penetrate as ordinary frying. Apart from fat, fish generally has a much smaller calorific value than meat. It has, however, a liberal protein content; indeed, herring and cod provide a good source of first-class protein.

Soups consist of water in which meat, bones or vegetables have been boiled and if clear consist only of salts and tasty extractives apart from the variable amount of gelatine they may contain. They supply important salts (especially potassium) but are not foods and are efficacious in stimulating the gastric juice. The same may be said of beef tea and many meat extracts from which clear soups are made.

Condiments. These play a valuable part in stimulating the digestive processes by increasing the palatability and desirability of the food and by acting directly on the stomach. They are to be avoided when any conditions such as ulcer or chronic inflammation are present.

Alcohol as an adjunct to food has advantages and disadvantages according to the individual concerned.

There can be no doubt of its beneficial action as a digestive. Dilute alcohol is a strong stimulant of gastric secretion and tends to promote a sense of well-being which is beneficial to the digestive processes generally. These considerations are commonly of value in invalids whose digestion may be subnormal and in whom worries may be exaggerated. There is no advantage in champagne or brandy over other wines or spirits of similar alcoholic strength.

On the other hand, the irritation caused especially by cocktails or spirits taken on an empty stomach may lead to inflammatory states of the gastric mucous membrane. This may amount to acute gastritis with vomiting but more commonly it leads to a low-grade dyspepsia which may long pass unrecognised. The taking of large quantities of alcohol has been shown to have a marked effect on the liver which may result in the destruction of liver cells. Eventually the blood supply through the organ may become obstructed resulting in abdominal dropsy (ascites).

Tea and Coffee. The use of these in moderate quantities does not appear to be harmful. They both depend for their stimulant action on their caffeine content and in this there is little difference between them. Caffeine is a nerve stimulant. It therefore makes the brain more active and increases the heart rate. There is great individual variation in the reaction to the drug. In sensitive persons sleep may be prevented and the heart unduly stimulated. On the other hand, caffeine reduces the sense of fatigue and may promote sleep in overtired persons. Coffee has the disadvantage of containing fat and when roasted is a gastric irritant. It is, therefore, disadvantageous in dyspepsia and hyperacidity. The disadvantage of tea is explained by its tannin content. Tannin is a protein precipitant and has an astringent action on the lining of the stomach. It gives the bitter taste to tea which has been long infused—the tannin content does not depend on the quality of the tea. Tea freshly made contains little tannin and this may be precipitated by the addition of milk. When infused tea has to be stored, it should be kept in contact with the leaves for three or four minutes only. Coco-cola is also a caffeine-containing beverage.

CHAPTER XX

DIGESTION AND METABOLISM

The various foodstuffs upon which we depend for nourishment do not commonly exist in a form in which they can be absorbed from the alimentary canal into the blood stream. They are usually protected and insoluble but become so changed by the process of digestion that they are readily absorbed.

The process involved is twofold, namely, mechanical and chemical, the latter being much the more important.

The food when first taken into the mouth is chewed and so broken up. During the chewing it is mixed with saliva and swallowed into the stomach where digestion commences and is continued in the intestine.

The process of digestion is carried out by the digestive juices which consist of acids and alkalies whose action is greatly hastened by the action of ferments or enzymes. Each variety of food is digested by different enzymes, of which the pepsin of the stomach is probably the best known. This process of digestion is purely chemical, for if the suitable substances are mixed together and kept at body temperature in a test tube digestion takes place in the ordinary way.

The digestive juices are secreted by glands. Glands exist in the digestive and respiratory tracts and in the skin for the purpose of manufacturing from the blood, substances which have special functions. In the respiratory tract they secrete mucus; in the skin, sweat.

The glands themselves are sometimes just enfoldings of the mucous membrane lining the canal but often they are branched and elaborate, with ducts which open to the surface.

Enzymes

In relation to digestion we referred to ferments or enzymes, but it should be realised that these remarkable substances play a fundamental part in practically all the chemical processes which take place in the body. Strong hydrochloric acid will break down protein quite quickly but the dilute acid of the stomach would do so very slowly, were it not for the action of the pepsin which acts as a catalyst. A catalyst is a substance which facilitates a chemical reaction without necessarily taking part in it. We are familiar with certain substances which if held in ordinary coal gas or petrol vapour will cause them to ignite in air. There are gas-lighters on this principle which do not need a flint.

The importance of enzymes in the breakdown of foodstuffs in the digestive tract has long been known and it has been referred to in relation to blood clotting, but it is now known that they are of importance in relation to such diverse activities as the oxidation of substances in the tissues, the calcification of bone, the breakdown and building up of glycogen by the liver and the rapid destruction of acetylcholine. Yet we do not at present know what exactly they are nor how they act. Like vitamins, they used to be looked upon as animate because they are easily inactivated by boiling but now many have been isolated in crystalline form.

Digestion

In the Mouth. Here the food is broken up by chewing and mixed with the saliva which has the dual function of lubrication and digestion. Saliva is secreted by the various glands which open into the mouth, especially the salivary glands. The mucous of the saliva acts as a lubricant and facilitates swallowing while the digestion of starch is initiated by its *diastase* or *ptyalin,* which converts boiled starch first to dextrin then to maltose. Natural starch if merely moistened and kept warm is converted into malt by the diastase of the husk. This is the first process in the making of beer or whisky. The saliva is secreted largely as a result of the anticipation and taste of food as may be well seen if food is shown to a dog. It may also secrete saliva if it sees, hears or feels a sensation which by experience is associated with the taking of food. This is known as a "conditioned reflex."

In the Stomach. After swallowing the food enters the stomach which is primarily a container, but in it is begun the digestion of protein, and the digestion of starch by the saliva is continued.

Samples of *gastric juice* can be obtained through a small rubber tube which strangely enough is quite easy to swallow and through which the juice is withdrawn by means of a syringe. The factors affecting its secretion are studied by withdrawing samples from time to time. It is found to contain a number of substances of which the most important are:

1. Hydrochloric acid and the enzyme pepsin which begin the digestion of proteins by converting them into proteoses and peptones.

2. Rennin—another enzyme, which curdles milk.

3. Lipase is present but is probably regurgitated from the duodenum.

4. Mucus, which has a lubricant and protective function.

5. A nerve-nourishing factor without which degeneration of the spinal cord is liable to occur.

6. A blood-forming factor without which the formation of the red cells is inadequate and death may occur from pernicious anaemia. It is now known that this substance is concerned with the absorption of vitamin B_{12}.

7. Salts, especially sodium chloride.

The secretion of gastric juice. Normally there is a very dilute juice in the stomach, but if a test meal of tea and toast is given there is a copious secretion of pepsin and hydrochloric acid which may rise from 0·01 to 0·2 per cent. by the end of an hour and a half, after which it becomes neutralised by alkali produced by the pyloric end of the stomach and regurgitated from the duodenum. It is also diluted by the secretion of a weak sodium chloride solution. If the neutralisation or dilution does not take place the subject is liable to gastric or duodenal ulcer.

The gastric juice is produced by the oxyntic cells of the body of the stomach, but in many persons who suffer from acidity these appear to be excessive in number.

Gastric secretion is believed to be brought about by three phases which, of course, overlap.

The first is cephalic and nervous and is the result of impulses reaching the vagus centre from the senses of sight, smell and taste of food. The impulses pass down to the stomach by the vagus nerves.

The second process is gastric and chemical and is due to the action of the food itself on the pyloric antrum of the stomach. If an extract of this part is injected into the blood stream, a secretion of gastric juice is produced, and it is therefore believed that the hormone *gastrin* is normally released into the blood by the foods, especially meat extracts and dextrin from the digestion of starch. Mere distension of the stomach may also cause a release. Alcohol and especially sodium bicarbonate (baking soda) are stimulants. The latter is specially important as it is often taken to neutralise excessive acidity. For this purpose the divalent salts of magnesium (oxide) and calcium (carbonate) are best.

Emotional states which may increase or decrease the secretion according to their nature also act via these nerves. Severe stress or physical exercises reduces the secretion of the juice but depression may lead to an over-secretion. In many persons it is now recognised that there is a high resting secretion when the subject is asleep, that is when the sympathetic activity is largely in abeyance and the parasympathetic predominates. This night secretion is easily prevented by atropine.

In the Duodenum. This upper part of the small intestine is of special importance in digestion because there are poured into it the digestive juices elaborated by the pancreas and which by virtue of its enzymes and sodium bicarbonate, plays such a large part in digestion. The duodenum also receives the bile from the gall-bladder and liver which has an important role in regard to the absorption of fats and all fat soluble vitamins. In the wall of this part of the intestine are the glands of Brünner which secrete an alkaline juice and it also produces the hormones *secretin* and *pancreozymin* which are responsible for pancreatic secretion.

Digestion by the Pancreatic Juice.

Pancreatic juice is composed of water, organic solids, and inorganic salts and is strongly alkaline in reaction.

The organic constituents are made up of the enzymes, chiefly the trypsin group, the trypsinogen group which requires activation by the intestinal juice (see Enzymes), amylase and lipase. The inorganic constituents are salts, especially sodium bicarbonate. *The trypsin* group is composed of several powerful proteolytic enzymes which split proteins, proteoses and pep-tones into polypeptides and then into their constituent amino-acids. These enzymes, because of the diverse nature of their action, digest more resistant proteins than pepsin, such as fibrin, gelatin and casein.

Amylase acts on carbohydrates, converting them into dextrin and maltose. It is much more powerful than ptyalin and can act on unboiled starch.

Lipase splits fats into fatty acids and glycerol. The fatty acids unite with glycerol to form soaps which greatly facilitate the absorption of fat. The soaps form a film on the surface of the fat globules which prevents them running together; the fats are thus suspended or emulsified, a process which is greatly facilitated by the action of bile.

Secretion of pancreatic juice is due principally to two hormones, *secretin* and *pancreozymin*, which are found in the wall of the duodenum but stimulation of the vagus nerves will bring about a secretion. When the stomach contents pass into the duodenum, peristaltic waves are initiated which relax the sphincter of Oddi and bile passes into the duodenum. Through the agency of bile salts secretin is absorbed into the blood and is carried round to the pancreas causing it to produce a copious flow of sodium bicarbonate and water. It has been found that the vagus and the hormone pancreozymin are responsible for the secretion of the pancreatic enzymes.

Digestion by the Succus Entericus.

The succus entericus is secreted by the glands of Lieberkühn in the small intestine. The presence of food in the intestine stimulates its secretion as also do the hormones secretin and histamine. The following enzymes are found in the succus entericus:

Erepsin which acts on proteoses and peptones produced at earlier stages and converts them into amino-acids.

The succus entericus converts disaccharides into monosaccharides through the agency of three enzymes—*invertase* which converts sucrose (cane sugar) into glucose and fructose; *maltase* which converts maltose into glucose; and *lactase* which converts lactose into galactose. The latter is converted into glucose in the liver.

In addition, the succus entericus secretes an activator of the pancreatic juice called *enterokinase* which is not an enzyme, but pancreatic juice cannot digest proteins without it.

At this stage it might be useful to summarise the various enzymes secreted by the digestive organs with a brief indication of their functions:

Mouth
Ptyalin converts boiled starch into maltose (in the stomach).

Stomach
Pepsin with HCl converts proteins into peptones.

Rennin clots milk.

Gastric lipase converts fats into fatty acids and glycerol (feeble action when compared with pancreatic lipase).

Pancreas
Trypsin with alkali converts proteins through a number of stages to amino-acids.

Amylase converts carbohydrates into glucose.

Pancreatic lipase (with the assistance of bile) converts fats into fatty acids and glycerol.

Intestine
Enterokinase converts trypsinogen, which is inactive, into trypsin.

Erepsin converts peptones into amino-acids.

Maltase converts maltose into glucose.

Invertase inverts cane-sugar into glucose and laevulose.

Lactase converts lactose into glucose and galactose.

Absorption and Functions of the Small Intestine

The digested foodstuffs are spread out over the very large surface of the small intestine, a surface which is increased not only by the folds in the mucous membrane but by its millions of villi.

Little absorption takes place in the stomach. There is absorption chiefly of water from the large intestine but the absorption of the products of the digested food occurs almost entirely from the small intestine, from which amino-acids, glucose and 40 per cent. of the fats are carried by the blood vessels which are tributaries of the portal vein to the liver, and the remaining 60 per cent. of the fats are carried into the lacteals and so into the thoracic duct.

The exact process by which absorption takes place is incompletely understood but we may assume that the process of diffusion plays a part, that is the substances simply pass from a region where they are concentrated, viz., the lumen of the intestine, to one in which they are less so, viz., the blood. At the same time it can be shown that there is some selectivity for glucose passes through more rapidly than any other carbohydrate.

Water is probably absorbed by osmosis, the plasma of the blood taking up water as salt does in a moist atmosphere. Salt solutions stronger than that of the blood are first diluted and then absorbed.

It seems possible that the activity of the villi is important. These minute finger-like processes can be seen under the microscope to be constantly contracting and relaxing and in so doing they probably squeeze some of their contents into the blood stream.

Metabolism

Metabolism of Carbohydrates.* All carbohydrates, in whatever form they may be taken and through whatever intermediate stages they may pass, are finally converted into glucose, and used as a source of energy and heat and are eventually oxidised into CO_2 and water. For the breakdown phosphorus is needed. The total amount of glycogen stored in the body is about 600 grams; 350 grams in the muscles and 250 grams in the liver. Six hundred grams of glycogen give 3,000 Calories which is sufficient energy for one day. If excess carbohydrate or protein is taken, the carbon and hydrogen are stored as glycogen (animal starch) in the liver.

For the complete utilisation of carbohydrates, *insulin*, a hormone produced by the islets of Langerhans in the pancreas is necessary and in its absence the condition of diabetes mellitus occurs. Diabetes is characterised by the appearance of glucose in the urine, because the unused glucose accumulates in the blood. It was formerly a fatal condition because of the faulty oxidation of fat (see later) which is produced, but now it is successfully treated by the injection of insulin obtained from the pancreas of animals. If an excess of insulin is injected, the glucose is converted into glycogen in the liver and muscles, causing a fall of blood sugar which may end in death.

Glucose appears in the urine whenever its level in the blood rises above

* For the composition of carbohydrates see p. 399.

180 mg. per 100 c.c. Normally it is between 75 and 100 mg. but after eating carbohydrates, indeed if sufficient is taken, glucose may appear in the urine (alimentary glycosuria).

Metabolism of Fats.* The fat in the body may be derived not only from the fats in the diet but also from carbohydrates and to a less extent from protein. Fat is taken up in the intestinal villi partly as fatty acid and glycerol and partly as neutral fat, but however absorbed it appears in the lacteals as neutral fat. Only 60 per cent. of the fat is absorbed into the lacteals the remainder passes to the liver via the portal vein. Fat is either burnt as fuel or is stored in the fat depots as a source of energy. It is the most economical method of storing energy for 1 gram of fat when burnt produces 9·3 calories of heat. Fat is a source of the vitamins A, D, E and K.

Fat in the fat depots contains 95 per cent. of saturated fatty acids. Liver fat is less saturated and one of the functions of the liver is to desaturate fats and this is the normal preliminary to their oxidation.

The fat burnt is converted into carbon dioxide and water, and for this adequate carbohydrate breakdown is essential. In diabetes, when carbohydrate utilisation is faulty, the products of abnormal fat metabolism (β hydroxybutyric acid, aceto-acetic acid and acetone) may accumulate in the blood and poison the patient.

Metabolism of proteins. (For the composition of proteins see p. 401.) Proteins are needed for growth and repair and those that are not wanted for this purpose are used as a source of energy. Protein alone among the foodstuffs provides the amino-acids essential for the construction of new tissue. Amino-acids are also required to build up substances essential for the normal function and well-being of the body, e.g., the hormones, the enzymes and the bile acids. The remaining amino-acids which are not used for this purpose are deaminated in the liver, i.e. they lose their nitrogenous part which is converted into urea by the liver and excreted by the kidney, the non-nitrogenous portions are used as a source of energy and are eventually burnt, the end products being CO_2 and water.

The modern method of labelling artificially made amino-acids with isotopes has shown that the proteins so readily move around the body that there may be a protein pool from which the body draws as needed. All the proteins seem to undergo a complete turnover every 160 days, but those in the blood and liver are changed every 20 days. Labelled nitrogen given in an amino acid distributes itself very rapidly throughout the whole body.

The nitrogen of protein metabolism is excreted in the urine, especially as urea and ammonium salts. Nitrogen excretion in the urine may be taken as an indication of the volume of protein metabolism occurring in the body.

Certain amino-acids, known as " essential amino-acids," are especially important as they cannot be built by the animal body and must be supplied in the diet. Thus when tissue has to be rebuilt as the result of pregnancy and lactation or after injuries which lead to much protein loss or in recovery from wasting diseases and particularly in the formation of new tissue during the period of growth, these amino-acids are essential (see p. 401).

* For the composition of fats see p. 400.

This is also true after injuries. For some unexplained reason injuries lead to great stimulation of tissue breakdown as seen by a greatly increased excretion of nitrogen and potassium in the urine.

Nucleo-proteins contain nucleic acid which is derived from the nuclei of cells and is present in quantity in cellular organs, e.g., liver, kidney, sweetbreads, etc.

These nucleo-proteins are first split into nuclein and protein by the gastric juice. By the action of the pancreatic juice the protein is converted into peptone and amino-acids and the nuclein into nucleic acid and protein. The final products which pass into the blood are the amino-acids from the protein part and purines, pyramidines, phosphoric acid and hexose (or pentose) from the nucleic acid, which are converted by the liver into uric acid and excreted by the kidneys.

The biological value of proteins. This term was originally applied to the power of proteins to permit the growth of young animals, but it may now be used in a much wider sense. The proteins of other animals contain all the substances necessary for the general nourishment of our bodies. They contain all the mineral elements we require especially potassium and the vitamins. We have already remarked on the need of vitamin B_{12} for the formation of the red blood cells. For general purposes the order of biological value is generally considered to be—eggs, milk, meat, wholemeal bread, potato, oats, corn, white flour and beans.

Functions of the Large Intestine.

Mechanical function. The large intestine stores the faeces and then evacuates them.

Absorptive function. Although digestion and most of the absorption are complete by the time the food reaches the large intestine, the contents of the intestine are still quite fluid. As they pass through the colon absorption of water takes place, hence the longer the faeces remain in the bowel the drier they become. This is evident in constipation.

Because of its absorptive powers it is possible to feed a patient per rectum, but these feeds are confined to readily absorbable substances in solution such as glucose, although even this is absorbed but slowly. Anaesthetics are sometimes given per rectum, e.g., avertin.

Secretive function. Mucus is secreted as the result of mechanical stimulation by the goblet cells and acts as a lubricant. Lack of this is one of the commonest causes of constipation.

Excretive function. The large intestine excretes substances which are not easily excreted by the kidney, such as the salts of heavy metals.

Bacterial action. The bacteria of the human colon do not appear to have much functional value except the production of the important vitamin B. In herbivorous animals, in which the large intestine is very large, they are, however, responsible for the breakdown of the carbohydrate cellulose of plants which is their chief source of energy.

The Movements of the Alimentary Canal

These movements are most effectively studied in man by means of a barium or bismuth meal. The insoluble salts of these metals are added to some simple food like cornflour and render the meal opaque to X-rays; their course along the alimentary canal may, therefore, be followed readily.

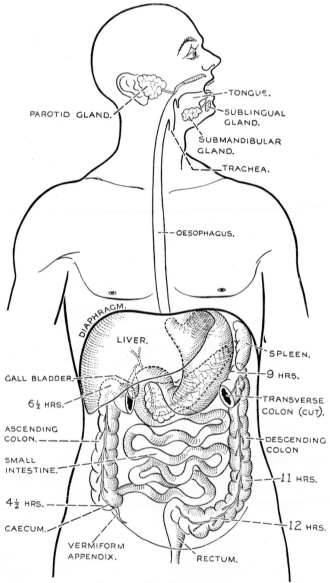

FIG. 290.—The alimentary tract.

The times at which food reaches the various parts of the large intestine are indicated.

By this means it can be shown that food begins to leave the stomach almost immediately it enters, but takes 3 to 5 hours to reach the caecum. It takes about 1½–2 hours more to reach the hepatic flexure and another 1½–2 hours to reach the splenic flexure, but it may remain many hours in the descending and pelvic colons. If not evacuated a reverse peristalsis may carry it backwards from the rectum to the pelvic colon where it is stored.

Swallowing. When food is taken into the mouth it is pushed by the tongue and cheeks into the back of the throat where it sets up a reflex or automatic contraction of the muscles of the pharynx. This drives it rapidly into the oesophagus down which it is forced by a wave of contraction or peristaltic movement which is not under voluntary control. As it reaches the opening into the stomach, both this orifice and the portion of the stomach in its neighbourhood relax and the food enters. Dry food may pass very slowly down the oesophagus and stick at the entrance of the stomach until it is forced into that organ by peristaltic waves which may cause considerable pain.

The Movements of the Stomach

The stomach acts for the most part as a container and, apart from exerting gentle pressure on its contents, does not move very much. If the food is not too fluid it tends to form layers in the upper part of the stomach and this is an advantage from the point of view of digestion, as it allows salivary digestion to continue without being interrupted by the acid of the stomach.

The pyloric portion of the stomach is, however, very active and is sometimes known as the pyloric mill. There, food is mixed and wafted gently through the pyloric sphincter guarding the exit from the stomach. The pain in one form of indigestion is caused when the pyloric portion of the stomach tries to drive a large mass of food into the duodenum. Sticky foods (such as badly cooked pastry or suet puddings, new bread and the like) tend to form large masses and are, therefore, particularly likely to cause this form of indigestion. In this connection it should be pointed out that the term "indigestion," as used popularly, usually refers to pains in the region of the stomach. Many articles of diet, such as the cellulose which forms the fibrous structure and skins of plants, are quite undigested by man but they do not usually cause indigestion.

Food, especially if it is fluid and alkaline, begins to leave the stomach almost at once and usually the organ is empty three hours after a meal has entered. Hard pieces of material may remain for many hours and, if large enough, indefinitely, while fluids pass through readily.

Movements of the Small Intestine

The chief movements of this part of the alimentary canal are peristalsis, segmentation and pendular movements.

Peristalsis consist essentially of a wave of contraction which is preceded by a wave of relaxation and is a movement by which the contents of many tubes throughout the body are moved along. The chief stimulus for peristaltic action is the stretching of the muscular wall of the intestines by the food and in this connection it should be remembered that food which produces a large residue, e.g., cellulose, is an important factor in causing this onward movement of the contents of the bowels, hence the importance of including in the diet substances such as wholemeal bread or bran, fruit, vegetables, etc. These also cause an increased secretion of mucus by the colon.

Segmentation consists of ring-like constrictions of the intestinal wall which divide the contents into sausage-like segments. This churns up the food so that it becomes thoroughly mixed. Segmentation does not produce an onward movement of the intestinal contents and is thus quite different from peristalsis.

Pendular movements are likewise not designed to propel the food on-wards but augment the action of segmentation. They effect side to side movement of the intestines which further helps to mix the contents thoroughly.

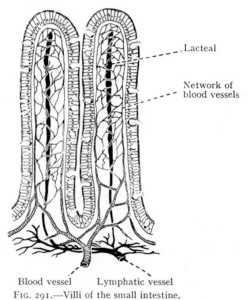

Lacteal

Network of blood vessels

Blood vessel   Lymphatic vessel

Fig. 291.—Villi of the small intestine.

In addition to these movements of the intestines as a whole, the villi are said to exercise a pumping action, referred to in regard to absorption. For this a hormone, called *villikinin*, is said to be responsible.

Movements of the Large Intestine

A barium meal is seen to reach the ileocaecal valve of the large intestine in four and a half hours, and various points on its subsequent route are indicated in fig. 290. These times are important as delay or accumulation indicates obstruction. When food reaches the rectum a desire for defaeca-tion is produced, but if this is ignored there is reverse peristalsis and the contents pass back into the colon when they lose more water and become hard. Such neglect is a common cause of constipation.

The movements of the large intestine are mainly due to peristalsis and are

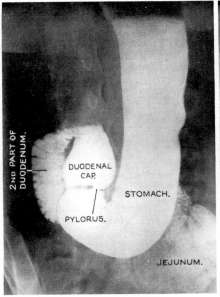

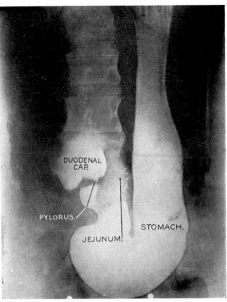

Average shape, size and position of normal stomach immediately after a meal. Note the narrow pylorus, the regular filling of the duodenal cap and the irregular contours of the 2nd part of duodenum to the left and of jejunal coils to the right.

Long, low stomach immediately after a meal showing peristaltic wave in the pre-pyloric area.

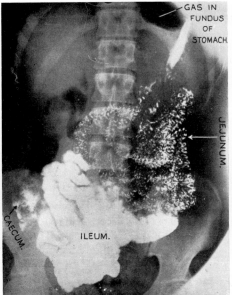

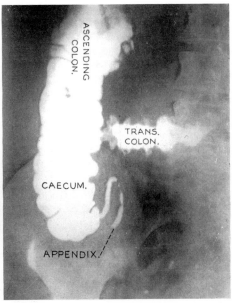

Radiograph 3 hours after meal showing pattern of the barium contents of jejunal and ileal coils.

Radiograph 9 hours after meal showing barium in appendix (which shows peristalsis), caecum, ascending and transverse colon.

Fig. 292.

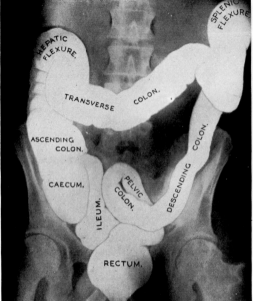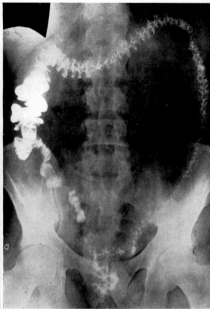

Radiograph showing disposition of large intestine which has been filled with a barium enema.

Radiograph showing same patient after the enema has been voided (note mucosal pattern).

FIG. 292 (contd.).

increased when food is taken into the stomach for at the same time the ileo-caecal valve relaxes and food, which at this point is quite fluid, passes from the small intestine.   These reflexes, known as the gastro-colic and ileo-colic reflexes, give rise to the increased desire to defaecate after breakfast, but this is in part caused by the assumption of the erect posture on rising from bed.

Usually the bowel is evacuated daily but individuals vary enormously in this respect.   Bulky food with an indigestible residue not only induces peristalsis but, as we have seen, causes an increased secretion of mucus which acts as a lubricant for the bowel.

The General Control of Digestion

Although in the absence of the nervous connections, digestion will continue because of the influence of chemical stimuli, normally it is controlled by the autonomic nerves.   All parts of the canal are supplied by sympathetic nerves which inhibit its activity.   The evidence is very complete that in intense mental emotion or severe exercise all the digestive processes are at a standstill.   The mouth becomes dry from lack of salivary secretion and this may be considered typical of what is occurring down the alimentary canal. Peristalsis is inhibited and if we judge by analogy it would seem that the pyloric and ileocaecal sphincters are closed so that the food is held up.   All these actions may be produced by adrenaline which we know acts like the sympathetic.   Although food is held up in the stomach and protein digestion inhibited it has been shown by experiment that the digestion of starch is continued by any saliva which may have been swallowed.

The action of the parasympathetic is, so far as glands are concerned, to increase the pouring out especially of the enzymatic part of the digestive juices and the secretion of mucus. In regard to movement its action appears to be to increase the movements of the alimentary canal, that is both contraction and relaxation. Thus we see that in exercise the role of the sympathetic and vagus in regard to digestion are the reverse of what they are in relation to the circulation. These facts are of importance because in convalescence vagal action is commonly very small and digestion is impaired. Therefore a light and easily digestible diet is desirable and indeed is in common use in hospitals especially in any state when the body temperature is raised. In such circumstances the subject very seldom desires food and has to be tempted to take a minimum, but digestion may be stimulated by the judicious use of meat extracts and dilute alcohol.

Thirst

Lack of sufficient fluid leads, as we all know, to a drying of the back of the tongue known as thirst. This is a local condition as is shown by the fact that it is abolished by painting the tongue with cocaine but it may be produced in a variety of ways. If a strong solution of salt or sugar or alcohol is taken it exerts an osmotic action on the tongue and abstracts water from the sensitive nerve endings concerned and this produces the thirst. If, however, there has been an excessive loss of water from the body, as in sweating on a hot day, the blood becomes more concentrated and the proteins of the blood exert a higher osmotic action and reduce the secretion of saliva and in turn produce a dryness of the mouth. In such circumstances thirst acts as an important safeguard against dehydration of the body.

Hunger

The exact cause of hunger is still a subject of debate. If a balloon attached to a tambour is swallowed and made to record on a drum, it can be shown that hunger is associated with contractions of the stomach, but if these are accurately timed it is observed that the hunger pain occurs between the contractions. The pain may also be produced by increasing the pressure in the balloon. Sensations in the stomach are produced by reducing the amount of sugar in the blood by means of insulin, but diabetics say they differ from hunger pains and it is found that they do not correspond to the hunger contractions.

It would seem, therefore, that lack of food somehow increases the tension in the stomach and this brings on both the hunger contractions and hunger pains, but there is a considerable psychological element concerned, for the extent to which hunger pains are experienced depends very largely on the habit of the subject and has very little relationship to the intake of food. Patients often show a disinclination for food which is distressing, while many well-nourished persons feel very hungry if they miss a single meal. There is now increasing evidence that there is an appetite centre in the brain.

28—A.PH.

CHAPTER XXI

THE LIVER

The liver receives via the portal vein all the digested carbohydrates, the proteins and about 40 per cent. of the fats (the remainder of the fats are carried into the bloodstream via the thoracic duct).

The liver is composed of a large number of small lobules which can be seen with the naked eye when fresh liver is cut across. Each lobule is composed of *columns of liver cells* arranged in a radial manner around a central vein (fig. 293).

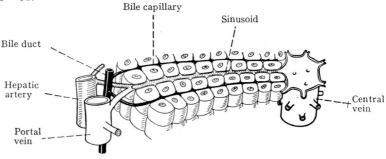

FIG. 293.

At the periphery of each lobule are the *interlobular veins* which are the terminal branches of the portal vein, the *interlobular bile ducts* and the terminal branches of the *hepatic artery* all embedded in areolar tissue. These branches of the hepatic artery open into the interlobular veins. The latter pass into vessels called *sinusoids* which run between the columns of liver cells carrying oxygenated blood from the hepatic artery and nutritious blood from the portal vein to the liver substance. In the walls of the sinusoids are the *stellate cells of Kupffer* which are part of the reticulo-endothelial system and have already been referred to (p. 353). The bile capillaries like the sinusoids are bounded on either side by the liver cells (fig. 293).

As the blood passes between the liver cells certain substances are removed from the plasma and are acted on by the liver cells. They are then converted into substances which can be used by the tissues of the body or into waste products which can be excreted. The liver cells also collect the bile salts and bile pigments which are then transferred to the adjacent biliary vessels. Not all the bile pigments are formed in the liver, they may be formed wherever red blood cells are broken down, e.g., in the spleen.

The blood from the sinusoids passes to the *central veins* and then into the sublobular veins which unite to form the *hepatic veins* and these open into the *inferior vena cava.*

The bile finds its way into the interlobular bile ducts, whence it passes into the hepatic ducts and so into the common bile duct and duodenum.

The liver is therefore a great chemical laboratory converting the products of digestion into substances which can be more easily used by the body. In addition it is a store-house, it manufactures and it detoxicates. The chemistry of these processes is too complex for a book of this kind but we shall group together the functions of the liver in an endeavour to understand its role in the body.

Action on carbohydrates. Should any soluble carbohydrates such as fructose or galactose be absorbed it converts them into glucose. It forms glucose from the non-nitrogenous portion of the amino-acids. If too much glucose is absorbed or made; the liver under the influence of insulin stores it in the form of glycogen from which it can be reconverted readily into glucose.

Action on fatty acids. It desaturates fatty acids, that is, it so acts upon the long chain of fatty acids of which fats are composed that they are more easily oxidised.

Action on amino-acids. It deaminises amino-acids, that is, it removes their amino or NH_2 group from those amino-acids which are not needed for repair of the body and converts them into urea, uric acid and ammonium salts. The carbon and some of the hydrogen from the remainder are used as fuel.

The liver is responsible for the *formation of bile.*

It manufactures *fibrinogen* and, under the influence of vitamin K, *prothrombin* which are essential for the clotting of blood. *Heparin* which prevents blood from clotting is made partly in the liver and is now known to be liberated from the mast cells of the connective tissue.

In the embryo it manufactures red cells but in post-natal life it destroys them. It does, however, play an important part in *blood formation* for it stores the *haemopoietic factor* which is derived from the extrinsic factor (red meat in the food) and the intrinsic factor of the gastric juice.

We have already referred to the liver as a store-house, for it *stores iron* (from the red cells which it has broken down); *fibrinogen* (which is mobilised in haemorrhage); *vitamin D,* hence liver oils are used in the cure of rickets; and *vitamin A* which is important in maintaining the health of the mucous membranes throughout the body.

The liver has *a detoxicating function* in that it can neutralise to some degree the effects of poisons which may have been absorbed from the alimentary canal.

The liver, as the result of its many activities, is kept almost constantly at work and so is secondary only to the muscles as the *source of heat* in the body.

THE BILE AND GALL BLADDER

The bile made by the liver is collected by the ducts of the gland (the hepatic ducts) and stored in the gall bladder. The gall bladder is a small sac lying under the liver and appearing just below it at the outer border of the right rectus muscle. The duct of the gall bladder joins the hepatic duct to form the common bile duct which, with the duct of the pancreas, enters the duodenum at the ampulla of the bile duct (fig. 220).

The sphincter of Oddi which, as we have seen, is situated at the distal end of the common bile duct is not circular as was believed but consists of longitudinal and oblique fibres which are capable of retracting the duodenal papilla and in that way closing the orifice. As the duct passes obliquely through the duodenal wall regurgitation from the alimentary canal is prevented.

We have seen that the hormone *secretin* stimulates the secretion of the pancreas and it is this same hormone together with the reabsorbed bile salts which stimulate the liver cells to form bile. Bile is secreted continuously but especially during digestion. When the stomach is empty, the sphincter of Oddi is closed, and then the bile is stored in the gall bladder where it becomes more concentrated and mucus is added to it. When food, especially fats, enters the duodenum the sphincter opens and the gall bladder contracts and bile pours into the duodenum activating the pancreatic enzyme lipase and facilitating the digestion of fats. Contraction of the gall bladder is believed to be brought about by a hormone called *cholecystokinin* which is absorbed into the blood stream from the wall of the duodenum.

The composition of the bile. About 500 to 1000 c.c. of bile are secreted daily. It is coloured by the pigments bilirubin and biliverdin and according to the concentration in the bile its colour may vary from yellow to brown or green. It is alkaline in reaction and has a very bitter taste. In addition to the pigments, it contains bile salts—sodium glycocholate and sodium taurocholate, mucus in varying amount and small quantities of fats, soaps, lecithin, cholesterol and mineral salts, especially calcium carbonate and phosphate. Gall stones which are precipitated from the bile acid are formed chiefly by cholesterol. The movements and potency of the gall bladder and ducts can be studied radiographically after the taking or injection of tetra-iodophenol which is excreted in the bile and is opaque to X-rays.

The bile pigments. When the effete red cells are broken down the iron is separated from the haemoglobin and stored in the bone marrow, liver and spleen. This iron-free haemoglobin *biliverdin* (green in colour) is converted into *bilirubin* by the reticulo-endothelial system, especially in the liver, and appears in the bile as such. In the intestine bilirubin is converted into *urobilinogen*, some of which is reabsorbed and appears in the urine in small quantities as *urobilin*. Some, however, is converted into *stercobilin*, the dark pigment which gives the faeces their colour.

Sometimes as the result of obstruction of the bile ducts (e.g., by a stone) the bile pigments accumulate in the blood. The patient then becomes jaundiced and it is not difficult to understand that in these cases the faeces are pale (clay-coloured stools) from lack of stercobilin and the urine is dark because it contains bile which has filtered into the urinary tubules from the blood. A less severe jaundice is seen in pernicious anaemia when there is an excessive breakdown of red blood cells.

The bile salts are the sodium salts of the bile-acids, glycocholic acid which is derived from the amino-acid glycine and cholic acid, a derivation of cholesterol and taurocholic acid which comes from taurine derived from the amino-acid cystine. Cholesterol is derived from the cell envelopes of the dead cells of the body. It follows, therefore, that a high protein diet increases the secretion of bile salts.

The functions of the bile

1. It aids the digestion of fats by facilitating the action of the pancreatic enzyme lipase.

2. It aids the absorption of fats by suspending fat in fine particles in the form of an emulsion.

3. Bile salts stimulate bile secretion.

4. It stimulates the peristalsis of the large intestine.

5. It retards the growth of bacteria in the intestine.

6. It forms water-soluble complexes of fatty acids of the fat-soluble vitamins and of cholesterol.

7. It facilitates the absorption of vitamin K.

8. In it is excreted cholesterol, iron, copper and calcium and many drugs.

9. It tends to be regurgitated into the empty stomach where its alkalinity helps to neutralise the normal acidity of that organ.

CHAPTER XXII

EXCRETION

Excretion is the process by which the body gets rid of waste matter. From what has been said regarding the general design of the body it is evident that the chief waste products are carbon dioxide (CO_2) and water (H_2O). In addition there is excretion of excess substances which have been taken in the diet, notably salts and nitrogenous compounds. The latter also result from the wear and tear of body proteins. The carbon dioxide is excreted by the lungs; water, salts and nitrogenous substances largely by the kidneys. The skin and to a much less extent the large intestine are also excretory organs. The lungs have been dealt with elsewhere and we shall now consider the other routes by which excretion takes place.

The Urinary Apparatus

The urinary apparatus consists of the kidneys, the ureters, the bladder and the urethra.

The *kidneys* help to maintain the composition of the blood constant by excreting urine which consists of water in which is dissolved a large number of substances. By far the most important are the products of protein metabolism but in addition the urine contains various salts in solution.

Structure of the kidneys. Each kidney is composed of about a million or more nephrons, each consisting of a glomerulus and tubule (fig. 294). The *glomeruli* lie in the renal cortex and each is formed by a tuft of capillaries invaginated by the blind end of a tubule. The invagination is known as the *capsule of Bowman* and the capsule with its contained capillaries is called a *Malpighian body*. The tubule leaves the body at the neck and is followed by the *first convoluted tubule* in which the epithelium is thick and the lumen narrow. Then comes a straight part of the tubule which descends into the medulla of the kidney as the *descending tubule of Henle* in which the cells are flat and the lumen wide. The next feature is the *loop of Henle* and this is succeeded by the *ascending tubule of Henle* in which, again, the epithelium is thick and the lumen narrow. This is followed by the *second convoluted tubule* which opens into a *junctional tubule* and this in turn opens into a *collecting tubule*. A number of these collecting tubules open into one of the *ducts of Bellini* which can be seen opening at the apex of a pyramid into one of the lesser calyces in the renal pelvis.

The arteries supplying the glomeruli are branches of the renal arteries and are called *afferent arteries*. From the glomerular capillaries, *efferent vessels* pass to supply the tubules (fig. 294), the capillaries surrounding which drain into veins which are tributaries of the renal vein. Since the arterial blood has to pass through the small capillaries of the glomeruli, it follows that the pressure of the blood in the afferent arteries forming a glomerulus will be much greater than that in the efferent vessels supplying the tubules, a factor which facilitates filtration in the glomerulus and re-absorption from the tubules ; indeed the process is very like the re-absorption of tissue fluid at the venous end of a capillary elsewhere.

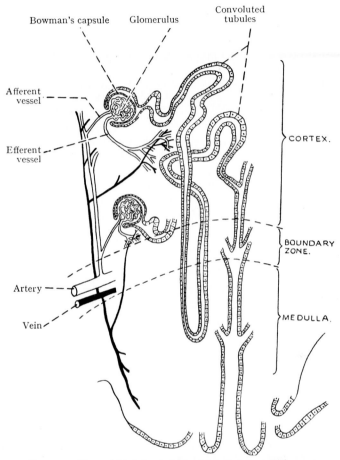

FIG. 294.—The renal tubules and blood vessels (schematic).

Formation of the Urine. Urine is formed by a process of filtration from the capillaries through the flattened epithelial cells of Bowman's capsule. A fall in the arterial blood pressure or a rise in the osmotic pressure of the blood decreases the volume of urine and conversely an increase in the pressure of the blood or a fall in the osmotic pressure (e.g. by drinking) causes an increase in the volume of urine. The filtrate is comparable to tissue fluid and is composed of dilute blood plasma minus its proteins which, since they have a large molecule, cannot pass through the capillary walls. It has been possible to put a minute hollow needle into the glomerulus and to draw off a few drops of the filtrate which has been found to contain all the soluble substances found in the blood plasma, including sugar.

This filtrate passes down the renal tubules and in so doing the urine is concentrated by two processes. There is a re-absorption of water and sugar, and various substances are added. This concentration is due largely to the vital activity of the cells of the tubules which have the function of selective re-absorption.

Substances with a fixed concentration in the blood such as sugar and chlorides are re-absorbed from the filtrate and returned to the blood. They are known as *threshold substances*. Other substances which are not re-absorbed, and are therefore fully excreted, are called *non-threshold substances*. A comparison of the compositions of the chief constituents of blood plasma with that of urine (see table) indicates the extent to which each has been concentrated.

It has now been shown that the concentration of urine is not so simple as used to be thought and that the interstitial tissue between the tubules of the kidney plays an important part.

The thick-walled ascending loop of Henle secretes sodium into the interstitium from which it not only passes into the circulation but draws water from the descending and collecting tubules. The urine becomes therefore increasingly concentrated as it passes towards the medulla where the salt content of the tissues is much greater than that of the cortex. Thus the benefit of the curious anatomical distribution of the tubules in the kidney becomes clearer.

The substances added to the urine in the tubules are urea, acid sodium phosphate, ammonium salts, uric acid and creatinine.

Composition of the Urine. The urine consists largely of water in which is dissolved a number of substances, the most abundant being urea and sodium chloride. It also contains uric acid, creatinine and ammonium salts. Of these only ammonium salts and acid phosphates are formed in the kidney, the rest are merely excreted by that organ.

	Blood-plasma per cent.	Urine per cent.
Total solids	10	4·0
Proteins	7·5–9	0
Chloride	0·37	0·6
Urea	0·03	2·0
Sugar	0·10	0
Uric acid	0·003	0·05
Creatinine	0·001	0·1
Ammonium salts	0·001	0·04

In certain circumstances the salts in the urine may form crystals. This so-called gravel causes irritation of the urinary passages and the formation of stones. These may be formed of uric acid, oxalates but most commonly of phosphate. The latter may be passed also as an amorphous precipitate which causes the urine to become cloudy or even milky in appearance. Such a precipitation of phosphates is very liable to occur in the alkaline urine which follows the intake of large quantities of green vegetables and fruit. This precipitate can be dissolved if acetic acid is added to the urine.

Urea, as we have seen, is formed from the breakdown of amino-acids resulting from protein metabolism and the table shows it to be more concentrated in the urine than in the blood. The smell of stale urine is due to bacteria converting urea into ammonium carbonate. The *ammonium salts* in the urine are also derived from the amino-acids but since they have a higher concentration in the urine than in the blood it follows that some are synthesised in the kidney. *Uric acid*, which is present in very small amounts, is formed in the liver as an end-product of nucleo-protein metabolism. In alkaline urine it occurs as urates. *Creatinine* is an end-product from the metabolism of muscle and is not affected by the diet. It is derived from creatine, a normal constituent of muscle which is formed in the liver from amino-acids.

Volume of Urine. A normal adult excretes about 50 ozs. (1500 ml.) of urine daily but this amount is very variable, for it is influenced by the fluid intake and by the fluid output in the form of sweat, expired air and faeces. When the blood is tending to become concentrated because of loss of water, the increased osmotic pressure acts in two ways—directly by reducing filtration through the glomeruli and indirectly by acting on osmo-receptors probably in the hypothalamus causing the posterior lobe of the hypophysis to secrete an antidiuretic hormone which apparently acts on the kidney tubules increasing the re-absorption of water. Emotion and exercise probably cause a reduction in the amount of urine produced by causing this hormone to be secreted.

The specific gravity of the urine varies from 1015 to 1025, according to its concentration. It is reduced if large quantities of water are taken and is raised after much sweating, in fever and in diabetes mellitus when there is sugar in the urine. Use is made of these facts in estimating the efficiency of the kidney. Ability to pass large quantities of urine after taking a litre of water indicates that the glomeruli are efficient while the ability to produce a concentrated night urine indicates that the tubules are efficient. This simple test has largely replaced the more elaborate tests.

The colour of the urine is due chiefly to *urochrome*, a yellow pigment of unknown chemical composition, but other pigments, such as *urobilin* from bile, also are present.

The Reaction of Urine. The urine is slightly acid to litmus paper because of the acid sodium phosphate it contains, but tends to become less so or even alkaline during the morning. This so-called "alkaline tide" may be due to an increase in respiration or to an increase in the secretion of the gastric juice since both these are means by which the body can get rid of, or use, excess acid in the blood. The reaction of fresh urine depends principally on the diet, for green vegetables and most fruits make it alkaline because the organic acids they contain are converted into carbonates, while meat, fats and whole cereals make it acid. Acidity of the urine is also increased by exercise owing to the formation of lactic acid. The kidney is thus the chief organ for maintaining the reaction of the blood as a slightly alkaline fluid. Urine rapidly becomes alkaline on standing, because of the liberation of ammonia from urea by bacteria.

Micturition. In the infant the emptying of the bladder is reflex or automatic. When the bladder becomes distended nerve impulses pass up the spinal cord to centres for bladder reflexes in the mid-brain whence impulses are sent to the bladder causing its muscular wall to contract and its sphincters to relax.

Later these reflex centres come under the influence of the cerebral cortex and the child acquires voluntary control. If for any reason the bladder is not emptied when the first sensations occur, the organ relaxes, the pressure within it falls and the sensations pass off temporarily. In conditions of excitement and in inflammation of the bladder, there is an increased frequency. Micturition in the adult is therefore due to a release of the lower centres from the higher inhibition. In damage to the upper part of the spinal cord voluntary control is lost. At first there is retention with overflow, but later if the lumbar region of the spinal cord has not been damaged, micturition again becomes purely reflex, depending on the degree of distension of the bladder.

Excretion by the Large Intestine

The excretion of the large intestine known as the faeces does not, as is popularly imagined, consist solely of undigested food residue.

For the most part its solid matter consists of epithelial scales from the lining of the intestine which, like the skin, are constantly being renewed, and of bacteria which are the normal inhabitants of the large intestine and which, in the herbivorous animals, are responsible for the digestion of the cellulose framework of plants.

Although it is probably advantageous to empty the bowel every day, many people do not do so without any apparent harm. More harm may be done by the excessive use of purgatives.

The faeces also contain the excretions of the colon itself, namely, any excess metallic salts which may have been absorbed into the blood. The major portion of the usual faecal mass, however, consists of water which varies with the amount of fluid taken in the food and the extent to which it has been absorbed into the blood stream. This in turn depends on the time it has taken to pass through the colon and on the amount of mucus secreted by the large intestine. The longer the faeces stay in the colon the drier they become, and if the mucous secretion is inadequate the hard faecal masses produced are difficult to excrete.

Excretion by the Skin

The excretion of the skin is chiefly water which contains substances formerly dissolved in the blood in small amounts. If, however, there is excessive sweating, as there may be in a hot environment, an excess of blood salts (especially sodium chloride) may be lost by the skin causing serious symptoms and even death. A similar state of affairs occurs in severe diarrhoea, in vomiting and as the result of the excessive drinking of water. In such circumstances it is essential to drink salt solution instead of water. The skin may also excrete a large variety of drugs if they are administered.

CHAPTER XXIII

THE SKIN AND REGULATION OF BODY TEMPERATURE

The Function of the Skin

The skin has a number of functions—protective, sensory, respiratory, absorptive, storage of blood, secretory, heat regulating and excretory. The latter has been dealt with elsewhere (p. 430) but it will be necessary to elaborate on the remaining functions.

Protection. The surface of the body is protected by the skin which consists essentially of layers of epithelial cells which are constantly being replaced. Growth takes place in the deeper layers which consist of typical polygonal cells with nuclei but gradually they become flattened and lose their nuclei as the surface is reached. The more superficial layers are but scales of cornified cells which have become hardened before being shed. These superficial cells are very liable to be removed too rapidly by frequent massage, hence the importance of reducing friction to a minimum. The various layers of epithelial cells have, for convenience, been given different names as they pass to the surface (*vide* p. 18). The most important of these is the stratum lucidum. This layer gives rise to the nails which are formed by an intensification of the hardening process. The outer layer of the skin which peels off in blisters is known as the epidermis. In areas subject to friction such as the palms of the hands and the soles of the feet, the epidermis is specially thickened.

The loose attachment of the skin enhances its protective value by causing blows to glance. This protection is further increased on the head by the presence of hair.

Sensation. Nerve fibres which often end in special nerve endings (see p. 20) are to be seen in the skin. These are responsible for initiating the impulses which give rise to skin sensations such as touch, temperature and pain. When the superficial layers of the skin are removed by blisters or by friction, the nerve endings are exposed and sensation is abnormally increased. Slight degrees of warmth may then be registered as pain. The sensory function of the skin is in a large measure protective, for when its numerous nerve endings are stimulated protective responses follow. In some animals sensation is increased by the possession of hairs or vibrissae, e.g., the whiskers of cats, which have specialised nerve endings at their bases.

Respiration. The respiratory function of the skin in man is negligible, but in thin-skinned animals, e.g., the frog, it may be sufficient to keep the animal alive.

Absorption. The most important substance which is normally absorbed from the skin is vitamin D. This vitamin is manufactured in the skin from a sterol by the action of the ultra-violet light of the sun. The skin also absorbs oily substances if they are massaged into the skin and it is possible for certain drugs, e.g., mercury or the turpentine of embrocation, to be absorbed in this way. Many drugs may, however, be ionised through the skin and this is common physiotherapeutic practice. In this procedure an electrode is placed on the skin over the area to be medicated and another at a distance. When a current is passed through the body it carries the drug with it.

Blood Storage. Blood is stored in the subpapillary plexuses of the dermis ready for use in an emergency. If the skin is soaked in oil the tips of these subpapillary plexuses can be seen under the microscope in the form of loops. They should be compressed if massage is to be of any value. One of the signs of haemorrhage is that the subject looks pale owing to the fact that the blood has been shifted from the peripheral skin. This is effected by sympathetic stimulation resulting in a vaso-constriction of the peripheral vessels. The same mechanism comes into play in cold, anger, fear and infections; also whenever extra blood is needed in the muscles and other organs. The evidence is now very complete that the capillaries shut down by virtue of their elasticity when their internal pressure falls below the critical closing pressure. When the blood pressure falls in fainting, or when there is increased sympathetic activity, the skin also becomes pale. Another cause of pallor is insufficient blood pigment (anaemia).

Secretion. The secretion of the skin is twofold. It secretes a clear watery fluid (the sweat) and an oily fluid (the sebum) which is the natural lubricant for the hairs. The sweat has a slightly bactericidal action.

The Secretion of Sweat

The sweat glands are most abundant in man on the brow, the palms and the soles.

The glands which produce it lie in the deeper layers of the skin and have long corkscrew-like ducts which pass through the more superficial layers to the surface (fig. 26). When the sweat glands are studied in more detail they may be divided into two types: (1) the *apocrine* or *large glands* which are derived from the hair follicles and which include the ceruminal glands of the ear, those of the eyelid, and the mammary glands. The change of the mammary gland from a sweat gland to one which produces milk is an interesting study in evolution; (2) the small or *eccrine glands* which are derived from the epidermis and scattered all over the body. The distribution of the large glands varies very much from individual to individual and from race to race. They are said to be, in many instances, of sexual significance and to become less so as we ascend the evolutionary scale. In humans the small sweat glands predominate, and the large glands are restricted to the face, ears, axillae and the sexual areas.

As long as the sweat is small in amount it is evaporated from the surface at once; this is called *insensible perspiration*. There is, however, some evidence that the insensible perspiration is not secreted but diffused as water vapour through the epithelium, for it is present in those persons in whom there is a congenital absence of sweat glands. As soon as sweating is increased or evaporation prevented, drops appear on the surface of the skin. This is known as *sensible perspiration*. The relation of these two varies with atmospheric conditions; the drier and hotter the air, the greater is the proportion of insensible to sensible perspiration. The total amount of sweat secreted by a man is about 450 c.c. in the twenty-four hours, but it may rise to 10,000 c.c. in extremely hot dry atmospheres, especially if exercise is taken and plenty of water drunk.

The control of sweat secretion. There are probably two types of sweat secretion, the hot or thermal sweat and the mental or cold sweat, but whether the mechanisms for them are different has not been determined.

Thermal sweating is generalised and occurs when the body temperature is raised by increased metabolism, commonly that of muscular exercise or when the external temperature is high. It is not present, however, on the palms of the hands and soles of the feet. It is brought about through the operation of the heat-regulating mechanism.

The application of heat to a part of the body may, however, cause local sweating by direct action on the glands or by a local reflex. Sweating is accompanied by a dilatation of the blood vessels of the region, presumably the result of the production of metabolic products.

Mental sweating, on the other hand, predominates on the palms and soles, but is also present in the head and neck and elsewhere. It occurs in many different kinds of emotion, even doing mental arithmetic. It may be produced experimentally by touching any very hot object, such as an electric globe, with the finger for a few seconds. The term mental is held to include that produced by sensory stimulation. There are, however, great individual variations in some otherwise normal persons. The sweat may be very profuse and drip from the hands or more commonly the face.

In muscular exercise the sweating is both thermal and mental. Sweating is reduced by cold, which at the same time reduces the cutaneous circulation. It is also reduced by dehydration, whether the result of deprivation of fluid intake or by sweating itself. When the latter occurs, and this is common in hot countries, the taking of a glass of cold water which dilutes the blood produces a profuse sweating.

The exact nervous mechanisms concerned in sweating are not completely understood, and different animals appear to vary appreciably. A very dry skin suggests a thyroid deficiency.

Composition of sweat. Sweat has a specific gravity of 1005 and is composed chiefly of water in which is about 1·2 per cent. solids. The solids are composed of epidermal scales and salts, of which the most abundant is sodium chloride and a minute quantity of urea which is quickly transformed into ammonium carbonate previously referred to. Sweat is normally acid in reaction due, as in the urine, to the presence of acid sodium phosphate but if the sweating is profuse it is neutral or even alkaline. It has a characteristic odour which varies in different parts of the body and is due to volatile fatty acids, and sometimes to ammonium carbonate.

THE MAINTENANCE OF BODY TEMPERATURE

This depends on the amount of heat produced and the amount of heat lost. *Heat is produced* by the activity of all tissues. By far the largest heat producing organs in the body are the muscles and muscle tone is increased throughout the body sometimes accompanied by shivering in conditions of extreme cold. Even at rest the activity of certain organs especially the heart, the respiratory muscle and the digestive glands (liver) produce over 1000 calories of heat.

Heat is lost by the respiratory tract, by the skin and by the excretions.

Respiration is rapid and shallow in the dog and sheep which do not sweat when they are overheated and at the same time there is an increased salivation which keeps the tongue moist. The protrusion of the tongue also facilitates heat loss.

The skin regulates its heat loss by changing the amount of blood passing through it. If the body is overheated, there is a general vaso-dilatation of the skin-vessels especially the arterioles and in some areas there is an opening up of the arterio-venous anastomoses so that the blood is more rapidly passed through the surface vessels. In these circumstances the body loses a greater amount of heat by *radiation*, i.e., the passage of heat rays; by *conduction*, i.e., by warming the objects with which it comes in contact and by *convection*, i.e., by warming the air passing over it but more especially by *evaporation*.

When the body temperature tends to rise, the sweat glands secrete and the evaporation of the sweat causes cooling. The amount of evaporation depends on the humidity of the atmosphere. We are familiar with the increased accumulation of sweat which occurs on a hot moist day. The hot day, however, has the advantage over the cold day in that the relative humidity of the air is decreased. The atmosphere varies in its cooling power according to the rapidity with which the air in the intermediate vicinity of the body is changed. Local cooling of a part may occur especially from cold convection currents (draughts) and may result in painful rheumatic states which call for physiotherapy. These states probably result from a reduction of the circulation through the part, which leads to the accumulation of toxins normally removed and there is subsequently an attraction of leucocytes and water which cause the stiffness. Any local bacteria may contribute.

When the temperature of the blood reaching the brain is above normal the *heat regulating centre*, which is believed to be in the hypothalamus, is stimulated. This brings into operation the processes just described to increase heat loss. At the same time there is a reduction of muscle tone and a lack of desire to do muscular work which produces heat. Physical exercise, therefore, should be performed whenever possible in a dry, cool atmosphere which favours evaporation and heat loss from the skin and at the same time gives a sense of well-being by stimulating it.

Heat is conserved when the body tends to become cold. The opposite changes occur to those enumerated above, while in addition shivering occurs and so additional heat is produced. These changes are also brought about by nervous reflexes before the actual cooling of the blood takes place and heat is thereby conserved. Thus it can be shown that cooling of the hand causes constriction of vessels elsewhere in the body, especially of the respiratory tract. Unaccustomed cold, therefore, may cause such a reduction of the blood supply to the respiratory tract that any bacteria which it may be harbouring are able to invade and an infection, usually the common cold, results.

In *fever* the regulation of the body temperature is upset by the toxins produced by the invading organisms. The probable explanation is that there is a reduction in the volume of the circulating blood resulting in a constriction of the skin vessels and a retention of heat. Once the body temperature has risen there is an increased heat production, but that this alone is not responsible is seen by the fact that there is no comparable rise of temperature when additional heat is produced in other ways, e.g., by exercise or in hyperthyroidism. In fever the heat regulating centre appears, therefore, to be set at a higher level than normally, but it still responds to changes in the external environment.

Body temperature is normally maintained between 95° and 98·4° Fahrenheit and is determined by the amount of heat gained and heat lost. It is highest between 5 p.m. and 10 p.m. and lowest in the early hours in the morning. The most accurate readings are obtained by placing a thermometer in the rectum but the armpit or the mouth are more convenient. The latter, however, may vary considerably. It is increased if hot fluids have been taken a short time before and decreased by recent breathing through the mouth on a cold day. Although a thermometer may record in half a minute, several minutes may be necessary to get an accurate reading. Observations with recording apparatus (thermopiles) thrust into tissues indicate that superficial parts, especially of the limbs, may be several degrees below blood temperature.

Fever is of paramount importance in medicine as it is almost invariably an indication of bacterial invasion. Many substances in common use, such as aspirin and phenacetin, temporarily reduce body temperature by causing a dilatation of skin vessels and a dilution of the blood. It should, however, be realised that it is not necessarily an advantage to reduce fever unless it is excessive, for fever is in some measure protective, since antibodies are more actively produced at a higher than at a lower body temperature. The increased metabolism which accompanies the fever also assists the body to deal more adequately with the infective agents, for the faster moving blood mobilises the leucocytes which kill the invading organisms.

The *sensation of warmth*, however, bears no relation to body temperature. After a hot bath or after taking alcohol the skin vessels are dilated and we have a sensation of warmth, but actually the body temperature may have fallen. In infections we may feel shivery because of the withdrawal of blood from the skin although the body temperature is above normal.

These facts show that the sensation of temperature depends on the nerve endings in the skin which are dependent on the temperature of the outside air and on the amount of blood flowing through the skin.

The sensation of heat of the skin bears little relation, therefore, to the temperature of the muscles underneath. If we heat a limb at the fire, the skin may feel very warm yet the tissues below may be normal. Short-wave therapy or high-frequency electric currents may heat the underlying structures, although the skin feels scarcely warm.

If all the blood vessels to the skin are opened up the skin is flushed and is warm to the touch.   If, on the other hand, the vessels are closed down the skin is pale and cold.

Sometimes, however, as in fever, the skin capillaries are shut down so that the skin is pale but the arterioles are open so that the blood circulates very rapidly through the skin.   In such circumstances the skin, although pale, is warm.

The Colour of the Skin

The skin of Northern Europeans when deprived of blood is quite pale as in fainting and haemorrhage, but normally it is a familiar pink colour as a result of the blood circulating through it.   If many vessels are dilated it becomes flushed.   This is well seen in blushing and in exercise.   In some persons this is a permanent state which results from the irritation of the rays of the sun or the wind and the rain.   Alcohol also tends to produce similar effects.   In cold weather these permanently dilated vessels tend to become blue or cyanosed because of the constriction of the arterioles and venules and slowing of the circulation in the superficial capillaries.   Then the blood loses most of its oxygen and becomes bluish.   Even in normal persons this may be occasionally seen, especially in the extremities, and may be demonstrated by simply occluding the blood supply to a part.   A generalised cyanosis occurs when the blood as a whole is deficient in oxygen and occurs typically if there is any interference with respiration, such as may occur as a result of too deep anaesthesia or drowning.

In jaundice the skin is yellow because of the circulation of bile in the skin capillaries.   In various other states other pigments may circulate and affect skin colour.

In some races the skin is pigmented.   In the case of Africans the pigment melanin, made from the amino-acid tyrosine, is deposited in the superficial layers of the skin.   This pigment is present in larger quantities where the skin is subjected to irritation, such as on the nipples and sexual organs.   It is the pigment of moles.

The Response of the Skin to irritation and injury

The skin shows a remarkable variety of responses to the application of physical or chemical agents and with many of these most people are familiar. Irritants not sufficient to remove its superficial layers bring about a simple reddening from a dilatation of the superficial capillaries.   This occurs typically as the result of rubbing, the application of hot water and a variety of chemical agents, notably turpentine, cantharides, dilute acids and alkalies. Some skins are much more sensitive to irritants than others and it cannot be over-emphasised that many attempts to cure a skin irritation fail because the chemical applied is too strong and actually keeps up the stimulation. Many of the most successful ointments do little more than give simple protection to the injured area and keep out extraneous infection.   The evidence is very complete that the irritants bring about the release of a chemical substance known as *H-substance* because of the resemblance of its action to histamine, the chief point of the evidence being that the duration of the reddening produced mechanically may be increased by reducing the circulation through the part.

The use of the antihistamine drugs has shown that the substances are not histamine. Histamine is released from the mast cells of the body into the blood in allergy and causes urticaria which is relieved by antihistamine.

The fundamental reactions are perhaps best seen when the skin of the arm is stroked, but not cut, with a not too sharp object. There may be first a contraction of the capillaries from mechanical stimulation which causes the appearance of a white line. This is followed by a *triple response* which may be imitated by the injection of histamine. This response consists of (1) a *red streak* which is due to the release of the H-substance and (2) a little later a *generalised flush* is seen which is evidently due to a reflex dilatation of arterioles for it is abolished if the nerves to the part are paralysed by the injection of novocaine. (3) There is evidence that the underlying vessels are also dilated (p. 366). If the irritation is more severe a *blister* appears and is commonly seen as the effect of an ill-fitting shoe or splint, or as a result of the application of hot fluids or hot-water bottles to anaesthetised patients. This is the result of the further action of the H-substance which not only dilates the capillaries but causes them to be more permeable so that water from the blood passes out under the superficial layers of the skin which become separated and may be shed. Whether or not any irritation proceeds to the wheal stage depends not only on the severity but also on the sensitivity of the patient. Mere stroking will cause whealing in some persons.

The effect of cold is more complex and is seen in varying degrees in frostbite. At first the vessels are constricted but if the application is temporary this is followed by a flush, the result of liberation of the H-substance in small amounts.

In prolonged cold the condition proceeds to a further stage, e.g., the feet may become oedematous because of the exudation from the blood into the tissues. This may be still further aggravated by actual freezing of the skin, the cells of which may die just as do the cells of plants because of the expansion of the frozen water inside them. Mild degrees of cooling of a limb are, however, sometimes taken advantage of in surgery. When the main vessels to a limb are damaged, cooling of the part reduces its metabolism, that is, the active oxidation processes within it, and time is thus given for new blood vessels to grow. Cold also reduces the liberation of oxygen by the blood and also the sensitivity of the skin which is therefore very liable to injury.

Prolonged but less intense irritation of the skin brings about a series of changes which appear to be protective but these changes may also follow severe injury. The laying down of pigment is common and is seen following damage to the skin and typically in sunburn and freckles (see the effect of light). Skin which does not bronze is most liable to be burnt by sunlight. In addition there is an increased growth of the skin with a hardening

29—A.PH.

of its layers, such as is seen on the hands of those who do hard manual work. The hardening and prevention of the normal desquamation of the superficial layers may be brought about by the application of spirit, a procedure commonly adopted for the prevention of bedsores which result from local stoppage of the circulation in those confined to bed, especially in the paralysed in whom the trophic or nourishment controlling action of the nerves is lost. In such patients areas of skin, especially over the buttocks and shoulder blades, may die altogether, and large raw areas, very liable to infection, may result. The condition is to be prevented by facilitating the circulation in parts most likely to be affected, by changing the areas on which the patient rests.

Sustained irritation and blistering on the hairy parts of the body causes an increased growth of hair and use is made of the fact in the treatment of baldness and to produce hair over the hoofs of horses.

The Application of Heat to the Body

Heat may be applied to the body in three ways, by radiation, by convection and by conduction. A large number of appliances have been designed to supply heat artificially according to whether it is desired to heat the body as a whole or merely to heat it locally.

Generalised heating is obtained by baths of great variety but the efficiency of all may be judged by the extent to which they raise body temperature and cause sweating. Baths of semi-solid material, such as peat, retain their heat longer than water, but the latter is not otherwise inferior to any other baths except that its temperature is more difficult to control and the skin may become sodden from prolonged immersion. For this reason electrically heated and hot vapour baths (e.g., pyrexia baths) are often preferred.

The raising of body temperature has many advantages. The most generalised effect is that all the cells of the body become more active since all chemical reactions take place better when the agents concerned are warmed; we all know that sugar dissolves better in hot tea than in cold. This principle governs all the body reactions which counteract bacteria. In addition the circulation of the blood is greatly hastened when the body temperature is raised, with the result that the white blood corpuscles which are the scavengers of the body are swept into the circulation. There is also a generalised dilatation of blood vessels. The latter, however, is not an altogether unqualified blessing, since it tends to cause a fall of blood pressure and may as we have said lead to fainting. Normally the effects of skin dilatation are prevented by compensatory vascular constriction in other areas. How far the general absorption of H-substance (histamine-like substance) from the skin occurs and is beneficial is not known, but this does not seem likely as the typical headaches produced by histamine when injected into the body do not occur although headaches after sunbathing are common. It is possible, too, that frequent generalised dilatation of vessels leads to an increase of blood volume.

Localised heating is, where possible, much more satisfactory and has in fact been used since earliest times. From the physiological point of view a maximum local dilatation of vessels is obtained in the region where it is needed, since it is not counteracted by vasodilatation elsewhere until at least the body temperature rises and then it is confined largely to the skin and respiratory tract. The increase of local chemical activity and the flushing of the part tend to hasten repair and remove any toxic substances which may be present. The relaxation, especially of muscle, which it produces also alleviates pain.

The means of applying heat are diverse. The poultice, the fomentation and localised baths are not necessarily bettered by more elaborate apparatus except for convenience, but it is not always realised that what are commonly known as infra-red rays are simply heat rays. An ordinary fire, electric or gas, radiates all the heat rays available by any other apparatus. (See the effect of radiation below.)

The great difficulty in applying heat is that it stimulates the hot spots of the skin and causes pain before the heat has adequately penetrated. In heating deep tissue the same principles apply as in cooking "a joint" in which slow heating is, as every cook knows, more effective in penetration than rapid heating which merely burns the surface without raising the interior sufficiently to coagulate the protein. It is in this that high frequency alternating electric currents (*diathermy* or *short wave*) are advantageous. The heat is produced by the current in the tissues overcoming their resistance as in the resistance of a wire of an electric fire, but it alternates so rapidly that it does not stimulate muscles or cause ionisation of salts in the tissues.

The Effect of Radiations on the Body

Great use is made of radiations in physiotherapy and although their fundamental nature is uncertain we have much knowledge regarding their activities. It is now known that such apparently dissimilar agents as heat, light, X-rays and wireless waves are all fundamentally similar. They may be considered to be electromagnetic vibrations in an hypothetical ether just as sound is due to vibrations of air.

If sunlight is passed through a glass prism it is split up into its component colours or spectrum similar to those which are seen in a rainbow when light is split up by raindrops. The colours seen are red, yellow, green, blue and violet, in that order. It can, however, be demonstrated photographically and otherwise that at each end of this visible spectrum there are invisible rays which can produce effects. Thus below the red rays we have the *infra-red* or *heat rays* which are emitted from a dark, hot body and which we can feel, while beyond the violet are the *ultra-violet rays*. These are emitted also by the sun and, although not visible in the ordinary way, can be shown to produce effects on a photographic plate.

Red rays penetrate better than rays at the other end of the spectrum and hence the use of red as a danger signal, but the same is still more true of the infra-red heat rays. It is, therefore, possible, by means of photographic plates sensitive to infra-red rays, to photograph through cloud. *Radiant heat* will penetrate even cold glass. Thus we may feel the radiant heat if we hold the hand close to an electric light bulb immediately after the light is switched on but while the bulb is still cold to the touch.

It has, however, become possible to produce by apparatus, rays which are much beyond those of the visible spectrum in both directions. Above the ultra-violet are *soft X-rays* which do not penetrate well, and higher still are the *hard X-rays* which have such remarkable powers of penetration that the shadows of bones and the like which they cast can be photographed. The shorter X-rays are like the R-rays emitted by radio-active bodies such as radium. Far below the infra-red rays are the Hertzian waves used in wireless.

The different kinds of rays can be defined by the distance from crest to crest of two waves and we are familiar with the term wavelength in relation to wireless. Some of the radiations are of much more importance in physiotherapy than others, especially in a country where the radiations of the sun are such an uncertain and variable quantity.

Ultra-violet light. This is emitted by the sun and is even more reflected from a blue sky. It can be produced artificially by an ordinary arc lamp or a mercury vapour lamp, such as is used in some street lighting. If applied to the skin it produces the effect of sunlight, that is, it irritates and may cause, if applied suddenly, the so-called "triple response" with inflammation, whealing and blistering and this is particularly true of a hot skin, for cooling reduces the action. If applied more gradually typical bronzing of the skin occurs, and this protects against blistering. The application of ultra-violet light by stimulating the skin gives a very considerable sense of well-being. Ultra-violet light penetrates only about 1 mm. but this appears to be sufficient to bring about the irradiation of the ergosterol in the skin and in plants and to cause the production of vitamin D thereby, which is so important in the calcification of bones and teeth. Ultra-violet light is also very lethal to bacteria and many insects (e.g., bed bugs).

The lack of penetrating power of ultra-violet light affects human beings who live indoors and in smoky towns, with the result that they are liable to suffer from deficiency of vitamin D and rickets unless they obtain the vitamin in animal fats or green vegetables. Even ordinary glass prevents the passage of ultra-violet light, and many transparent materials which allow it to pass when new, fail to do so as they become older, a point which is of considerable importance in regard to the construction of buildings.

Repair of the Skin and Other Tissues

When a part is damaged by injury or disease it tends to repair itself, and this power of repair is one of the most important to the physiotherapist whose function is to assist the process. All tissues do not, however, have this power of repair equally and it tends to be reduced by age. Senility, indeed, is characterised by a failure of the body to repair its normal wear and tear. Parts with a good circulation such as the face and mouth heal much more rapidly than the lower limbs.

An idea of what occurs in repair is obtained from a study of simple cuts in the skin. If the skin is cut a variety of changes ensue and these are facilitated if the edges of the wound are brought into apposition by stitching. At first the space between the edges is filled by blood clot which adheres to the side. Threads of fibrin tend to form bridges along which new blood vessels rapidly grow and soon the clot becomes organised or full of living cells. This highly vascular tissue is the first stage of repair. Cells known as fibroblasts appear and lay down fibrous tissue which is a replacement tissue holding the wound together while the epithelium rapidly regenerates on the surface. Such healing is known as healing by first intention and for it vitamin C is essential for the activity of the fibroblasts which form the fibrous tissue.

If bacteria have gained access to the wound, as is usual in accidents, they are at once attacked by vast numbers of white corpuscles which reach the area from the blood stream. If the bacteria are numerous or virulent they may kill the leucocytes and these, together with dead tissue cells and exuded tissue fluid, form pus which usually becomes sealed off to form a localised abscess and if not too large in amount is eventually absorbed but it may burst on the surface. Some organisms, e.g., haemolytic streptococci, have the power of producing fibrolysins which dissolve the coagulated fibrin which retains them and, therefore, they tend to spread rather than to remain localised. Such infection delays the healing wounds by causing much greater reaction than would occur in a sterile injury such as a simple fracture of a bone and a large amount of scar (fibrous) tissue may result. The use of modern antibiotics to counteract bacteria has revolutionised the progress of repair.

In rapid healing the scar tissue is negligible in amount, but in a large scar there may at first be a keloid or excess of scar tissue which subsequently contracts causing deformity and, it may be, restriction of movement. For this reason all scars such as those made at surgical operations become less conspicuous but this process may take years. If the scar is exposed to tension, e.g., a scar on the abdominal wall, it may stretch.

When, however, a large amount of skin has been lost, or the wound remains open for any reason, healing by granulation occurs, the term granulation tissue being given to a mass of highly vascular tissue which bleeds easily and which is really a mass of new capillaries. If it becomes excessive it is known as "proud flesh." Healing by granulation occurs after a severe burn, but in this condition the growth of the epithelium from the sides of the wound would be so slow that skin grafting is resorted to. This consists normally of transplanting minute pieces of skin to act as growth centres but in plastic surgery large areas of skin are transplanted.

As we have said, different tissues repair unequally.

Epithelial tissue repairs easily, the epithelial cells grow out from the normal skin or mucous membrane or from skin grafts when they are used. New epithelium is at first very thin, giving the wound a bluish appearance and may be only a cell or two thick. It is, therefore, very easily damaged and requires protection. The endothelium of blood vessels grows very quickly on any surface coated with blood. It will even grow on the inner walls of "arteries" made from nylon.

Muscular tissue is not replaced except in the blood vessels themselves, therefore, if a muscle is damaged its repair is by fibrous tissue but any remaining muscle fibres grow in size and may take over the duties of the parts lost.

Bones are rejoined if the broken ends are brought into apposition, but if not, the junction is by fibrous tissue and a false joint may result. Commonly the ends are kept in proper position by splints and osteoblasts or bone producing cells rapidly grow from the periosteum into the granulation tissue and join the bones in a manner somewhat reminiscent of a plumber's joint, the new bone or callous being much larger than the original bone. It may later become more normal but commonly the increased thickness remains.

Glandular tissue repairs rapidly and some glands, such as the liver and kidney, adapt their growth to the needs of the body.

Nerve tissue. Students should at this stage read the section on the structure of nerves. Nerve cells when damaged are not replaced but it is often possible for existing nerve cells to take over the function of those lost. Peripheral nerve fibres, on the other hand, regenerate freely and grow into any new tissue which may be formed.

When a nerve is cut or crushed its distal or peripheral end rapidly degenerates and ceases to conduct nerve impulses in about three days. The axis cylinder breaks down anatomically and chemically and turns into droplets of fat until finally the nerve becomes a functionless cord (fig. 299). The central end at about the beginning of the second week, on the other hand, sprouts and each axis cylinder as it flows out splits into a number of fine fibrils which pass into the surrounding tissues. Meantime chains of Schwann cells from the neurilemma of the peripheral stump also grow out and may succeed in bridging the gap between the two ends if they are not too far apart. The process is facilitated by suturing the cut ends. Then the regenerating fibrils grow rapidly at about 3 mm. per day into the persistent neurilemmal tubes and are thus led to their destinations. Each tube may at first have many fibrils, even as many as 25, but eventually only one remains. It is evident that whether or not the fibrils from any given nerve cell reach their original destination is largely a matter of chance, hence it is that functional recovery is seldom complete although much may be done by a process of relearning. Recovery is more complete, therefore, if the nerve is merely crushed and not cut. Provided the muscles have been prevented from degeneration, recovery takes place, as a rule, in from three months to two years, depending on the length of nerve involved. Sensation is at first quite crude (protopathic sensation) and does not convey detailed information as to the exact nature and site of the stimulation, but slowly more accurate (epicritic) sensation returns. There is no regeneration in the brain and spinal cord, partly, no doubt, because of the absence of neurilemmal sheaths.

The recovery period is of the greatest importance to physiotherapists, for the electrical stimulation and massage of muscles prevents their degeneration until new nerve fibres have grown into them. If this degeneration is allowed to proceed the muscles lose their cross-striation, become granular and eventually nothing is left but fibrous tissue.

The Skin and the Sense of Well-being

There seems to be little doubt that the sense of well-being in the average healthy person depends very largely on skin stimulation. This is experienced on a dry day on which the evaporation from the skin is good, but also occurs as the result of baths and sea-bathing and in these rough towelling increases the effect. In the latter the minute amount of salt which remains on the skin is slightly irritating—an important fact for those who have sensitive skins. The tonic effect of general massage and ultra-violet light or sun-bathing are also well recognized.

How the sense of well-being is produced is somewhat problematical, but it may depend on the receiving of a large number of sensory impulses into the nervous system, or on the production of minute amounts of H-substance in the skin as indicated on page 437. The absorption of this substance into the body is known to bring about a secretion of adrenaline from the suprarenal bodies, and this generally accelerates body processes, particularly that of the circulation.

Clothing

The value of clothing in keeping the body warm has been much studied of recent years. It is now clear that its major requirement is to insulate the body from surrounding cold air by surrounding the body with a layer of hot air. Quilted garments, especially when covered with almost impervious material to keep out the wind, are therefore the most efficient, but completely impervious materials of rubber or plastic have the disadvantage that they retain moisture and tend to become wet inside. This is not so important in really cold climates. Several layers of light meshed clothing are as warm as thick heavy garments. Wool has the advantage that unlike cotton its fibres have an elastic quality which prevent them from matting when they become moist with perspiration. In accurate work on this subject the unit of "one clo" has been introduced.

One clo is the thermal insulation of normal clothes which will maintain a resting-sitting man whose metabolism is 50 kcal/sq.m/hr. comfortable indefinitely in an environment of 21° C. (70° F.) with a relative humidity of 50 per cent. and air movement of 20 ft./min.

There is little doubt that clothing has been neglected by physiotherapists who apply heat to injured parts and do not insist that they are subsequently well protected, for it has been amply shown that localised chilling of tissues, especially of the limbs, readily occurs.

The Constancy of the Internal Environment

The regulation of body temperature is a good example of how the body regulates the conditions in which the tissues live and function. Thus we find that there are a number of mechanisms which maintain the composition of the blood approximately constant. We have seen that the heart is remarkably sensitive to any alteration in the fluid with which it is supplied.

In most cases when there is an adequate diet, the body varies the amount of substances lost by the excretions especially in the urine but it may also vary the amount absorbed from the intestine as in the case of iron.

In some cases the body has stores of important substances such as calcium in the bones; sodium in the skin, muscles and bones; potassium in all living cells; water in the tissue spaces; sugar in the liver and so on. In case of necessity the blood can draw on these stores and may at the same time reduce loss from the body by controlling excretion. Thus the kidney by neutralising and excreting acids as neutral salts and the lungs by excreting carbon dioxide play an important part in maintaining the slight alkalinity of the blood, in spite of the fact that during exercise, considerable amounts of lactic acid are liberated by the muscles.

By far the most important stores are those required for physical exercise. We have already remarked on the stores of high energy phosphate for immediate need but for greater needs the carbohydrate glycogen is stored in the liver and muscle, while fat is stored generally, especially in the subcutaneous tissues and the abdominal viscera. Oxygen is one of the few substances not stored and death occurs in a few minutes if it is not available to burn carbon.

CHAPTER XXIV

THE DUCTLESS GLANDS

In relation to digestion we have seen that there exist glands which manufacture from the blood, secretions which they pour into the digestive tract. There exists also a number of glands without ducts called the endocrine or ductless glands, which perform a similar action, but their secretions (hormones) are poured directly into the blood and usually have a generalised effect on the body. They produce the chemical regulation of the body additional to that supplied by the diet.

The Thyroid Gland

This gland consists of two lobes which lie on each side of the trachea and are united by an isthmus. It is made up of large vesicles filled with colloid and is surrounded by a fibrous capsule within which the parathyroid glands also lie.

The thyroid gland secretes a hormone called *thyroxine* which is a combination of iodine with the amino-acid tyrosine. An iodine deficiency causes

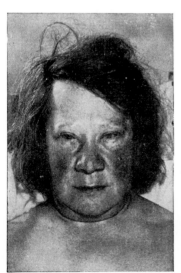 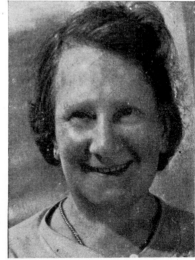

FIG. 295.—A case of myxoedema before and after treatment.
(*Savill's " Clinical Medicine."*)

enlargement of the gland (simple goitre) due to an accumulation of colloid, not necessarily associated with symptoms, but iodine is usually contained in the soil in sufficient amount for our needs. It is present in certain vegetables, and in milk and eggs. The absorption of iodine from the alimentary canal may, however, be prevented by bacteria and certain vegetables and

445

by the chalk of hard waters. The prevalence of goitre in chalky districts such as Derbyshire has led to the condition being called Derbyshire neck.

The thyroid gland controls the metabolic rate (i.e., the rate at which the body fires burn) and the rate of division of developing cells.

If then there is a thyroid deficiency—*hypothyroidism*—in adult life the patient becomes slow in mind and body. Since the metabolic rate is slow a less active circulation is necessary. In addition the heart metabolism itself is reduced and the rate of the heart is, therefore, slow. There is an accumulation of fuel in the form of fat, the skin becomes dry, the subcutaneous tissues degenerate, the hair tends to fall out and the patient may become denuded of hair over the whole body. The mental processes are slowed down. The condition is known as *myxoedema* and is considerably relieved by the administration of the dried gland or *thyroxine*, its active principle.

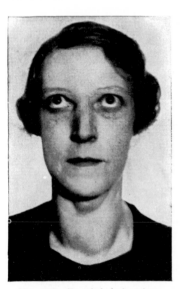

FIG. 296.—Exophthalmic goitre.
(*Photograph lent by Sir Thomas Dunhill.*)

Deficiency in thyroid activity is not uncommon in women after 50 and is in part responsible for the "middle-age spread."

If the deficiency is present in infants a condition known as *cretinism* is produced. It is essentially the same as that seen in adults but in addition there is dwarfism. Skeletal growth is stunted, the sexual organs do not develop, the brain does not grow and so the child is an idiot.

If the thyroid becomes over-active— *hyperthyroidism* — the metabolic rate is raised considerably, the patient quickly burns up fuel and uses excessive oxygen. The result is that he loses weight; sweats profusely; his heart rate is so enormously increased that he may die of cardiac exhaustion; nervous activity is increased and the patient is easily excited. Sometimes the eyes protrude and the condition is then known as exophthalmic goitre. The condition is relieved by removal of a portion of the gland and may be ameliorated by the administration of thiouracil which prevents the iodine being utilised. The gland may become over active as the result of over activity of the hypophysis. In the diagnosis of diseases of the thyroid gland, the taking of the metabolic rate (see p. 394) is most important, but the power of the thyroid to take up radioactive iodine and later to excrete it in the urine is now considered to be just as valuable. The estimations are done with a Geiger counter.

The Parathyroid Glands

These are four small bodies lying behind the thyroid gland. They are concerned with maintaining the calcium of the blood at a constant level and are essential to life. If the parathyroids are removed, calcium accumulates in the bones and the level of blood calcium falls. This causes an irritability of the nerves, tetany and death in convulsions. These symptoms are at once relieved by the injection of calcium or parathyroid extract which restores the level of calcium in the blood. Excessive secretion such as occurs in tumours of the parathyroids leads to excessive withdrawal of calcium and softening of the bones, just as occurs in rickets when there is faulty absorption of calcium from the intestine as a result of a deficiency in vitamin D. Calcium is necessary for a large number of processes (see p. 402).

The Suprarenal or Adrenal Glands

These glands lie on the upper part of the kidneys and, functionally, each is divisible into two parts, a *cortex* on the outside and a central *medulla*.

The *adrenal cortex* produces a large number of corticoids which are apparently secreted during a great variety of conditions such as stress, cold, haemorrhage, oxygen lack, and surgical operations and in such circumstances the body may be depleted of its hormones apparently. Some but especially aldosterol appear to have a direct control over the power of the kidney to retain sodium chloride, for if the cortex is removed in animals or diseased in man (Addison's disease) death results because of an excessive loss of sodium in the urine. This is prevented by giving extracts of the gland. The best known substance extracted from the adrenal cortex is *cortisone*, which has a dramatic effect in reducing inflammatory reactions, but it does not abate the growth of bacteria which may cause these reactions. Indeed, it actually reduces the number of white blood cells and in this way the resistance to the infection is lowered. It ameliorates but does not cure rheumatoid arthritis for which massage and movement are very valuable when the acute phase has passed off. It is also of great benefit in the treatment of asthma, but a patient so treated may show evidence of water retention and the so-called moon face.

Excessive activity of the adrenal cortex leads to abnormally rapid sexual development in young males and in women to virilism characterised by a masculination or development of the male secondary sexual characteristics, such as hair on the face and deepening of the voice.

The adrenal cortex also stores ascorbic acid (vitamin C) which is also lost during stress. This substance we have seen is intimately concerned with the making of fibrous tissue and the healing of wounds (see p. 397).

The adrenal medulla is not essential to life but produces two hormones, *adrenaline* and *nor-adrenaline* (sometimes called sympathin), which greatly increase the physical efficiency of the body. Adrenaline brings about a major transfer of blood from the skin and abdomen to the muscles. It accelerates the heart, raises the blood sugar by depleting the liver, increases the metabolic rate and very slightly the respiratory rate and it dilates the pupil. It is greatly used to dilate the bronchioles in asthma and to constrict the blood vessels in acute allergy. It is now believed that a substance almost identical with, if not actually nor-adrenaline, is liberated at sympathetic nerve-endings and is responsible for the maintenance of vascular tone.

Nor-adrenaline and adrenaline are secreted also in conditions of stress, especially in emotion and on exposure to cold. They are probably responsible for the pallor of fright by constricting the blood vessels in the skin. They appear in increased amounts in the blood in exercise.

When the adrenals are diseased (Addison's disease) there is very great physical weakness and low blood pressure.

The Hypophysis or Pituitary Body

This little organ, about the size of a hazel nut, lies embedded in the sphenoid bone at the base of the skull. It is connected to the inferior surface of the brain by means of a stalk through which it receives its nerve supply. Its importance is out of all proportion to its size for it is the controlling factor in most endocrine activity. It has been aptly and neatly described as "the leader of the endocrine orchestra."

It is divided into several parts of which the anterior and posterior lobes are the most important.

The *anterior lobe* produces a large variety of hormones.

1. A *growth hormone* which is responsible for the growth of the skeleton. If produced in excess in a young person giantism is produced. If deficient there is dwarfism. In an adult it produces a great thickening of bone of the extremities and face (acromegaly). A dwarf so produced, unlike that which results from deficient thyroid, is lively and is commonly seen in circuses.

2. *Thyrotrophic hormone* which controls the thyroid gland.

3. *Metabolic hormones* which affect metabolism, abnormalities of which may lead to abnormal adiposity or thinness.

4. *Gonadotrophic hormones* which control the development and activity of the testes and ovaries. They control both the internal secretions responsible for the secondary sexual characteristics and the production of sperms and ova in the male and female respectively. They are also responsible for the cyclic changes which take place in the uterus and are responsible for menstruation in the female.

5. *Lactogenic hormone* which is responsible for the secretion of milk in the mammary gland already prepared by the gonadotrophic hormones.

6. *Adrenocortico-trophic hormone* (A.C.T.H.) which is one of the most active substances known and as its name suggests, stimulates the adrenal cortex. There is good evidence that it is secreted during stress of various kinds (see adrenal cortex). It is specially important as it has been suggested that lack of its secretion, as the result of exhaustion or lack of stimulation in adult life may lead to rheumatoid arthritis. When the concentration of the hormone in the blood falls, the pituitary is stimulated to secrete more.

7. A *diuretic hormone.* There is some evidence that there is also produced a hormone which stimulates the production of urine.

The *posterior lobe* produces two hormones:

1. Vasopressin or the **antidiuretic hormone** which is stimulated if the blood becomes concentrated and which is reduced if its dilution is increased. This conserves the excretion of water. It apparently acts by varying the amount

of sodium chloride excreted by the kidney. The hormone is also secreted during mental stress.

Presumably as a preparation for exercise, it constricts blood vessels of the skin and intestines and drives their blood into the muscles. In its absence excessive very dilute urine is secreted (diabetes insipidus). It has now been shown to be a mixture of amino acids.

2. An *oxytocic factor** can also be extracted which is particularly active in stimulating the smooth muscle of the uterus. It is often used to control post-partum haemorrhage and by producing quick delivery it is of great value to obstetricians.

How exactly the pituitary is stimulated to produce the various hormones is incompletely understood.

The Thymus

The thymus is a large gland in children which extends from the lower border of the thyroid gland in the neck, to the pericardium of the heart in the thorax. Its function is not known but it atrophies at puberty and is believed to retard sexual activity until skeletal growth has reached a mature stage.

The Islets of Langerhans

The islets of Langerhans constitute a ductless gland which lies within the substance of the pancreas. They secrete the hormone *insulin* which is necessary for the proper utilisation of carbohydrates, and if there is disease of the pancreas affecting the islets *diabetes mellitus* results. This disease is successfully treated by injecting insulin which facilitates the use of sugar and so a fall in the level of the blood sugar ensues. (See carbohydrate metabolism, p. 413.)

Mast Cells and Anaphylaxis

Mast cells are unicellular glands, somewhat like fat basophyl cells, scattered throughout the body but located in the skin, the liver and especially in the lungs. When suitably stimulated they liberate histamine, which is an intense dilator of capillaries and constrictor of smooth muscle; heparin, which is an anticoagulant; and serotonin, also a constrictor of smooth muscle. Release of these substances occurs in anaphylaxis, a curious response of the body to a wide variety of foreign proteins such as articles of diet, pollens and moulds including penicillin. It is now believed that many pains which physiotherapists are called upon to treat may be due to similar local reactions in injured tissues.

The Testes and Ovaries

In addition to producing sperms and ova the testes and ovaries produce internal secretions which are responsible for the changes that occur at puberty. These are described on page 466.

* Known commercially as "pituitrin."

CHAPTER XXV

THE NERVOUS SYSTEM

The function of the nervous system is to transmit messages from one part of the body to another. It has been likened to a telephone system. The impulses pass into exchanges or nerve centres which may pass them on to other centres or direct to various muscles or organs which are to be activated.

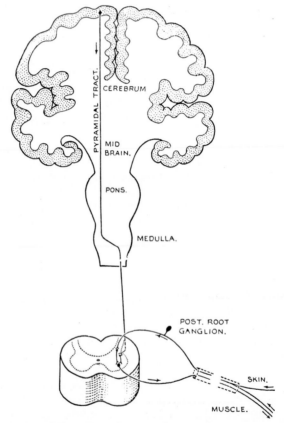

Fig. 297.—Diagram to illustrate a reflex arc and the course of the pyramidal tracts. The sectioned spinal cord has been deliberately enlarged.

An internuncial neurone connecting the pyramidal tract with an anterior horn cell and another connecting a posterior horn cell with an anterior horn cell are shown, but it must be realised that there are many hundreds of these connecting links.

We have already seen that the *structural unit* of the system is the neurone, that is, a cell with its processes by which it is linked to other cells. The *physiological unit*, on the other hand, is the *reflex* which in its simplest form consists of an afferent (ingoing) and efferent (outgoing) neurone.

The General Function of a Nervous System

A study of the nervous system of lowly animals, of the reactions of human beings whose systems are diseased or injured and of animals whose brains have been removed indicates that a primary function of the nervous system is to protect the body from injury by withdrawing the hurt part from the offending object. This function is seen in all nervous systems from the lowest animal to man. Even if the brain is separated from the spinal cord the latter still continues to have this function even in man.

The next important function of the nervous system is that which makes locomotion possible. This is seen in the lowliest animals which have legs. First there are developed reflexes by which the legs automatically resist the effect of gravity and do not bend under the weight of the body. For this function the next highest part of the nervous system, the medulla, is necessary. Associated with standing is walking and the co-ordination of muscular activity by which balance is maintained. Again a further set of reflexes are developed through a still higher part of the brain stem, the pons and mid-brain for even reflex walking can occur in the absence of the cerebrum. At the same time, since locomotion necessitates a greatly increased supply of nourishment and of oxygen, there are developed, especially in the medulla and the pons, mechanisms which control respiration and the circulation of the blood which thereby becomes much more efficient and are capable of supplying greater amounts of these to the muscles. We have already referred to the circulation and respiration as servants of the muscles.

For consciousness the cerebrum is necessary. It not only receives nervous impulses but compares them with what has been received before and thus enables the individual to appreciate their significance. But as we shall see even the response to what has been learnt becomes very largely a reflex or automatic activity. We know how habits both of action and of thought become so fixed that they are difficult to alter.

The most important thing a human being learns compared with, say, a dog is language by which he becomes aware of the experiences of others, while eventually in the highest form of human brain there is developed the power of imagination and of forming concepts or ideas quite beyond the powers of the animals. Some of these functions of the nervous system are now described in more detail.

The Humoral Nature of Nervous Action

On p. 337 we have seen that motor nerves act by liberating acetylcholine. This has now been shown to be the general pattern of nervous activity. The vagus has been shown to slow the heart by a similar liberation, and now it appears that the sympathetic acts likewise by liberating a second substance, nor-adrenaline, at sympathetic nerve endings just as it causes the suprarenal gland to liberate adrenaline. It has been shown too that transmission at sympathetic synopses is also dependent on the local production of acetylcholine, and there is some evidence that it is also concerned with sympathetic transmission in the central nervous system. The action of certain drugs suggests that acetylcholine may not be the only substance liberated, at least in the brain.

Reflex Movement and the Reflex Arc.

Reflex movements are those which are made independently of the will but through the operation of pathways to and from the central nervous system. These pathways constitute *the reflex arc*. By their operation the body is protected and kept in normal posture automatically and the higher parts of the brain and consciousness are relieved to some extent of such duties. Their presence is of great importance in physiotherapy as they are responsible for much protective spasm of muscle in and around injured parts. Many more activities of the body occur as the result of reflexes than is generally recognised. The closure of the eyelid when the eye is threatened, or the withdrawal of the hand if it is pricked even in a sleeping person, are typical examples. They are found in the body of an animal after its head has been removed under anaesthesia, provided excessive loss of blood has been prevented by occluding the cerebral blood vessels. It is also necessary to apply artificial respiration, for such a procedure cuts off the essential respiratory centre. Reflexes are also found in the legs even if the subject has lost all voluntary control from damage to the spinal cord above the lumbar region.

The reflex arc (fig. 297) consists of an afferent pathway, which enters the C.N.S. along a posterior root of the spinal cord, then passes to an anterior root and then along an efferent pathway to the muscle concerned. There may be one or more intermediate or internuncial pathways connecting the posterior with the anterior root. The neurone, consisting of a nerve cell with its afferent and efferent processes, is the anatomical unit of the nervous system, but the physiological unit is the reflex. The presence or absence of reflexes is an important diagnostic aid.

In the reflex arc there are one or more *synapses* by which the neurones communicate with each other and these are specially important, as they determine the direction of impulses; for an impulse, although it can travel in both directions in a nerve, can pass through a synapse only in one direction. Synapses might be described as the switches in the nervous system. Some idea of the number of synapses in a reflex is obtained by finding the time taken for an impulse to pass from the posterior to the anterior (sensory to the motor) nerves.

A nerve impulse takes longer to pass across a synapse than to pass along a nerve, but this synaptic delay is greatly reduced by repetition. The reflex is said to be facilitated or canalised and on this process of *facilitation* probably depends the acquisition of habits and skill in the learning of new movements, and it is therefore important in rehabilitation after injury.

This resistance of synapses is also important as it determines the extent of the spread of reflexes. Thus a reflex protective withdrawal movement is brought about if the forefoot is stimulated, but it can be shown by studying action potentials in the spinal cord that although a few impulses reach the lumbar region, the hind legs do not move because the synaptic resistance is too high. When, however, the stimulus is greater, more impulses react, the lumbar cells are stimulated and the hind leg also moves. In strychnine poisoning or in tetanus (lock-jaw), due to action of the toxin of the tetanus bacillus, there is a great reduction of this resistance with the result that quite small stimuli set up very severe and general reactions.

It is at the synapse also that a build up of an excitatory state occurs and small stimuli are summated, and it seems likely that there is an accumulation of acetylcholine for reflexes are enhanced by eserine (see p. 337), which prevents the destruction of acetylcholine. This probably is why there is an *after-discharge* in a reflex, that is the muscle contraction it brings about does not stop abruptly when the stimulus ceases, like a muscle twitch.

There are many varieties of reflex.

The protective reflexes are most important in body defence and all are polysynaptic. Many afferent impulses and synapses probably take part and this is responsible for the reflex being sustained. They are initiated by noxious stimuli such as a prick or a burn. They become greatly exaggerated in animals when the brains have been removed and in disease in man if the higher centres are cut off by disease or injury This exaggeration brings about the rigidity of limbs which physiotherapists are sometimes called to treat. A protective reflex of this kind causes rigidity of the abdominal wall in abdominal inflammation and especially around joints when they are injured. The protective reflexes are essentially flexor in type and cause the limb to be withdrawn from the noxious object and as they involve the spinal cord only, they are known as spinal reflexes.

Postural reflexes are those responsible for the posture of the body. A postural reflex is responsible for maintaining the extension of the knee joint when we stand. In this case the afferent impulses arise in the sensory stretch receptors of the extensor muscle of the thigh when it is stretched by the weight of the body tending to bend the knee, but there is a long afferent pathway to the vestibular nucleus in the medulla oblongata in the brain and a long efferent path, via the vestibulo-spinal tracts to the anterior horn cells of the lumbar region of the spinal cord and to the extensor muscles. Because of the way they originate they are sometimes called "*stretch reflexes,*" or shortening reactions. If the brain above the vestibular nucleus is removed the exaggeration of the reflex causes the limb to pass into a state known as decerebrate rigidity. Such rigidity occurs in birth palsies when the brain is injured and after cerebral haemorrhage. This is now thought to be due to the withdrawal of the inhibitory influence of the reticular formation in the lower brain stem (see p. 459).

The contraction of a muscle when its tendon is tapped is essentially part of a postural reflex, but it has also a shortened pathway through the spinal cord only and its presence or absence is valuable in indicating the site of injury or disease. A typical postural reflex is *the knee-jerk* which occurs when the patellar tendon is tapped but a similar reflex can be elicited from many muscle tendons. The knee-jerk which occurs in spinal man is of much shorter duration than the normal. Thus absence of the knee-jerk produced by tapping the patellar tendon indicates disease of the pathway responsible for the jerk. It is therefore absent when poliomyelitis (infantile paralysis) or injury affects the anterior horns of the lumbar region of the spinal cord or when the afferent path is damaged by syphilis (tabes dorsalis) or if the afferent nerves are damaged by neuritis. The absence of the knee-jerk indicates a *lower motor neurone lesion.* On the other hand the knee-jerk may become exaggerated in lesions affecting the pathways from the brain to the cord. This is known as an *upper motor neurone lesion.* It is of value in the diagnosis of a unilateral lesion for in many excitable persons the knee-jerk is brisker than in others.

Ankle Clonus. This reflex is commonly absent in normal persons but in an upper motor lesion it may be very evident. It is elicited by pressing up the foot sharply to stretch the calf muscles. Provided the pressure on the foot is maintained, the muscles contract clonically, i.e., with intermittent contractions.

The Tone of Muscle and Reciprocal Innervation

If we place a hand over a muscle we feel it to be firmly elastic. This state of tone is because the muscle is always in a state of slight contraction. Such muscle-tone depends on the integrity of the spinal reflex arcs and is lost if the reflex arcs are damaged. Then the muscle becomes flabby and in the case of the leg the limb becomes flail-like. This is seen typically after anterior poliomyelitis. Muscle also becomes flabby through disuse when it accumulates fat.

When a muscle contracts voluntarily or reflexly, however, there is an active relaxation of the opposing muscle which then becomes flabby to the touch. For example, when the brachialis is contracted the triceps of the arm is relaxed. In a decerebrate animal this reciprocal elongation of the opposing muscle may be recorded. How exactly this is brought about is still a puzzle, for it is evident that there must be some inhibition of the centres responsible for the maintenance of normal tone.

The Plantar (Babinski) Reflex. If the sole of the foot is scratched with a blunt instrument the foot executes a grasping-like movement, the toes being flexed. This is part of the postural mechanism of walking. If such a stimulus is applied to a patient with a pyramidal lesion there is a dorsiflexion, especially of the great toe, and a fanning of the other toes. Here we see that the postural response has become replaced by the typical protective spinal reflex which would withdraw the foot from the stimulus. The presence of the dorsiflexion is known as Babinski's sign, an important point in the diagnosis of disease of the pyramidal tract (upper motor neurone lesion). It is, however, present in deep sleep and in children who have not walked (see Voluntary Movement). Stimulation with a *sharp* object always causes a typical withdrawal response.

Reflex Standing and Postural Reactions

The maintenance of the erect posture depends on a variety of impulses which arise especially from the eyes and the vestibule of the inner ear and from the muscles of the legs.

Impulses from the muscles have already been described in relation to postural reflexes which depend on the stretching of tendons.

Impulses from the eyes. The importance of these impulses can be shown by standing *steadily* with the eyes closed. This can be done easily but if one leg is lifted the procedure becomes more difficult, indeed, some persons cannot do it at all. For a similar reason, patients whose other balance mechanisms are deficient tend to become unstable or lose their balance entirely when they close their eyes or lose their visual impulses for other reasons. Thus a patient who has disease of the posterior nerve roots (loco-motor ataxia) tends to fall forward when, with his eyes shut, he stoops to wash

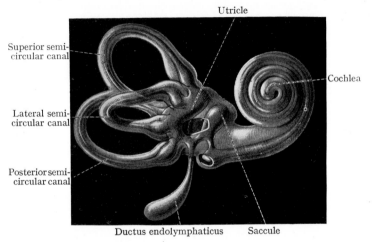

Utricle

Superior semi-circular canal

Cochlea

Lateral semi-circular canal

Posterior semi-circular canal

Ductus endolymphaticus   Saccule

FIG. 298.—The internal ear.

The figure shows the bony labyrinth inside which is the membranous labyrinth. The vestibule is the central portion of the bony labyrinth lying between the cochlea and the semicircular canals.

his face, and finds difficulty in walking in the dark. Commonly he cannot stand steadily with his eyes shut and his feet together (Rhomberg's sign). The same phenomena occur in patients suffering from disease of the ear which has destroyed the vestibule (see below). Patients who have had atropine put into their eyes to facilitate examination by an oculist may have similar diffi-culties because they cannot focus objects properly and we are familiar with the fact that many normal persons feel giddy when looking from a height. Many other similar examples could be given.

Impulses from the vestibule. These are a most elaborate set of complex reflexes which relate the posture of one part of the body to another. First, there are the *vestibular reflexes* by which the position of the head is related to the earth. In the inner ear are two small otolithic chambers, the utricle and saccule, in which small grains of chalk hang on sensitive hairs and these send impulses to the vestibular nucleus in the pons regarding the position of the head, and as a result the appropriate muscles of the neck are contracted to keep the head in the erect position.

If these little chambers get destroyed, as they may do from an extension of the common septic disease of the middle ear (otitis media), the patient is liable to suffer from giddiness but gradually he uses his eyes more and more and the symptoms may pass off. The vestibular reflexes may be thrown out of action by spinning the body round rapidly. This also causes giddiness. Closely allied to the otolithic cavities are the semicircular canals. There are three of these, one in each plane, and when the head is moved, the fluid which they contain stimulates delicate hair cells at one end and we become aware of the movement. Another set of *righting reflexes* relates the position of the trunk to the head. Thus when an animal rises from the ground righting reflexes from the vestibule carry the head the right way up, then the tension on the neck muscles causes the body to come into alignment with the head. All these reflexes become much more efficient with use.

The *lengthening reactions of muscle* are the opposite to the shortening reactions described previously. If too great a force is applied to the rigid muscles of decerebrate rigidity there is not a shortening reaction but the reverse, the muscle at once relaxes as a result of impulses which are set up from specialised receptors in the muscle, thus the muscle is protected against too great a strain. This appears to be a protective mechanism which normally prevents us from contracting our muscles too forcibly and tearing them from the bones. We are unable to use our muscles to a maximum degree except under conditions of severe stress. It is by getting rid of these lengthening reactions that the lunatic acquires his great strength but he may tear his muscles in so doing. The point of importance in physiotherapy is that people with debilitated muscles may damage themselves if asked to perform too strenuous an exercise.

Conditioned Reflexes and Learning

These are reflexes which become established as the result of experience.

The famous experiment is that of teaching a dog that it will get food when a bell rings. Eventually it will secrete saliva when the bell sounds although the food is not presented and it can be shown that the reaction is firmly implanted in the nervous system.

There seems little doubt that many of our reactions become fixed as the result of a similar process.

Of the actual process concerned we as yet know little but we do know that any stimulus which for conscious or unconscious reasons gives rise to a given response gradually becomes more fixed by repetition. It can be shown that the time taken to respond becomes shorter and that there is a reduction in the time taken for the impulse to pass across synapses. Once fixed, conditioned responses are very difficult to eradicate.

The establishment of conditioned reflexes not only requires repetition but time for their development, a fact of special importance in recovery from injury involving permanent damage, for patients tend to become depressed until they grow accustomed to new conditions.

From the point of view of physiotherapists it is important to realise that pain on movement may also become conditioned or a habit. Thus a patient may have learned by bitter experience that a certain movement produces pain, and even after the injury has healed the pain may persist. A similar reaction is seen in dogs and there seems little doubt that successful treatment, by a vast number of methods which go by different names, suggestion, faith healing, physical therapy, etc., really act psychologically, by suggesting to the patient that as a result of their application the afflicted part may be moved without pain. The fact, however, that such methods cure patients is sufficient justification for their use, and although they do not do so in the way they profess, they may be the most satisfactory way of treating certain patients.

The fact that a large variety of pains following injury may be caused to disappear by the injection of a local anaesthetic, which acts only for a short time, is probably due to the dissipation of some such conditioned reflex or the relief of muscle tension. The possibility of treating cases in this way has been recognised only comparatively recently.

THE FUNCTION OF THE CEREBRUM

The cerebrum or fore-brain is the most recently developed part of the brain and is concerned with the higher nervous activities of which we are conscious. By studying the effects of disease, by removing parts in animals and by noting the effects of electrical stimulation of the brain it has been possible to determine that different parts of the brain have special functions. These are best studied in fig. 158 in which are seen the areas for general sensation, for hearing, for seeing, and for the control of the movement of the voluntary muscles. Damage to the motor area of the brain which may occur in injury, most commonly at birth, brings about a typical upper motor neurone lesion with loss of voluntary movement, exaggerated reflexes and spastic muscles of the opposite limbs. It is to be noted in regard to the detailed function of the cerebrum, unlike that of the cerebellum, that each side of the brain is connected with the opposite side of the body except where the muscles which we normally use in pairs are concerned, e.g., those of the forehead and the trunk which are innervated from both sides. The motor area of the brain is connected with the anterior horn cells of the spinal cord by the cerebrospinal (pyramidal) tracts. If these tracts are damaged, paralysis results on the opposite side of the body. This occurs most commonly as the result of cerebral haemorrhage (stroke) due to the bursting of a blood vessel deep in the cerebral hemisphere in the region of the internal capsule.

The function of the cerebrum is primarily to correlate old and new experiences and to determine what line of action, if any, is to be taken. On the cerebrum, too, depends our higher thinking powers so that disease of this part may lead to various forms of lunacy.

Sensation

The ordinary sensations such as pain, temperature and touch are set up by the stimulation of nerve-endings at the termination of the afferent nerves.

All these senses are present in the skin, but in the muscle only pain and a sense of position are present.

There are specialised nerve-endings with a peculiar histological structure for the sensation of touch and temperature, but pain appears to be set up by extremes of temperature and by the stimulation of free endings, i.e., nerve fibres without the specialised endings, but in the case of the skin, removal of the superficial layers results in warmth being appreciated as pain. In areas such as the cornea of the eye, where there are only free endings, pain only is felt.

The impulses set up by any stimulation pass into the sensory nerves by the posterior nerve roots for the body, and by the 5th cranial nerve for most of the head. Those for pain and temperature and part of touch (tactile localisation and sensibility) pass up the spinothalamic tract of the opposite side to the thalamus, the crossing taking place soon after the impulses enter the cord. The impulses which give information regarding the position of the muscles and joints (the muscle joint sense), together with the remainder of touch (tactile discrimination), pass up in the posterior columns (fasciculus gracilis and cuneatus), cross in the medulla and thence to the thalamus. From the thalamus there is a further relay to the cortex of the cerebrum just behind the central fissure. In the thalamus there is an appreciation of crude sensation, i.e., of heat, cold and pain, but fine sensation such as the finer grades of temperature and touch and the localisation of sensation depend upon the impulses reaching the cerebral cortex, for these sensations are lost if this area is damaged.

In disease or injury of the spinal cord we may, therefore, obtain some curious distribution of sensory loss. In syringomyelia, a disease which affects the centre of the cord and, therefore, involves the spinothalamic tracts conveying pain and temperature change, a man may be quite able to hold a cigarette in his fingers but be unaware when it burns them. A patient with an injury to one half of the spinal cord may, for a similar reason, lose the sensation of pain and temperature on the opposite side below the injury while it is normal on the same side, but touch and muscle sense which have not yet crossed are absent only on the injured side. It is best to work out the changes produced with the aid of a diagram such as fig. 165.

Of recent years it has been possible to trace the sensory impulses in the nervous system by recording the electrical changes which are set up as they pass along the pathways.

The difference between touch and pain is seen when a needle is placed in the paw of an anaesthetised animal and the action potentials recorded from the nerve from the part. When the skin is simply touched a short burst of impulses is recorded but if the paw is pricked there is a much larger burst. The evidence suggests that the intensity of the sensation depends on the frequency of impulses set up. There does not, however, seem to be any hard and fast line between impulses which set up pain and any other sensation.

Pain in muscle may be set up if the blood supply to a muscle is cut off by a tight ligature, or a sphygmomanometer cuff applied to the arm at a pressure above the arterial pressure. This causes severe pain which is increased if the muscles of the forearm are exercised. The duration of the exercise appears to be more important than the tension produced and the pain continues as long as the occlusion of the artery is maintained. These facts led to the suggestion that a pain (P) substance accumulates during the occlusion. This pain substance may be lactic acid which is known to be produced in such circumstances. One of the most severe pains known to man is that which occurs from occlusion of a coronary artery to the heart muscle.

In muscle, which is a special consideration of the physiotherapist, it has been possible to discover four distinct groups of endings (fig. 20).

(i) Flower-spray endings on the muscle spindles which are responsible for recording length. They indicate position.

(ii) The annulo-spiral fibres also on the muscle spindles which only record severe stretch or tetanus. They initiate, therefore, the impulses which record the pain of cramp.

(iii) The tendon organs which record absolute stretch not rate of stretch. They initiate postural reflexes.

(iv) The nerve-endings in the fascia.

These are, of course, all quite different from the motor end-plates which are concerned with movement.

Adaptation at nerve-endings is of great importance in sensation. Thus, when a needle is forced into the skin there is at first pain and a burst of impulses (which can be recorded electrically in an anaesthetised animal) passes up the sensory nerves. If the needle is kept still it ceases to produce impulses and is no longer painful. Such adaptation takes place in almost all nerve endings and is of great practical importance, as injuries cease to be painful for similar reasons. We are familiar with adaptation in regard to the wearing of spectacles or false teeth. Adaptation does not take place to any extent at the nerve-endings of muscles on which our posture depends.

Pain in muscle has already been discussed in relation to fatigue, when it was seen that there is evidence that the pain arising in a muscle when its circulation is deficient is due to the accumulation of chemical substances.

The reticular sensory pathway

The introduction of electrical methods for studying nervous pathways shows that sensations pass up the spinal cord and brain stem by the reticular formation. This is a network of nerve fibres which lie between the main tracks and along which impulses pass relatively slowly. The importance of this pathway is that in anaesthesia and during narcosis it becomes "silent," although impulses reach the thalamus and cerebrum by the ordinary fast route. It would appear that the reticular pathway is responsible for the awareness of sensation which hitherto has been credited to the thalamus and it explains why subjects without parts of the cerebrum are less incapacitated than might be expected.

Varieties of pain

The character of pain varies according to the circumstances in which it arises. A throbbing pain is commonly the result of an engorgement of a septic part such as a septic tooth or a finger. The tension causes the beat of the neighbouring blood vessel to be communicated to the nerve endings.

The pain of colic such as occurs in the alimentary tract and other tubes of the body is characteristically intermittent because it depends on the contractions of smooth muscle. This is very important in diagnosis. By contrast, a needle prick is a sharp stab.

The pain of arterial occlusion is continuous. Pain due to irritation of nerves fluctuates irregularly but continues for long periods.

Pain in the alimentary canal may be related to food. That due to ulcer of the stomach occurs on taking food but that of duodenal ulcer is more severe when the stomach is empty. Spasm of the colon, on the other hand, occurs 4 or 6 hours after the last meal, when the food has reached the large intestine. Pain due to inflammation of the pleura is made worse by respiration and in the same way pain on movement may help to localise its cause. So also may tapping or palpation of the part.

The appreciation of sensation

Sensation is not, however, so simple as at first sight appears, especially in injury and disease. Normally if a pin is thrust into the little finger we feel pain in that finger but we may also produce sensations in the little finger by stimulating the ulnar nerve at the elbow, indeed, if the arm is removed at the elbow the patient may complain of pain in the amputated hand if by chance the nerves which formerly went to the fingers are stimulated. This is known as *referred pain*. Similarly we have no experience of impulses which arise from many internal organs, so if impulses do arise the pain is referred to that part of the body supplied by the same spinal root and from which we have had experience of sensation. We have already mentioned that pain in the hip may be referred to the knee and vice versa, pain from the gall bladder may be felt between the shoulders, pain originating in the ureter may radiate down the inner side of the thigh or into the testis, while pain caused by obstruction of the coronary artery (angina) radiates into the left arm and so on.

Another important variety of pain is that which may be conveniently called *conditioned or association pain*. A patient has been injured and unavoidably certain movements set up impulses which cause pain, but gradually the injury is recovered from but the movement still produces the pain. This variety of pain is commonly noted after injury if the subject has some good reason for still desiring to consider himself an invalid (e.g., if a pension depends on it). The difficulty is that there has been an injury and the patient in the last resort is the sole judge as to whether or not he feels the pain.

It cannot be over-emphasised that all sensation is a mental phenomenon. Two persons looking at or listening to the same thing do not necessarily see or hear the same thing. What they appreciate depends upon their circumstances or the *mental state* at the time. Hippocrates, the father of Medicine, pointed out two thousand years ago that if we are hurt in two places, one injury is likely to predominate.

We are familiar with the apparent variability of toothache and sometimes in games a severe hurt may be received without our knowledge.

Normally we ignore a large number of impulses which reach the nervous system such as the minor movements of the intestines, the beating of the carotid artery in the region of the ear, the passage of the blood corpuscles in the vessels in front of the retina of the eye, but in certain circumstances we may become aware of them and complain, e.g., of discomfort in the abdomen, buzzing in the ears or spots before the eyes.

Abnormal sensations are liable to occur if the patient is "run down" as a result of disease, especially infections, and often they are dispelled by a reassurance from the doctor.

The opposite state of affairs can also occur in the condition of hysteria in which the patient believes that he is unable to exercise certain functions; he may believe that he has lost all sensation in some part of his body, he may imagine he is paralysed or that he is deaf. Any disability can be simulated and only an accurate knowledge of anatomy, physiology and pathology makes correct diagnosis possible.

Such patients are in a state of auto-suggestion or self-hypnotism and as we all know under hypnotism all sensation or movements can be abolished temporarily.

It is not, however, to be imagined that such patients are necessarily feigning or "playing the old soldier" for they may become chronic invalids and a great trial, not only to their friends but also to themselves, if this state is allowed to proceed without treatment. In many cases physiotherapy is of great benefit as a therapeutic adjunct for it gives the patient the idea that he is being cured thereby. He would, however, probably resent any suggestion that his state is largely mental, although the doctor may be able to prove that such is the case. At this stage it should be emphasised that the physiotherapist may do great disservice to the patient by suggesting that the complaint is not real and he must be prepared to accept the credit even when he knows that it is not fully justified.

Voluntary Movement

A very large amount of the activity of the nervous system is seen in the performance of voluntary movement.

This is usually done because of some stimulus from the outside world which gives us the idea to make the movement at a given time.

The cerebrum which stores our memories of past sensations and activities then decides what action is to be taken and passes on an impulse to the appropriate part of the motor area. It is here, conventionally, that the activity is considered to commence, because from this point the pathways of the impulse are accurately known.

It is, however, not generally appreciated that in order to move a limb, for example in a given direction, we must know what exactly is the position of the limb at rest. We become aware of this from impulses which are constantly being "fed back" to the cerebrum from the sensory nerve endings in the joints and the muscles themselves.

The more purposeful or skilled the movement the more it depends on sensory impulses. Thus the movement is partly controlled by the results of the movements observed with the eyes or other sensations which the movement may give rise to. For certain accurate movements, such as writing or needlework, the eyes are essential while the degree of muscle tension and amount of muscle contraction is delicately adjusted to the task. This we easily appreciate if we try to do accurate work with the eyes shut.

Slowly with repetition, owing to the process of facilitation at synapses (see page 452), special pathways are laid down so that the skilled movements become more accurate. We easily recognise this if we try to use a knife and fork in the unaccustomed hands.

In complicated movements the cerebellum and its pathways appear to play a considerable part, for if they are damaged, such movements lose their accustomed smoothness and become coarse or ataxic.

Walking in man is at first a voluntary movement, but in quite a short time it becomes automatic. In animals it would seem that it is automatic or reflex from the beginning, for if a decerebrate animal is placed in the standing position on a moving platform it will move its legs according to the speed of the platform, just as we put a foot forward if a push from behind throws us off balance.

Little is known as to how this is brought about, but we know that if in such an animal one leg is forcibly bent, the other will extend.

When the sensory pathways in the spinal cord of man are damaged or diseased, walking becomes tabetic or stamping because the nervous system does not have sufficient information regarding the position of the limbs; while if the cerebellum is diseased, the patient may tend to lurch to the side of the injury.

The power of voluntary movement is lost whenever there is any interference with the pathways from the brain. This is a common variety of paralysis. In hysteria, however, there may be a functional loss of movement. The patient thinks he cannot move a part and does not, although there is no physical damage to pathways. There may, however, be temporary blocks at cerebral synapses and the patient may be tricked into performing movements unintentionally. He may, for example, claim that he has lost his voice yet is quite able to say "ah" which is the fundamental action in speaking. It should, however, be emphasised that such a loss of function is not a deliberate fraud as at first sight appears but is due to a little understood loss of function which responds remarkably well to immediate treatment on psychological lines.

A study of the anatomy of the spinal nerve roots shows how it is possible for a patient to lose the power of voluntary movement without there being necessarily any change in sensation. The reverse is true to some extent only because afferent impulses are necessary for the execution of perfect movements. If, however, a mixed nerve is cut, both movements and sensations are lost but the overlap of the sensory nerves makes the latter loss less than would be expected. Loss of voluntary movement is not accompanied by a loss of the reflexes from the part unless the reflex arcs are destroyed; indeed, as we have seen, the reflexes may actually be increased if the upper motor neurone is destroyed and the reflex arcs are intact.

Even if the motor area of one side is removed (as in an operation for tumour) there is often, after a time, remarkably little impairment of movement. The subject may be able to walk reasonably well presumably because the remainder of the cortex takes over the function of the parts lost. Removal of the sensory area is, however, much more disabling and function is seldom regained. This shows the great importance of sensation in performing all movements and indicates that physiotherapy is likely to be most beneficial in purely motor lesions.

The Function of the Cerebellum

The cerebellum is informed of the position of the muscles and joints by impulses from various afferent nerve-endings, especially the muscle spindles and tendon organs. The impulses pass by the posterior nerve roots to the spinal cord and thence after synapsing pass to thoracic nuclei which give rise to the cerebellar tracts. These are uncrossed and pass up the same side of the spinal cord to the cerebellum. Here they are related in a manner not understood, with impulses from the cerebral cortex and the red nucleus.

We see then that afferent impulses from the muscles play a larger part in the performance of normal movement than might at first be suspected.

As would be expected any disease or damage to the cerebellum or to any of the nerve pathways connected with it leads to muscular inco-ordination which shows itself in a variety of ways, such as lack of normal balance and inability to perform smoothly and accurately the more complex muscular actions such as touching the tip of the nose with the index finger. The patient when walking tends to fall to the affected side, because there is also a lack of tone of the muscles on that side. It will be evident, too, that so far as the movement of the head is concerned, the cerebellum is kept informed by impulses which reach it from the semicircular canals (fig. 298).

Thus we see that faulty voluntary movement may result from damage to the central nervous system in a variety of ways by damage to the pathways to the spinal cord, the pathways to the cerebellum and cerebrum and those from the cerebrum to the spinal cord.

The Effects of Damage to the Motor Pathways

Damage to the upper motor neurones, we have already seen, not only leads to paralysis but after a period of shock there is a recovery and then an exaggeration of reflexes with an excessive tone and spasticity of the muscles in the affected part. The muscles remain normal but undergo some disuse atrophy. Recovery is usually negligible although some may occur from other areas of the brain taking over a new function. True regeneration does not occur in the central nervous system but it does occur in the peripheral nerves.

Degeneration of nerve. Damage to the lower motor neurone, which occurs most commonly from injury to a nerve, is of more importance to physiotherapists as recovery will certainly occur if the continuity of the nerve is preserved, and if the muscles are not allowed to degenerate too far, for then disuse atrophy proceeds rapidly. When a nerve is cut the parent cell is separated from the peripheral end and this after a few days commences to degenerate and ceases to conduct nerve impulses. The myelin sheath of the nerve fibres breaks up into fat-like droplets and the nerve now becomes stainable by various agents such as osmic acid. The axis cylinder dies and eventually the nerve becomes little more than a fibrous cord.

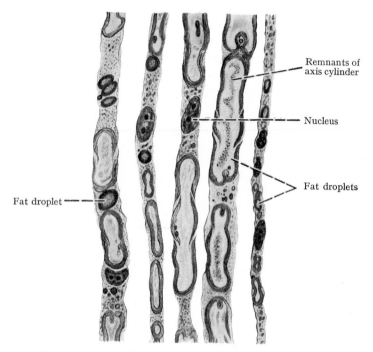

Remnants of axis cylinder

Nucleus

Fat droplets

Fat droplet

FIG. 299.—Degeneration occurring in a nerve four days after operation. (After Cajal.)

An index of the amount of degeneration is given by the R.D. or reaction of degeneration. The degenerating muscle at first becomes more easily stimulated directly, but later this applies especially to stimulation by a galvanic (i.e., a direct) current as distinct from the shorter faradic (i.e., an alternating) current induced by a transformer. The excessive irritability shows itself at the anode (positive pole) rather than at the kathode (negative pole). The R.D. is indicated thus ACC > KCC, i.e., anode closing contraction is greater than the kathode closing contraction. Although there exists the state of "irritable weakness" the contraction is propagated slowly and the galvanic response appears sluggish. Eventually all reaction disappears, that to the shorter faradic current going first. At this stage the degeneration is very advanced. In investigating the R.D. one of the electrodes is placed at a distance, e.g., on the back, while the other, which may be the anode or the kathode as desired, is applied to the motor point of the muscle (i.e., where the nerve enters it) and the minimum strength of stimulus just necessary to bring about contraction noted. (For regeneration of nerve, see Repair, p. 442. See also apparatus used for stimulation, p. 343).

The Effects of Stress

The term stress is now used in a wide sense and includes mental stress, any acute illness and especially physical injury produced accidentally or by surgical operation. The last two are of special interest to physiotherapists.

It has long been known that the adrenal medulla secretes adrenaline in these circumstances, but the retention of sodium and water which occurs indicates that the adrenal cortex also becomes very active. At the same time there is a great loss of potassium and of the products of protein breakdown in the urine.

All these changes lead to a general exhaustion and weakness which may last for days or months according to the duration of the stress. That from injury or surgical operation is fortunately usually short lived. All these changes emphasise the importance of supplying protein in adequate amounts during convalescence.

CHAPTER XXVI

REPRODUCTION AND GROWTH

Reproduction of the species takes place as a result of the union of the male and female elements in the reproductive passages of the female into which the male elements are ejected.

The Male Reproductive Organs (fig. 227)

The male elements, spermatozoa, are developed in the testes. From each testis the spermatozoa pass along the vas deferens into a seminal vesicle where they are stored. From the seminal vesicles they pass into the urethra. The penis is normally pendulous, but during sexual excitement it becomes rigid and erect because the sponge-like erectile tissue of which it is largely composed becomes engorged with blood. In such circumstances, the ejaculatory reflex is set up and the spermatic fluid ejected. This fluid contains the spermatozoa and also the secretions of the prostate and other smaller glands which both carry and protect the sperms. The latter, viewed under the microscope, are seen to be minute structures somewhat like tadpoles with large heads and mobile tails by means of which they propel themselves along the reproductive passages of the female. Should a sperm meet an ovum the two unite and thus the ovum becomes fertilised. Fertilisation usually takes place in the outer end of the uterine tube. Spermatozoa are very easily killed in the vagina, especially by dilute acids, but once they have gained access to the tubes may remain alive for some days.

In addition to producing spermatozoa, the testes are responsible for an internal secretion which causes the male secondary sex characteristics to manifest themselves (the growth of hair on the face and pubes, the breaking of the voice, etc.). These characteristics do not develop if the testes are removed before puberty. The development and activity of the testes are controlled by the hypophysis.

The Female Reproductive Organs (fig. 132)

The ovaries produce the ova. One ovum escapes from the surface of the ovary, on or about the fourteenth day after the onset of menstruation. It is picked up by the fimbriae of the uterine tube and so passes into the uterus. The shedding of an ovum from the ovary is known as *ovulation*. In addition to the production of the ova, the ovary is responsible for an internal secretion which causes the female secondary sex characteristics (the establishment of menstruation, growth of the breasts, development of pubic hair, etc.) to manifest themselves. These characteristics do not develop if the ovaries are removed before puberty. Like the testes their development and activity are controlled by the hypophysis.

The Structure of the Uterus

The uterus is a hollow muscular organ rich in blood vessels and lymphatics. The musculature of the uterus is called the *myometrium* and its epithelial lining the *endometrium*. The endometrium consists of columnar cells most of which are ciliated and all are secretory. The ciliary current is directed towards the vagina.

Changes in the Uterus during Menstruation and Pregnancy

Menstruation. Every twenty-eight days (variable) during reproductive life (say, between the ages of 14 and 45) a woman menstruates. The uterus is, however, always active, it is never in a resting phase.

Starting, for the purposes of description, at the 7th day of this 28-day cycle, the endometrium, under the influence of oestrogen from the Graafian follicle, is in *the proliferative stage*, which follows the phase of menstruation and repair.

On the 12 to 13th day of the cycle (fairly constant) *ovulation* occurs and from then until the 28th day the endometrium is under the influence of both *oestrogen* (which continues for a further 7 days) and *progesterone* from the corpus luteum and it enters the *premenstrual* or *progestational phase*. The features of this are that the thickness of the endometrium, as a whole, is markedly increased, the stroma (connective tissue), undergoes enlargement and decidual transformation, the glands become active, tortuous and sacculated and the capillaries, which have assumed a spiral shape, become engorged with blood. The endometrium generally is oedematous.

On the 28th day (or often before this) the secretion of progesterone ceases and is succeeded by oestrogen from the new Graafian follicle. *The menstrual phase* follows during which there is a general break down of the endometrium, and the engorged blood vessels and glands leak and bleeding occurs. The menstrual flow contains, in addition to blood and mucus, detached portions of the endometrium. The average loss is 50/150 ml. This phase continues for the next 7 days (variable) during which time the endometrium is repaired. The proliferative phase follows.

The activity of the Graafian follicle, which secretes oestrogen, and the corpus luteum, which secretes progesterone, is controlled by gonadotrophic hormones from the hypophysis.

Pregnancy. When the ovum is fertilised, the endometrium under the influence of oestrogen, and especially of progesterone, becomes thicker and the glands hypertrophy and proliferate. By this means the endometrium is converted into a *decidua*. The placenta will form at the point of contact between the ovum and the decidua and is partly foetal and partly maternal. The muscle fibres which constitute the body of the uterus increase in length, thickness and number. Eventually they enlarge to at least ten times their normal size so that the organ becomes almost entirely muscular.

During pregnancy, oestrogen and progesterone come from the placenta as well as the corpus luteum.

The Mechanism of Reproduction

The fertilised ovum becomes embedded in the wall of the uterus. In its earlier stages it is known as an *embyro*, later it is called a *foetus*. The wall of the uterus rapidly adapts itself for the reception of the embryo and eventually the *placenta* (afterbirth) is formed. This is a flat, fleshy, sponge-like organ composed partly of foetal tissue, called *villi* and partly of the maternal *decidua*. The villi are finger-like processes carrying embryonic blood vessels and between these processes are the intervillous spaces filled with maternal blood. Oxygen and nutritious products pass from the

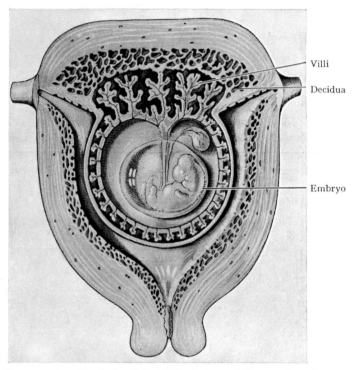

Villi

Decidua

Embryo

FIG. 300.—A sectional plan of the pregnant uterus at the second month.
(*Redrawn from Gray's " Anatomy."*) *From " Gynaecological and Obstetrical Anatomy " by Smout and Jacoby.*

mother's blood through the villi into the foetal blood vessels; waste products and carbon dioxide pass from these vessels into the maternal blood. The foetus is attached to the placenta by the umbilical cord containing the two umbilical arteries and the umbilical vein. These vessels carry the blood between foetus and placenta.

The uterus enlarges greatly during pregnancy until at the seventh month it reaches as high as the xiphoid process.

During pregnancy a number of other changes occur in the mother, notably a great enlargement of the breasts. At the time of birth the breasts are ready to give a supply of milk which is secreted by the glands contained within them. The glands are prepared under the stimulating influence of the anterior lobe of the hypophysis and of the corpus luteum. This structure develops in the ovary in the space previously occupied by an ovum. If the ovum is not fertilised the corpus luteum rapidly disappears, but if fertilisation takes place it enlarges enormously and acts like a ductless gland in producing a substance which is responsible for many changes that take place in the wall of the uterus and the mammary glands. All these changes are controlled by the hypophysis.

Birth

Normally at about the ninth month the various structures at the exit to the pelvis become soft. Eventually the cervix becomes soft, the uterus contracts very forcibly, and the child is expelled. But it is still attached to the placenta by the umbilical cord. Normally this is tied and cut, and the placenta is discharged a little later.

The Growth of the Body as a Whole

The growth of the body depends on a large number of factors, some of which are inherited and some of which are nutritional and environmental.

When a child is born its head is relatively the largest part of its body. Its legs are relatively short and are little longer than its arms. The lower part of the body increases very rapidly in size and the height of the child depends very largely on the length of its legs. The sitting height of different people is much less unequal than the standing height. Some individuals may be of normal height until thirteen or fourteen but stop growing at puberty, others continue until the epiphyses have joined (from 18–25 years). A few appear to be undersized from birth in spite of being adequately nourished.

Surveys of the effect of the milk ration in schools in poorer districts indicate that a considerable proportion of lack of growth is due to lack of nourishment, that is, to a deficiency of calories, proteins and vitamins. A study of animal growth shows that all these are important factors. It would seem that the amino-acids of the proteins are most important, some being more important than others, but if calories are inadequate, protein is wasted as essential fuel for the active child. It has been clearly proved by animal experiments that even if all other factors are supplied, animals will not grow unless vitamins A and B are supplied while vitamin D is essential for the calcification of bones. Vitamin C is important in repair as a whole in that it stimulates the formation of fibrous tissue.

The hormones have also been shown to play an important part in growth. The growth of the skeleton is determined by the hypophysis and the speed of growth of the tissue, generally, by the thyroid. If either is deficient dwarfism results and an overgrowth of the anterior lobe of the hypophysis produces giantism.

It would appear most likely that when nutrition is adequate failure to grow is due to hereditary factors acting through the hypophysis and possibly the thyroid, for in regard to the latter it has been shown that the feeding of thyroid although hastening growth, results in premature maturity.

Mental functions do not appear to be related to body growth.

Senility.   There comes a time variable in different individuals when the powers begin to fail.   This state is characterised by a failure to repair from injury or to resist infection, the circulation fails from senility of the heart or disease of the arteries, leading to mental deterioration, but mental and physical failure by no means run parallel.

Death.   Eventually for one reason or another death occurs.   It is considered to have taken place when respiration ceases or the heart stops beating.   Unconsciousness commonly but not necessarily precedes their failure. It is possible to keep the carcase of an animal alive for a few days even if we remove its head, provided we give it artificial respiration and tie the blood vessels to prevent loss of blood.   This emphasises that the respiratory mechanism is of all the most important.

At the beginning of the section on Physiology we noted that the circulation and respiration are the servants of the rest of the body, but, as in any society, when the servants fail all higher activities are curtailed.

DEMONSTRATIONS

It is most desirable that the following demonstrations should be shown to all students:—

1. The effect of various kinds of stimulation on nerve and muscle.
2. The beat of the isolated heart (frog and mammal).
3. The capillary circulation in the frog's web.
4. The utilisation of oxygen by isolated muscle during recovery and by man.
5. The effect of over-breathing and asphyxia (rebreathing from a bag).
6. The digestion of solid egg-white by pepsin and HCl.
7. The antigravity and protective reflexes in the frog.
8. An artificial scheme of the circulation of the blood.
9. The action of counter-irritants of heat and of novocaine.
10. A cinematograph film of X-rayed movements of the diaphragm and of joints, especially those of the foot.
11. The flow of lymph in an animal (Gilding's experiment).
12. The movements of the intestine.
13. The measurement of the metabolic rate.

CHAPTER XXVII

AN INTRODUCTION TO PATHOLOGY AND BACTERIOLOGY

The literal meaning of Pathology is the study of disease, and so in its widest sense it covers most of the study of medicine. In other words pathology is an attempt to understand the alterations which occur when our health deviates from the normal.

The study of the causes of disease is known as *aetiology*, and the factors which cause disease are called *pathogenic*.

The morbid (diseased) change in the functioning or structure of a tissue or organ is known as a *lesion*. *Disease* is a concept, established by extracting and totalling those characteristics of the sick person which differ from the normal. A disease cannot exist independently of a patient.

In clinical practice pathology is divided up into various special branches. *Morbid anatomy* is the naked eye or macroscopic examination of a body after death, or of an organ or part of the body removed at surgical operation. The examination of the dead body by dissection is known as *necropsy* or *autopsy* and more popularly as a *post mortem*. *Morbid histology* is the examination of abnormal tissues under the microscope, and a special aspect of this is *cellular pathology*, which is the study of alterations in cells. *Experimental pathology* is the study of diseases using the experimental method. *Chemical pathology* is the study of disordered chemical processes in living organisms, and *clinical haematology* the study of disease of the blood or blood-forming organs.

Clinical bacteriology, virology and parasitology are departments concerned with the study of these lowly forms of life which can invade and cause disease in human beings, and the effects of such invasions.

If the pathologist can discover and work out the cause of a disease, it is then possible to take rational steps to prevent it, and prevention rather than cure is the ultimate goal of medicine. If a patient becomes ill, knowledge of pathology will enable the medical attendant to interpret the symptoms and signs of the patient, and to carry out various laboratory tests upon the blood, urine, faeces, cerebro-spinal fluid, etc., on his bacterial flora, or to cut out a small piece of tissue for microscopical examination (*biopsy*).

It is impossible to treat a sick person rationally without first making a diagnosis, but with a diagnosis and a knowledge of the pathology of that disease the proper method of treatment can be applied.

The Causes of Disease

Diseases can be congenital or acquired. *Congenital diseases* are those which originate before birth and can be either: (i) *hereditary*, when they are due to the inheritance of abnormal chromosomes or abnormal genes (chromosomes are minute paired structures in the nuclei of cells, with the even smaller genes attached, and between them they determine the transmission of the

472

characteristics of the parents to their offspring, e.g., size, colour of eyes or skin, blood groups, etc., and also the sex of the foetus); or (ii) *developmental*, when they are due to environmental abnormalities in the uterus which result in the abnormal formation of the embryo.

Examples of diseases due to abnormal inheritance are colour-blindness, haemophilia, some cases of diabetes mellitus, congenital acholuric jaundice, and mongolism.

Congenital developmental diseases can result from deficiencies of essential dietary factors, or the presence of toxic substances in the maternal blood-stream which can be chemical (e.g., thalidomide babies), or due to living organisms (e.g., deformed babies born to some mothers who have suffered from German measles in the early months of pregnancy).

Diseases acquired after birth are usually environmental and are due either to deficiency in quantity or quality of essential substances necessary for the maintenance of life (oxygen, water or a proper diet), or the effect on the body of external agents which can be either inanimate (which in turn can be physical or chemical) or animate, that is to say various types of living organisms which can invade the living body and cause illness.

Illness due to deficiencies in diet are most strikingly typified by diseases due to lack of one or more of the vitamins, e.g., scurvy or rickets (see Chapter XIX). Physical agents which can cause disease include mechanical injury (*trauma*), heat, cold, actinic radiation (excessive sunlight), electrical currents and ionising radiations (x-rays).

Chemical agents include an immense range of substances which vary greatly in their degree of *toxicity*. Such substances may act locally at the site of contact, and others only after absorption into the body whether through the skin, or by swallowing, or inhaling into the air passages, etc. They may act immediately, or after a variable period (which may be years), and sometimes only after the development of an abnormal hypersensitivity of the tissues.

Animate agents of disease may be so small that they can be seen only under the light microscope (e.g., *bacteria*), or they may be much smaller and can be seen only by means of the electron microscope (*viruses*).

The causes of many diseases remain unknown. Such diseases are then said to be *idiopathic*, which is a convenient label to cloak ignorance.

In many diseases there are multiple aetiological factors. These may be initiating factors, or they may be contributory factors, such as a poor nutritional state, or a pre-existing structural abnormality, permitting a pathogenic organism to gain a foothold and cause illness.

Inflammation

Inflammation is the commonest and most basic of pathological reactions. The features of inflamed tissues are well known—redness, heat, swelling and pain and are the result of the local reaction of the tissues to injury. In living tissues, inflammation is a progressive reaction involving mainly the vascular and lymphatic structures, and this is accompanied or followed by reparative, healing processes.

The agents which cause inflammation may be trauma, chemical or physical agents, or pathogenic living organisms. The irritant agent causes direct injury to the cells of the body, which then in turn produce substances which cause the characteristic changes in the tissues.

As a general rule inflammation is a protective mechanism tending to localise or dispose of the injurious agent and also to prepare the inflamed area for repair.

The changes show a regular sequence of events which may be divided into six phases:

1. There is a transient constriction of the small blood vessels especially the capillaries.

2. This is followed by a dilatation of the blood vessels, particularly the arterioles, then the veins and last of all the capillaries. Due to this dilatation there is an increased blood flow, and this accounts for the redness and heat of inflamed areas, and partly for the swelling. Many small blood vessels in the area which are normally constricted tend to open up and dilate.

3. After a varying period, which may be about an hour, the walls of the blood vessels become more permeable, water and proteins from the plasma escape into the surrounding tissues, in consequence the blood becomes thicker and more viscous and thus the blood flow slows down.

4. The white blood cells accumulate around the endothelial lining of the blood vessels.

5. Throughout this process increasing amounts of blood plasma escape through the vessel wall which becomes increasingly permeable to the plasma proteins. This fluid, rich in protein, which escapes into the tissues is the *fluid exudate* and is largely responsible for the swelling of the inflamed areas. It often contains a large amount of fibrinogen which may be converted into fibrin by thrombokinase released by the damaged tissues.

6. The white cells in the blood stream, already at the periphery of the blood vessels, begin to migrate through the vessel walls in increasing numbers giving rise to a *cellular exudate*.

In really severe inflammation red blood cells may also escape through the damaged vessel wall, a process known as *diapedesis*, and the exudate in the tissues then becomes *haemorrhagic*. The fibrin in the clotted exudate tends to seal off the inflamed area, and with it the causal agent (e.g., bacteria) setting up the inflammation may be localised.

There is an increased lymph flow and this takes part of the exudate, both fluid and cellular, with it; and if bacteria are included, the inflammatory process may spread along the lymphatics giving rise to a *lymphangitis*. In some cases fibrin clots may form in the lymphatics, thus blocking them. This is another way of limiting the spread of the infection.

The Cells in Inflammation

The cell most strikingly involved in acute inflammation is the *polymorph*.

These escape from the blood vessels by their own amoeboid movements, squeezing between the endothelial cells forming the walls of capillaries.

At the same time as the local inflammatory reaction is going on there is usually an increase in the number of leucocytes in the circulation (*leucocytosis*). This results from stimulation of the white-cell-forming tissue in the bone marrow by substances produced in the inflamed area.

The function of these polymorphs is to engulf and destroy invading bacteria or tissue fragments, a process known as *phagocytosis*. They also produce various substances of an enzyme nature which can dissolve protein (e.g., damaged cells). There are other polymorphs, called *eosinophils* because they stain bright red with eosin, which are usually present in abundance in allergy and in diseases due to metazoan parasites (worms).

Lymphocytes also play a part in inflammatory processes. Their numbers are not usually increased in acute inflammations, except in infants and in the early stages of acute inflammation of the central nervous system. They are much more numerous in chronic conditions. These cells are not phagocytic but are probably concerned with the formation of substances known as *antibodies* which neutralise toxic substances.

A cell related to the lymphocyte is the *plasma cell*, and this is seen in chronic inflammatory cell exudates. It also produces antibodies. A white cell larger than the polymorphs and lymphocytes is the *macrophage*, which is very important in both acute and chronic inflammations. They are amoeboid and phagocytic. Being much larger than polymorphs they can ingest larger fragments and sometimes clump together to form one very large multi-nucleated giant cell which can then ingest even larger foreign bodies.

Types of Inflammation

All types of inflammation can be acute, subacute or chronic, depending upon the duration and severity of the process. The best classification of inflammation is according to the aetiology, but it is also useful to consider a few special types by the reaction they produce, as these are the terms often employed by doctors.

Serous inflammation—this is a type of inflammation characterised by a great outpouring of serous inflammatory exudate (e.g., a blister).

Fibrinous inflammation occurs when there are great shaggy masses of fibrin in the inflammatory exudate.

Haemorrhagic inflammation occurs where diapedesis of red blood cells is marked and usually occurs when the inflammation is due to a particularly virulent organism.

Purulent or suppurative inflammation is seen when pus is formed. Pus is a creamy fluid composed of broken down tissues with many polymorphs, many of which are dead and are then known as *pus cells*. If the pus becomes sealed off in an enclosed space, the lesion is known as an *abscess*.

Membranous inflammation is a severe type of fibrinous inflammation of epithelium when the toxic agent causing the inflammation is so powerful that it causes the death of the epithelium (e.g., in diphtheria).

Catarrhal inflammation is a mild form of inflammation of mucous membranes and is characterised by a considerable outpouring of mucus from the mucous-secreting cells (e.g., the common cold).

Regeneration and Repair

When an inflammatory process has been overcome, the body will attempt to restore the tissues to their original condition. If there has been little, or no, cell destruction during the inflammatory phase, the tissues may be restored exactly, a process known as *resolution*. If tissue destruction has taken place, other mechanisms are put in motion. Some tissues, e.g., skin may *regenerate* so that new cells exactly like the old dead ones are produced. More commonly, however, the destroyed tissues are replaced by simpler tissue, particularly scar tissue which is fibrous. This process is described in Chapter XXIII.

Bacteriology

Bacteria are minute unicellular organisms usually of simple structure. There is an enormous number of different types of bacteria but only a relatively small number cause disease in man or animals. Organisms which do not cause disease are said to be *non-pathogenic*, those which do are said to be *pathogenic*. In health the normal body harbours an immense number of bacteria on the skin and mucous membranes, and especially within the large intestine. These bacteria make up the normal "flora" of the body and they live on the secretions and waste products of the body. They are known as *commensals*. Sometimes a healthy person may harbour what to him is a commensal but in someone else may produce a disease. He is then known as a *carrier*.

Bacteria are classified by their appearance under the microscope and their staining properties, by the manner in which they grow in culture or in living tissues, by their biochemical activities and by various special tests using immunological techniques. Bacteria which are more or less spherical in shape are known as *cocci*. Rod-shaped bacteria are known as *bacilli*. If the rod is curved, the organism is called a *vibrio*; and a spiral-shaped organism is known as a *spirillum*. The diameter of an average type coccus is of the order of one micron, which is one-thousandth of a millimeter. Some bacteria show hair-like projections known as *flagellae*; others have a capsule of jelly-like material; and certain bacteria can produce a *spore*, which is a dormant form of the organism highly resistant to destruction (e.g., from prolonged boiling). Pathogenic bacteria produce *toxins*. Two types of toxin are described: 1. *exotoxins*, which diffuse out of living bacteria; 2. *endotoxins*, which are only released when the bacterium breaks up after the death of the organism. Bacterial toxins are some of the most poisonous substances known. *Viruses* are minute infective organisms much smaller than bacteria and can be seen only by electron microscopy. Viruses can grow in living cells only. They may be dormant in tissues for long periods, producing neither symptoms nor lesions, and may be excreted by the host causing infection in other persons, or may become virulent to the original host if for any reason his resistance

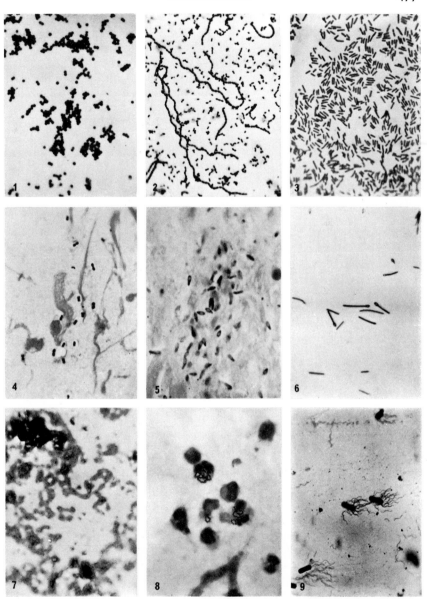

FIG. 301.—BACTERIA showing (1) staphylococci (2) streptococci (3) escherichia coli (bacillus coli) (4) pneumococci, which are diplococci and some of which are showing capsules (5) clostridium sporogenes with spores (6) clostridium tetani showing terminal spores (7) pneumococci stained to show capsules (8) phagocytosis of streptococci within polymorphs (9) bacilli showing flagella.

falls.   Most virus infections in man produce a high degree of long-lasting immunity, but the common cold and influenza are well-known exceptions. Some viruses are transmitted to man by insects—known as *vectors* (e.g., yellow fever transmitted by mosquitoes).

Viruses may be classified by the tissue in which they prefer to grow. **Neurotropic viruses** grow in nervous tissue (e.g., poliomyelitis).   **Dermato-tropic viruses** grow in the skin, e.g., chicken pox, measles, herpes simplex (cold on the lip), or smallpox. **Respiratory viruses** grow in the respiratory tissues (e.g., the common cold, influenza or virus pneumonia).   There is also a miscellaneous group which grows in parenchymatous organs, e.g., mumps in the salivary glands or infective hepatitis in the liver.

Antigens and Antibodies

The living body tends to reject foreign substances which gain entrance into it.   The body may produce specific substances, known as *antibodies*, which can combine with the foreign material, neutralise it if toxic, or facilitate its removal.   These foreign substances which can provoke antibody production are known as *antigens*.   Many bacteria and viruses produce antigens, and the production of antibodies by the host is one of the main methods of resistance to infection.   A host with enough antibody to neutralise the antigens of an invading organism is said to be *immune*.

Antibodies may be *agglutinins*, which causes clumping of antigens, these can then be more easily removed; *precipitins*, which precipitate soluble antigens; or *antitoxins*, which neutralise the poisonous effect of antigenic toxins.

Infection

Infection is the establishment and multiplication of pathogenic organisms in the body.   The infection may remain strictly localised (e.g., a boil), or it may spread locally (e.g., a *cellulitis*), or it may spread throughout the blood stream (*septicaemia*).

Many types of organisms can produce disease: viruses, bacteria, protozoa, fungi and worms.

These organisms can enter the body by various routes, called the *portal of entry*.   The infecting organism may: (i) penetrate the intact skin or con-junctiva; (ii) enter a wound in the skin or mucous membrane; (iii) may be inhaled; (iv) may be swallowed; (v) may enter via the urethra, vagina or anus.

Other organisms have a single portal of entry (e.g., typhoid fever results only from swallowing typhoid bacilli).   After a pathogenic organism has entered the body various factors influence the possibility of infection.

1. The Size of the Invasion

For any given organism a certain number is necessary to produce an infec-tion, and the larger the number the more severe the infection as a rule.

2. The Portal of Entry

Some organisms can produce an effect on certain tissues only, or may be more easily destroyed at some sites than others.   Thus more than 100 times the number of tubercle bacilli are necessary to cause an infection by mouth than by inhalation.

3. The Virulence of the Organism

Aggressiveness or invasiveness is the power of multiplying in the body despite the body's defences.

Toxigenicity is the power to produce toxins. Tetanus and diphtheria bacilli show high toxigenicity but are poorly invasive. The anthrax bacillus is very invasive but only slightly toxigenic.

4. Synergism between Organisms

For example, in deep wounds infected with a mixed collection of organisms, tetanus bacilli can grow more easily.

5. The Resistance or Immunity of the Host

May be natural or acquired, local or general. *Natural immunity* or *species immunity* can be illustrated by syphilis, gonorrhoea and cholera, all of which are exclusively human infections, while myxomatosis affects rabbits but not hares.

Acquired immunity. May be active—following an attack of the disease, or following artificial processes—e.g., vaccination.

Passive immunity. May result from inheritance, i.e., by the passing on of the defensive substances from the mother to her offspring *via* the placenta in utero or in the maternal milk; or may be produced by artificial means, e.g., the injection of antitetanic serum. General factors also influence the establishment of infection.

Nutrition. Poorly nourished persons have a poor resistance to many infections, and in famines many people die of infections rather than by starvation.

Exposure to cold may enhance respiratory infections.

Fatigue and surgical shock or other upsets of the circulation may increase the risk of infections.

Disinfection, sterilisation and asepsis. Disinfection and sterilisation refer to the treatment of objects so that living organisms are destroyed. The two terms have been used synonymously meaning the same thing, but are best separated by referring to chemical methods as disinfection and physical methods as sterilisation. *Chemical disinfection* can be carried out using many different types of disinfectant. Carbolic acid (phenol), which was the first antiseptic used by Lister; halogens such as chlorine or iodine: alcohols, ethylene dioxide or formaldehyde. The choice of disinfectant will depend upon the type of thing to be disinfected, as many disinfectants are poisonous to persons as well as the organisms. A special type of chemical disinfection known as *chemotherapy* is the use of, e.g., sulphonamides or antibiotics, which can be given to living patients and will destroy or inhibit the growth of harmful organisms without harming the patient.

Sterilisation is commonly carried out by heat, either moist or dry. Most organisms are rapidly killed at the temperature of boiling water, but bacterial spores may survive boiling for long periods. In consequence, sterilisation of instruments, dressings, etc., in hospital is carried out by *autoclaving*. This means heat treatment with steam under considerable pressure.

ATROPHY, HYPERTROPHY AND HYPERPLASIA

Atrophy

Atrophy is a decrease in the size of a cell, or of an organ, which was formerly of normal size. The term must be distinguished from *agenesis*, in which the tissue or organ has not developed at all in the foetus; *aplasia*, in which the tissue or organ appears in the foetus but then fails to develop to any effective size; and *hypoplasia*, in which there is only partial development and the tissue, or organ, remains smaller than normal in the fully-grown individual.

Atrophy results from inadequate nutrition. This may be generalised, as in starvation or wasting from disease or old age. It may be physiological, as in the shrinking of the uterus after childbirth or of the thymus after puberty. It may be due to disuse, as in the muscles of paralysed limbs or the remaining bone in an amputation stump, or it may occur in the secretory cells of a gland which is prevented from secreting by the blockage of the corresponding duct. Continuous localised pressure due to a tumour or distended blood vessel may cause *pressure atrophy*. *Endocrine atrophy* may result in organs dependent

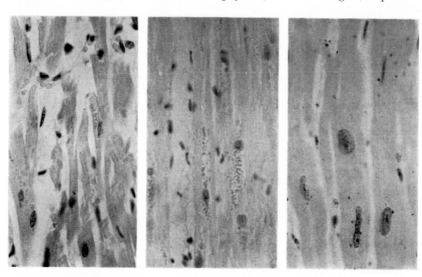

Fig. 302.—*Atrophy and Hypertrophy*. Comparative sections at the same magnification showing myocardial fibres which are (1) atrophied (2) normal (3) hypertrophied. In hypertrophy the nuclei as well as the fibres are hypertrophied.

upon endocrine stimulation, if this stimulation is cut off, e.g., atrophy of the thyroid, adrenals and gonads in cases where pituitary hormone production ceases.

Hypertrophy

An increase in the size of a cell, or of an organ if the increase is due to the hypertrophy of the constituent cells, is known as hypertrophy. An increase in the size of a tissue or organ due to an increase in the number of constituent cells is known as *hyperplasia*. The two conditions are often present together.

A good example of hypertrophy is seen in the muscles of weight-lifters. At the same time their bones and muscle attachments tend to become bigger mainly due to hyperplasia. The heart muscle hypertrophies if there is mechanical obstruction of the outflow from the heart due to narrowing of the aortic valve or because the peripheral blood pressure is raised. Other examples of hypertrophy of muscles are common, such as the muscle in the walls of arteries in cases of raised blood pressure, or of the bladder wall in cases of chronic obstruction to the outflow of urine. All these examples are cases of hypertrophy due to increased work.

Physiological hypertrophy occurs in the muscle of the uterine wall during pregnancy. Compensatory hypertrophy occurs when tissue is lost from disease or surgical removal. For example, if one lung or kidney is removed, the paired organ hypertrophies to take over the function of the other, as well as its own.

Hyperplasia rather than hypertrophy tends to occur in some tissues and organs under the same types of stimuli. Thus physiological hyperplasia occurs in the mammary glands during lactation, compensatory hyperplasia occurs in the liver or thyroid following loss of tissue in the organ, and work hyperplasia occurs in the bone marrow if there is need of increased blood production.

Hyperplasia and hypertrophy are processes which cease when the stimulus which caused them stops. If the multiplication of cells continues after the stimulus is withdrawn, a much more sinister process is occurring known as *neoplasia*.

OEDEMA

Oedema is the excessive accumulation of fluid in the tissues and can be localised or general. If it occurs in serous cavities, it is known as *hydrothorax*, or *pleural effusion* in the pleural cavities; as *hydropericardium* or *pericardial effusion* in the pericardium; and as *ascites* if present in the peritoneal cavity.

Oedema results from an upset in the factors which in health control the fluid interchange between the capillaries and tissues. These include capillary blood pressure forcing fluid out of the vessels into the tissue, which is normally balanced by the osmotic pressure of the plasma proteins drawing the fluid in again: by the degree of capillary permeability; by the power of the lymphatics to drain away excess tissue fluid; and by the amount of sodium ion retention in the extracellular fluid.

Hydrostatic pressure in the capillaries may be raised if the venous pressure rises due to the heart failing as an effective pump and causing venous congestion. In this case the oedema will be most marked in the dependent parts of the body, e.g., the ankles. This is known as *cardiac oedema*, and is also considerably aggravated by sodium retention. Localised rise in the venous, and hence the capillary pressure, may result from pressure on veins, as in the case of the pregnant uterus pressing on the iliac veins and resulting in oedema of the ankles.

The osmotic pressure of the plasma will fall if the level of the plasma proteins, especially the albumen, falls. This may be due to failure or formation of the serum albumen due to starvation causing *nutritional oedema* or disease, e.g., severe liver disease such as cirrhosis, or excessive loss of serum albumen in renal disease causing *nephrotic oedema*. Oedema due to a fall in serum albumen level will always be generalised and will be much less influenced by gravity than is cardiac oedema, so that it is equally developed in the non-dependent parts and may show itself first in the face.

Increased capillary permeability is seen in acute inflammation, causing *inflammatory oedema*. The inflammation may be the result of an allergic reaction, as in urticaria, and is usually, but not always, localised.

If the lymphatics draining a limb are all blocked by some disease process, or following surgical removal, as for example the surgical removal of the axillary lymph nodes during an operation for carcinoma of the breast, in some cases there results a form of chronic oedema of the limb.

DEGENERATIVE CHANGES

A cell can be either alive or dead, and if dead, is referred to as being *necrotic*, a term which can also be applied to a piece of tissue or an organ in which all the cells are dead.

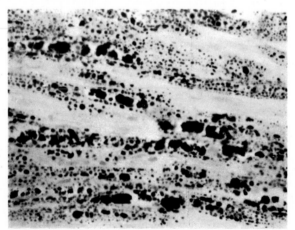

FIG. 303.—*Fatty Degeneration.* A section of heart muscle stained with osmic acid to show the fat droplets, stained black, situated in the muscle fibres. In normal myocardium there would be none of these droplets.

Before death occurs in a diseased cell it may show various degenerative changes. *Cloudy swelling* is the earliest degenerative change to be seen, and in it the cells, and the affected organ made up of the cells, become swollen and pale. If the process causing the degeneration continues, whether it be ischaemia, anaemia, deficient nutrition, bacterial toxaemia, physical trauma or poisoning, the cells may show *fatty degeneration.*

Abnormal fat droplets appear in the cell cytoplasm, and these tend to fuse. Both cloudy swelling and fatty degeneration particularly affect the more specialised and metabolically active organs, such as the heart, liver and kidneys.

In a cell which is damaged and dying, changes are also seen in the nuclei. The chromatin condenses to form a solid mass, a process known as *pyknosis.*

Necrotic cells, if they remain sterile, are usually broken down by enzyme action and liquefy. This process is known as *autolysis.* If infection with proteolytic bacteria takes place, *putrefaction* occurs, usually with the production of gas in the dead tissue. If putrefaction occurs in a gangrenous limb, the process is known as *wet gangrene*, as opposed to uninfected gangrene of a limb in which the dead tissues tend to dry up and shrivel, and the process is known as *dry gangrene.*

DISTURBANCES OF THE CIRCULATION

The healthy existence of living tissues depends heavily upon a normal flow of blood through the tissue. Disturbances of the blood flow may take various forms. A local increase in blood supply is known as *hyperaemia* or congestion. Hyperaemia may be active, when there is dilatation of the small blood vessels (vasodilatation), or passive, when there is obstruction to the normal outflow of blood, either due to local blockage of the veins draining the area or generalised venous congestion due to failure of the heart as a pump.

A local decrease in the blood supply is known as *ischaemia* and can be due to blocking of the arterial supply by something occluding the lumen of the artery, by blockage due to thickening of the artery walls, due to excessive muscular contraction in the artery wall, or due to tying off or twisting the arterial supply. The result of ischaemia will be an attempt by the body to restore the circulation through the ischaemic area by the opening up of small blood vessels from adjacent areas, thus establishing a collateral circulation. If this is unsuccessful, the ischaemic tissue may die and the area of dead tissue caused by the failure of the circulation to it is known as an *infarct.*

Infarction

Infarcts are most common in those organs or tissues which have poor collateral circulations, for example the heart muscle, the brain, the intestines, the spleen or the kidney. They are uncommon in organs with good collateral circulations like the stomach, the voluntary muscles or the liver, which has a double circulation. The lung also has a double circulation, and pulmonary infarcts only occur when there is already some difficulty of circulation as in heart failure.

Infarcts are usually pyramidal shaped with the apex pointing towards the arterial obstruction causing the infarct. Red and swollen at first, the infarct usually becomes pale in colour. Organisation by fibroblastic activity then occurs, and in time the infarct is replaced by a fibrous scar.

In the brain, infarcts liquefy and a cystic cavity is left eventually (softening of the brain).

Infarction of a limb may occur if the main artery is blocked, and the more proximal the blockage the more of the limb is involved.   The dead part of the limb is described as *gangrenous*.

Occasionally, due to the pressure of bandaging or to splinting which is too tight, there may be extensive emptying of small vessels in a muscle leading to

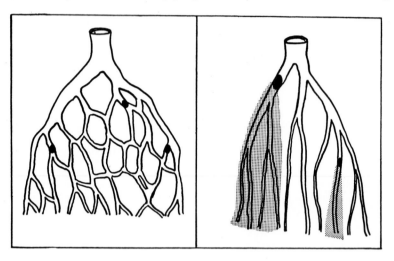

Fig. 304.—*Anastamosing and End Arteries*.   On the left is an anastamosing circulation in which blockage of a vessel in any of the three positions shown will not cause infarction, as the flow of blood can be maintained through collateral vessels.   On the right the arteries are end arteries and blockage at either of the points shown will cut off the blood flow to the area supplied by that branch, with subsequent infarction, represented by the stippling.

infarction.   The muscle fibres are then replaced by fibrous tissue leading to a condition known as *Volkmann's ischaemic contracture*.

Thrombosis

In normal health the blood in an individual remains fluid.   If blood is shed, due to an injury, etc., the bleeding is checked and stopped by contraction of the blood vessels and clotting of the blood, which seals off the damaged vessels.   Clotting of blood within the vessels during life, intravascular clotting, is always abnormal and is known as *thrombosis*.   The abnormal clot within the blood vessel or the heart is known as a *thrombus*.   There are three factors which singly or together may result in thrombosis:

(1) Changes in the lining of the blood vessel; (2) changes in the blood flow either of velocity or turbulence; (3) changes in the constituents of the blood. The endothelium lining the heart and blood vessels is water repellent and very smooth.   If it becomes roughened by disease or injury, it becomes sticky and blood platelets will adhere to it.   The adherent platelets can then set up the

process of blood coagulation, and fibrin becomes added, forming, with the blood cells trapped with it, a thrombus.

With a normally rapidly flowing circulation any thrombus which for any reason starts to form on the wall of a blood vessel would be swept away. If the flow of blood becomes sluggish, or even stagnant, for any reason, this mechanism does not apply. Also the blood platelets in a slowing circulation tend to be forced to the periphery as the heavier, larger, blood cells remain in mid-stream, where the flow is faster, by centrifugal force. An important cause of slowing of the blood stream in leg veins is confinement to bed, with subsequent lack of muscular movements to pump the enclosed blood back toward the heart, aided by the valves in the veins which permit blood flow towards the heart only.

Changes in the constituents of the blood are particularly seen after injuries or surgical operations when for a week or ten days the platelet count in the blood rises and the platelets become more adhesive, both to themselves and to vessel walls. Both these circumstances increase the liability to thrombosis, and when combined as they usually are by venous stasis due to resting in bed there is considerable risk of thrombosis in the leg veins. The danger of thrombosis in the leg veins is that the clot tends to become larger by further thrombosis at the proximal end, towards the heart, and may extend by propagation up the leg via the femoral vein to the iliac veins and even into the inferior vena cava. Part of this elongated clot may then break off and be swept by the blood stream to the heart and then block the pulmonary artery as it narrows on dividing up into its branches in the lung. Blocking of the pulmonary circulation in this way (*pulmonary embolism*) may be rapidly fatal, or in any case will make the patient very ill. A particulate foreign body free in the circulation is known as an *embolus* and in the case just described is a thrombotic embolus.

Embolism

Apart from detached portions of a thrombus other types of emboli occur.

Fat embolism. When bones are fractured, particularly the bigger bones, globules of fat from the bone marrow may enter the circulation. The same thing may occur in cases of extensive burns. These small globules of fat are liquid at body temperature but may still act as small solid objects which can block the capillary circulation of vital organs such as the brain or lungs and can cause severe illness and even death.

Air embolism. Air may be sucked into veins which are wounded and in which there is a negative pressure, e.g., the veins of the neck. It may also enter the circulation due to faulty blood transfusion or injury to the lung. It may also appear as bubbles in the blood of persons who have been working under increased atmospheric pressure, e.g., divers or caisson workers, who are decompressed too rapidly. The air dissolved in the blood comes out of solution. Bubbles of air in the blood tend to dissolve quite rapidly, but if the quantity of air is large, serious consequences may follow as very small bubbles tend to act as solid objects due to the effect of surface tension. They may, therefore, block the capillary circulation of vital organs, such as the brain or the heart, and cause death before there is time for the air to dissolve. Air in the blood stream will also form a frothy mass in the cavities of the heart. This froth is compressible during systole so that no blood is pumped out of the heart and the circulation fails. This is another mechanism by which air embolism may cause death.

Bacterial embolism. In the condition known as bacterial endocarditis large masses of bacteria grow on the affected heart valve. Clumps of bacteria may then break off and form emboli in the circulation. These clumps may be large enough to block arteries and so cause infarction particularly in the brain, the spleen and the kidneys.

Other kinds of emboli occur, including emboli of tumour cells, of animal parasites (particularly some sorts of small worm), amniotic fluid and squames during pregnancy, and even foreign bodies such as bullets.

Thrombotic emboli which are infected are particularly dangerous, and are known as *septic emboli*. If they cause infarction, the dead tissue has no resistance to infection and is an excellent culture medium for the growth of the infecting organisms. Septic infarcts result which may suppurate and thus form abscesses.

HEART FAILURE

The heart is a pump responsible for taking the blood from the veins and ejecting it *via* the aorta or the pulmonary artery through the greater or lesser circulation, respectively.

It may fail in this function either acutely or chronically for a variety of reasons. The form of failure may be either: (i) a failure to maintain an adequate flow of oxygenated blood through the arteries, usually due to a fall in cardiac output, and this is sometimes known as *forward failure*; or (ii) a failure to pump out all the blood being returned to it by the veins so that the venous pressure rises and blood accumulates in the veins, *backward failure*, or *congestive cardiac failure*. In many cases of heart failure both forms are present.

The causes of heart failure may be classified under several headings:

1. Inadequate return of blood to the heart via the veins.
2. Obstruction to the normal filling of the heart in diastole due to constriction of the pericardium.
3. Failure of the myocardium to contract properly.
4. Failure of the heart valves to work properly.
5. Obstruction to the normal outflow of blood.
6. A need for an abnormally increased blood flow.

Inadequate return of blood to the heart will result from haemorrhage and a fall in blood volume.

Constriction of the pericardium, so that the heart cannot fill properly, usually results from tuberculous pericarditis causing fibrous thickening and adherence, or from effusions of fluid in the pericardiac sac. Failure of the myocardium may be produced by many causes. The most dramatic is the sudden cutting off of its blood supply through one of the branches of the coronary artery as a result of a thrombosis occluding the lumen—*coronary thrombosis*. This may produce acute total failure and sudden death due to the heart stopping, or may greatly weaken the heart beat causing acute failure, particularly of the left ventricle, so that blood is dammed back in the pulmonary circulation causing acute congestion and oedema, and consequent shortness of breath. Gradual cutting off of the coronary circulation may result from *atheroma*, a degenerative disease of arteries in which there is laying down of fatty material beneath the endothelium which results in fibrosis in the wall of the artery, and narrowing of its lumen. With coronary atheroma present the flow of blood to the myocardium may be adequate to cope with rest conditions only, so that when the sufferer makes a physical effort demanding greater work from the heart, the myocardium is unable to respond and the patient suffers severe pain in the chest—*angina pectoris*. The myocardium may suffer from an inadequate oxygen supply due to severe anaemia or because the blood is not being adequately oxygenated in the lungs due to lung disease, or the myocardium may be diseased itself, due to acute rheumatism producing rheumatic myocarditis, or deficiency in vitamin B_1 causing beri-beri, or due to toxins in the circulating blood damaging it as in diphtheria. Fatty degeneration of the myocardium with subsequent weakness may result from many things: chronic anaemia, high fever, bacterial toxaemia and some kinds of poisoning, the most common being alcoholism. Occasionally the myocardium may fail due to injury, either penetrating, such as a bullet or knife wound, or non-penetrating, as when the driver of a motor car is crushed against the steering wheel. The myocardium may fail because it is beating too rapidly, and does not permit enough time in diastole for the cavities to refill, so that output falls. This will happen in uncontrolled thyrotoxicosis but more commonly in cases in which the heart beat is affected by disease of the conducting system. The commonest important variety of this is atrial fibrillation in which the atria beat so rapidly that the atrioventricular node is unable to keep pace. Thus the ventricles beat much too rapidly for efficient pumping, and the ventricular beats, and subsequently the arterial pulse, are irregular in timing and force.

Diseased heart valves may be either *stenosed*, i.e., having their orifice narrowed, or *incompetent*, i.e., they do not close fully so that blood can regurgitate back from whence it came. The commonest cause is acute rheumatic fever. The mitral valve is the one most commonly diseased, and then the aortic. The valves of the right heart are much less often affected apart from congenital stenosis of the pulmonary valve. Syphilis may cause aortic incompetence due to stretching of the valve ring, and in old age there may be calcification of the aortic valve producing both stenosis and incompetence. Bacteria may settle and grow on heart valves, usually after previous disease of the valve, causing a condition known as *bacterial endocarditis*. This may result in ulceration of the valve cusps and hence incompetence.

Obstruction to the normal outflow of blood may be due to stenosis of the aortic valve, congenital narrowing of the aorta due to coarctation, or to increased peripheral resistance as in high blood pressure, or from pulmonary embolism.

A need for an abnormally increased blood flow may be due to an abnormal shunt of blood from the arterial to the venous side, either congenital, as in a patent ductus arteriosus, or acquired, as in the case of an arterio-venous shunt due to injury, or in Paget's disease of bone.

Results of Heart Failure

In acute failure, notably from coronary thrombosis, pulmonary embolism or rupture of a valve cusp due to bacterial endocarditis, death may occur suddenly.

In chronic cases the heart will attempt to compensate and will first dilate and then hypertrophy. The different heart chambers will not necessarily hypertrophy equally depending upon the cause of the failure and the chamber upon which the increased load has mainly fallen.

In cases of heart failure in which there is a rise in venous pressure the organs will show passive congestion and cardiac oedema will occur.

NEOPLASIA

Neoplasia is the excessive, usually progressive, and apparently purposeless, overgrowth of tissue which proceeds without any regard to the surrounding tissues or the requirements of the organism as a whole. The mass of tissue in this process is known as a *neoplasm* or new growth.

While forming part of the body the neoplasm is not regulated by the ordinary physiological processes and it grows independently, acting as a parasite, drawing nourishment from the body but serving no useful function and often doing harm.

There is a small special group of neoplasms of developmental origin which grow only during the normal period of growth of the individual, known as hamartomata. These consist of abnormal masses of tissue produced by the excessive overgrowth of a particular tissue which is normally present at the site of the lesion. The commonest example is the angioma, an abnormal mass of blood or lymph vessels seen as the "port wine stain" of infants, or the cavernous haemangioma or lymphangioma. Another less common example is the outgrowth of a knob of bone on a long bone known as an hereditary exostosis.

Apart from hamartomata, neoplasms are divided into two classes: (i) benign or simple, (ii) malignant or cancerous. Commonly, neoplasms are referred to as tumours, but strictly speaking this is a term which means any abnormal mass of tissue and can be applied to lesions which are not neoplasms, for example cysts, abscesses, dilated blood vessels (aneurysms) or granulation tissue.

Neoplasms are commonly classified by adding the suffix -oma to the name of the type of tissue involved, especially in the case of simple neoplasms. Thus, a neoplasm of fibrous tissue, is called a *fibroma*, a neoplasm of muscle a *myoma*, a neoplasm of cartilage, a *chondroma*, a neoplasm of bone, an *osteoma*, a neoplasm of fat, a *lipoma*, and so on. A simple neoplasm of an epithelial tissue is either a *papilloma* from surface epithelium or an *adenoma* from glandular epithelium.

Malignant neoplasms are either *carcinoma*, if they arise from epithelial tissues, or *sarcoma*, if they arise from connective tissues, and may further be

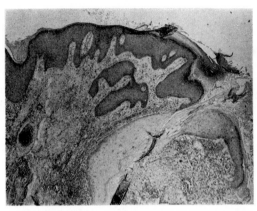

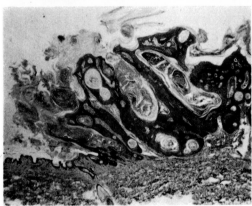

Fig. 305.—*Skin Carcinoma and Skin Papilloma.* Above is a section of skin carcinoma (squamous carcinoma) with columns and masses of malignant epidermal cells invading downwards into the dermis. Below is a benign skin papilloma with masses of epidermal cells heaped upwards and showing no invasion of the underlying dermis.

specified by giving the tissue or origin so that the comparable malignant neoplasms to the simple neoplasms given above are fibrosarcoma, myosarcoma, chondrosarcoma, osteosarcoma, liposarcoma, squamous carcinoma or adenocarcinoma.

Characteristics of Benign Neoplasms

These are usually composed of well-differentiated, mature cells which closely resemble normal cells. They grow slowly, expansively and equally in all directions and do not invade surrounding tissues so that there is a sharp line of demarcation (often a fibrous capsule) between them and the surrounding normal tissues. They never spread to other parts of the body and they remain strictly localised. Though they are called benign they may produce harmful and even fatal effects by a number of mechanisms:

Mechanical. As a result of its anatomical situation a single neoplasm may do harm, as when occurring within the cranial cavity and pressing on the brain, in the mouth preventing mastication, or within the chest or abdomen pressing on vital structures.

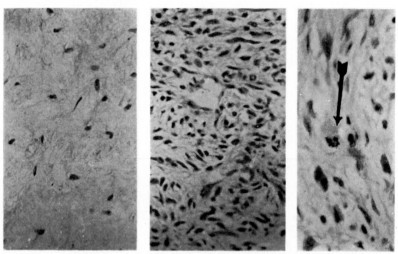

Fig. 306.—*Fibroma and Fibrosarcoma.* These high-power magnification sections show on the left a simple fibroma, and in the middle a malignant fibrosarcoma. In the fibroma the tissue is similar to normal fibrous tissue with scanty nuclei scattered amongst collagen fibres. The fibrosarcoma is very cellular and the nuclei are larger than normal. They show also active cell division by the presence of mitotic figures, an example of which is shown in the higher magnification picture on the right.

Accidental as a result of ulceration leading to infection or haemorrhage; or when twisted, with the cutting off of the blood supply; or when in the intestine, being pulled by peristalsis along the lumen of the gut, pulling the affected part of the intestine inside out, a process known as intussusception.

Hormone production. A neoplasm of endocrine tissue may produce an excess of hormone which may be harmful.

In addition, benign neoplasms may be disfiguring and might cause psychological difficulties in the case of sensitive patients.

Characteristics of Malignant Neoplasms

As compared with benign neoplasms malignant neoplasms are usually made up of imperfectly or atypically differentiated tissue. They often grow rapidly, which is both expansive and infiltrative. This means that columns of cells grow out into the surrounding tissues like projecting tentacles, and the formation of a capsule does not occur. Infiltrating neoplasms eventually grow beyond the bounds of the organ of origin and into the surrounding tissues or organs. Much more sinister still, pieces of malignant neoplasm may be broken off and carried as emboli in blood or lymph vessels or via other natural channels to settle and grow at a point distant from the primary growth. These seedlings are known as *metastases*, secondary growths or secondaries, and grow and spread like the primary growth. Often they multiply and may themselves metastasise in turn.

Carcinomata are much more common than sarcomata. Early spread of carcinoma tends to be via the lymphatics either by continuous infiltration along the lymphatic vessels, a process known as lymphatic permeation, or by emboli to the regional lymph nodes. This feature is of great importance in cancer surgery. The surgeon when cutting out a primary growth will try to excise all the related lymphatics in the hope that all parts of the neoplastic tissue are removed and that there will therefore be no recurrence.

Malignant neoplasms, if untreated, or if they cannot be completely removed by surgery, or destroyed by radiotherapy or chemotherapy, will usually progress, spread and metastasise until they kill the patient.

Malignant neoplasms (cancer) become more frequent in older people, and account for about one in six of all deaths in Britain.

The cause of some individual cancers is known. Some chemicals may produce cancers either at the point of application, e.g., tar cancers on the skin or at a distant point, and bladder cancer in workers in the aniline dye or rubber industries. Some cancers are genetically derived, and others may be produced from a large overdosage of irradiation from x-rays or radioactive substances, or from overdosage of ultraviolet light over a long period.

Neoplasms sometimes arise in old scars or areas where the tissues are chronically irritated. The most important example of this is bronchial carcinoma (lung cancer) arising in a bronchus. This form of cancer is becoming rapidly more common and killed 27,000 people in Britain in 1965. It has now been shown to be due in almost all cases to irritation of the bronchial mucosa as the result of cigarette smoking which must be classified as a dangerous habit from this cause alone, though it is known to be a contributory cause in a number of other serious illnesses (e.g., chronic bronchitis, coronary artery thrombosis and peptic ulcer).

Neoplasms of the reticulo-endothelial and lymphoid tissues form a special group, and often arise in many parts of the reticulo-endothelial or lymphoid system at once, unlike other malignant neoplasms which usually start in one place. Varieties seen are *Hodgkin's disease* and *lymphosarcoma* arising in lymphoid tissues and *leukaemia* of various kinds arising in the white blood cells and the white cell forming tissues.

GLOSSARY

Abduction, to draw away (Latin, ab = from, and ducere = to lead).

Accessorius, accessory (Latin).

Acetabulum, vinegar cup (Latin, acetum = vinegar).

Acromegaly, a disease of the hypophysis manifested as an enlargement of the hands, feet, etc. (from the Greek, akros = extremity, and megalos = great).

Acromion, the point of the shoulder (Greek, akros = point, and omos = shoulder).

Addison, English physician, 1793–1860.

Adrenaline, the hormone from the suprarenal medulla, called also epinephrine and adrenin (Latin, ad = to, and ren = kidney).

Adventitia, the outer coat of a blood vessel—literally "coming from without" (Latin).

Afferent, conveying from the periphery to the centre (Latin, ad = to, and ferre = to carry).

Ala, a wing (Latin).

Alveolus, a sac or socket (Latin).

Amylase, an enzyme converting starch into sugar (Greek, amylos = starch).

Anconeus, pertaining to the elbow (Greek, agkos = the bend of the arm).

Annular, ring-shaped (Latin, annulus = a ring).

Aponeurosis, a flat tendon (Greek, apo = from, and neuron = a tendon).

Appendix, an appendage (Latin, appendere = to hang upon).

Arachnoid, like a spider's web (Greek, arachnes = spider, and eidos = form).

Areolar, a small space (Latin, area = space).

Artery, a vessel conveying blood from the heart (Latin, arteria).

Articular, pertaining to a joint (Latin, articulatus = jointed).

Ase, a suffix indicating an enzyme.

Aspera, rough (Latin).

Asphyxia, a condition in which there is oxygen lack and an accumulation of carbon dioxide (Greek, a = not, and sphuxis = pulse).

Astragalus, the ankle bone (Greek) (Latin, talus).

Astringent, something which constricts the blood vessels (Latin, ad = to, and stringere = to bind).

Atlas, named after the Greek god who was supposed to support the universe.

Auricularis, pertaining to the ear (Latin, auricula = an ear).

Autonomic, self-controlling (Greek, autos = self, and nomos = law).

Axilla, armpit (Latin).

Axis, a pivot (Latin).

Babinski, French physician born 1857.

Bacillus, a germ, often shaped like a rod (from the Latin = a little stick).

Bell, Sir Charles Bell, surgeon, 1774–1842.

Betz, Russian anatomist, 1834–1894.

Bier German surgeon born 1861.

Bigelow, American surgeon, 1816–1890.

Bilirubin, the red pigment in bile (Latin, bilis = bile, and ruber = red).

Biliverdin, the green pigment in bile (Latin, bilis = bile, and viridis = green).

Broca, French surgeon, 1824–1880.

Bronchus, from the Greek, brogkhos = windpipe.

Buccinator, a trumpeter (Latin).

Burdach, German physiologist, 1776–1847.

Bursa, a sac (Greek).

Calcis, of the heel (Latin, calcar = a spur).

Callosum, thick (Latin).

Calorie, a unit of heat (Latin, calor = heat).

Canaliculus, a small canal (Latin).

Capillary, a minute vessel (Latin, capillaris = pertaining to the hair).

Capitulum, a small head (Latin, caput = head).

Capsule, an outer case (Latin, capsula = a little box).

Carotid, from the Greek, karos = deep sleep. Compression of the carotid arteries causes unconsciousness.

Cartilage, from the Latin, cartilago = cartilage.

Casein, from the Latin, caseus = cheese.

Catheter, a tube used to draw off fluids (Greek).

Caudate, having a tail (Latin, caudatus).

Cellulose, a carbohydrate forming the framework of plants (Latin, cellula = a little cell).

Cereal, derived from grain (Latin).

Cerebellum, the small brain (Latin).

Cerebrum, the main brain (Latin).

Cervical, from the Latin, cervix = neck.

Cholesterol, a chemical substance occurring in bile (and elsewhere) (Greek, chole = bile, and stereos = solid).

Chyle, emulsified fat in the lymph vessels in the intestine (Greek, chulos = juice).

Cilium, an eyelash (Latin).

Cisterna, cistern (Latin).

Clarke, J. L., English physician, 1817–1880.

Claustrum, a barrier (Latin).

Coccyx, from the Greek, kokkuks = cuckoo. The coccyx is said to resemble a cuckoo's bill.

Coeliac, pertaining to the belly (Greek, koilia = belly).

Condyle, from the Greek, condulos = knuckle.

Conniventes, converging (Latin).

Cornification, conversion into horn (Latin, cornu = a horn).

Coronal, from the Latin, corona = a crown.

Corpus, a body (Latin).

Corpuscle, a small body (Latin).

Cortex, the outer layer, e.g., the bark of a tree (Latin).

Creatine, derived from muscle (Greek, kreas = flesh).

Cricoid, shaped like a ring (Greek, cricos = a ring, and eidos = form).

Cruciate, shaped like a cross (Latin, crux = a cross).

Crureus, from the Latin, crus = leg.
Crus, a leg (Latin).
Cutaneous, pertaining to the skin (Latin, cutis = skin).
Cuneiform, from the Latin, cuneus = a wedge.

Defaecation, the discharge of faeces from the bowel (Latin).
Deferens, conveying away (Latin).
Deltoid, from the Greek, delta = a letter of the alphabet shaped thus *Δ*.
Dermis, from the Greek, derma = the skin.
Diabetes mellitus, a disease marked by excess sugar in the blood which is excreted in the urine (Greek, dia = through, and bainein = to go).
Diaphragm, a partition (Greek, dia = across, and phragma = a wall).
Diaphysis, the shaft of a growing bone (Greek, dia = across, phuein = to grow).
Diarthrosis, a movable joint (Greek, dia = through, and arthron = a joint).
Diastole, the stage or relaxation of the heart muscle, during which the ventricles are filled with blood (Greek, dia = through, and stellein = to send).
Digastric, from the Greek, dis = double, and gaster = belly.
Digital, from the Latin, digitus = a finger.
Duodenum, twelve (Latin)—so called because it is said to be twelve fingers' breadth in length.
Dura, hard (Latin)—dura mater = hard mother.
Dyspepsia, indigestion (Greek, dus = ill, and peptein = to digest).

Efferent, conveying from the centre to the periphery (Latin, ex = out of, and ferre = to carry).
Ellipsoid, ellipse = a regular oval (Greek).
Endo-, from the Greek, endon = within.
Endocrine, literally self-curing (Greek, endon = within, and krino = to sift).
Enzyme, an organic catalyst (Greek, en = in, and zume = leaven).
Ephedrine, a substance derived from a Chinese plant which raises the blood pressure and dilates the bronchioles.
Epi-, upon (Greek).
Epiphysis, the ends of a growing bone derived from secondary centres of ossification (Greek, epiphuein = to grow upon).
Epiploicae, the membrane of the intestines (Greek, epiplöon).
Epithelium, the covering of the skin and mucous membranes (from the Greek, epi = upon, and thele = nipple).
Equina, of or belonging to a horse (Latin)—cauda equina = a horse's tail.
Ergosterol, the sterol precursor of vitamin D, formed from the action of ultraviolet light; originally derived from ergot.
Erythrocyte, red blood corpuscle (Greek, erythros = red, and kutos = a cell).
Eustachius, Italian anatomist, 1520–1574.

Faeces, residue discharged from the bowel (Latin).
Falciform, sickle-shaped (falx = a sickle).
Fallopii, Fallopius, an Italian anatomist, 1523–1562.
Falx, a sickle (Latin).

Faradic, named after Michael Faraday, an English physicist, 1791–1867.

Fascia, a band (Latin).

Fauces, the space between mouth and pharynx (Latin).

Femur, the thigh (Latin).

Fibrin, a protein which plays an essential part in the clotting of blood (Latin, fibra = fibre).

Fibula, a buckle (Latin).

Filum, a thread (Latin).

Fimbriae, a fringe (Latin).

Flavum, from the Latin, flavus = yellow.

Foetus, the offspring in the womb after the 3rd month, up to this time it is called an embryo (Latin, fetus = an offspring).

Follicle, a small secretory sac (Latin, folliculus = a little bag).

Foramen, a window (Latin).

Fornix, an arch (Latin).

Fovea, a pit (Latin).

Galvanic, named after Luigi Galvani, an Italian physicist, 1737–1798.

Gasserian, Gasserius, an Italian anatomist, 1505–1577.

Gastric, pertaining to the stomach (Greek, gaster = belly).

Gastrocnemius, from the Greek, gaster = belly, and kneme = leg.

Gemellus, a twin (Latin).

Genu, a knee (Latin).

Gimbernat, Spanish surgeon, 1742–1790.

Ginglymus, a hinge joint (Greek, gigglumos = a hinge).

Glenoid, from the Greek, glene = cavity and eidos = form.

Glomerulus, a cluster of blood vessels found in the kidney (Latin, glomus = a ball).

Glottis, the aperture between the vocal cords (Greek).

Gluten, a sticky substance derived from the protein of wheat (Latin, gloia = glue).

Gluteus, from the Greek, gloutos = buttock.

Glycocholate, a bile salt derived from the amino-acid, glycine.

Glycogen, a carbohydrate obtained from glucose and stored in the liver and tissues (from the Greek, glucus = sweet, and gennan = to produce).

Goll, Swiss anatomist, 1829–1904.

Gracilis, slender (Latin).

Gulae, pertaining to the gullet (oesophagus).

Haemoglobin, the pigment of the blood containing iron in combination with the protein globin (Greek, haima = blood).

Haemopoietic, blood forming (Greek, haima = blood, and poiein = to make).

Hallux, from the Latin, hallex = great toe.

Hamstrings, the tendons at the back of the knee which flex the leg on the thigh (possibly a derivative of the Latin word, hamatum = bent).

Haversian, Havers, English anatomist, 1650–1702.

Heister, German anatomist, 1683–1758.

Hemiplegia, paralysis of one side of the body (Greek, hemi = half, and plege = a stroke or shock).

Heparin, a substance found in the liver which prevents the clotting of blood (Greek, hepar = liver).

Hepatic, pertaining to the liver (Greek, hepar = the liver).

Hering, German physiologist born 1866.

Hernia, the protrusion of an organ or tissue through an opening, known also as "rupture" (Latin).

Hilum, a trifle (Latin).

His, Wilhelm His, German physician born 1863.

Histamine, a vasodilator, derived from the amino-acid histidine.

Histology, the minute structure of the tissues (from the Greek, histos = web, and logos = discourse).

Hormone, an internal secretion carried in the blood stream which stimulates the activity of organs (Greek, hormanein = to excite).

Humerus, the arm bone (Latin) known in colloquial English as "the funny bone."

Hunter, John Hunter, most famous British anatomist, 1728–1793.

Hyaline, from the Greek, hyalos = glass.

Hypoglossal, situated under the tongue (Greek, hupo = under, and glossa = the tongue).

Ileum, the distal part of the small intestine (Greek, eilein = to twist or coil).

Iliacus, pertaining to the ilium (Latin).

Ilium, the hip bone (Latin).

Inguinal, pertaining to the groin (Latin).

Innominate, nameless (Latin, in = not, nomen = a name).

Insulin, a hormone from the islets of Langerhans in the pancreas (Latin, insula = an island).

Inter-, between (Latin), thus interossei = between the bones.

Intima, innermost (Latin).

Intra-, within (Latin).

Invertase, an intestinal ferment which inverts cane sugar.

Ischium, from the Greek, ischion = the hip.

Jejunum, empty (Latin, jejunus = fasting).

Jugular, from the Latin, jugulum = the neck.

Keratin, horn-like (Greek, keras = horn).

Kocher, Swiss surgeon, 1841–1917.

Labrum, a lip (Latin).

Lacerum, from the Latin, lacerare = to tear.

Laciniate, a fringe (Latin).

Lacrimal, pertaining to the tears (Latin, lacrima = a tear).

Lactose, the sugar of milk (Latin, lactare = to suckle).

Lacuna, a small pit (Latin, lacuna = a pit).

Lambdoid, from the Greek, lambda = a letter in the Greek alphabet shaped thus λ.

Lamella, a small plate (Latin, lamina = a plate).

Lamina, a plate (Latin).

Langerhans, German pathologist, 1847–1888.

Lata, from the Latin, latus = broad.

Latissimus, broadest (Latin).

Legume, the seeds of a plant having pods, e.g., peas and beans. These are known as pulses (Latin, legumen = pulse).

Lemniscus, from the Greek, lemniscos = fillet.

Lentiform, lens-shaped.

Leucocytes, white blood corpuscles (Greek, leukos = white, and kultos = a cell).

Linea alba, a white line (Latin).

Lingual, pertaining to the tongue (Latin, lingua = tongue).

Lingula, a small tongue (Latin).

Lipase, a pancreatic ferment which splits fats, sometimes called steapsin (Greek lipos = fat).

Lister, Lord Joseph Lister, English surgeon, 1827–1912 (upon whose researches antiseptic surgery was founded).

Lordosis, arching forward of the spine (Greek, lordoun = to bend).

Louis, French surgeon, 1723–1792.

Lumbar, pertaining to the loins.

Lumbrical, wormlike (Latin, lumbricus = a worm).

Luschka, German anatomist, 1820–1875.

Luteum, (corpus luteum) a yellow body left behind in the ovary after the discharge of the ovum (Latin, luteus = yellow).

Lymph, from the Latin, lympha = spring water.

Lymphocyte, a white blood corpuscle (Latin, lympha = spring water, and Greek, kultos = cell).

Lysine, an essential amino-acid derived from protein digestion.

Magendie, French physiologist, 1783–1855.

Mandible, from the Latin, mandere = to chew.

Manubrium, a handle (Latin).

Massage, from the Greek, massein = to knead.

Mastoid, nipple-shaped (Greek, mastos = breast, and eidos = form).

Mater, mother (Latin).

Matrix, the ground substance (Latin).

Maximus, greatest (Latin).

Meckel, German anatomist, 1714–1777.

Media, middle (Latin).

Median, situated in the mid-line (Latin), not to be confused with *medial* which means nearest to the mid-line.

Mediastinum, a median partition (Latin).

Medulla, marrow (Latin).

Medullated, from the Latin, medulla = marrow.

Meninges, membranes (Greek).

Meniscus, from the Greek, meniscos = a crescent.

Menstruation, the monthly discharge from the uterus (Latin, mensis = month).

Mesentery, from the Greek, mesos = middle, and enteron = bowel.

Meso-, middle (Greek, mesos).

Metabolism, the chemical changing of substances in the body (Greek, metabole = change).

Metacarpal, from the Greek, meta = after, and karpos = the wrist.

Micturition, from the Latin, micturire = to urinate.

Minimus, smallest (Latin).

Mitral, shaped like a bishop's mitre.

Monro, Alexander Monro (primus) Scottish anatomist, 1697–1767.

Morphology, the study of the form of the lower animals (Greek, morphe = form, and logos = discourse).

Multangulum, from the Latin multus = many, and angulum = angled.

Multifidus, split into parts (Latin, multus = many, and findere = to split).

Mylo-hyoid, from the Greek, mule = mill, and hyoid = U-shaped.

Myo-, pertaining to muscle (from the Greek, mus = muscle).

Neurilemma, from the Greek, neuron = a nerve, and lemma = a sheath.

Neuroglia, from the Greek, neuron = a nerve, and gloia = glue.

Nissl, German neurologist, 1860–1919.

Node, from the Latin, nodus = a knot (hence nodose).

Nuchae (nuchal), from the Latin, nucha = the neck.

Nucleus, a small round body (kernel) within a cell, without which the cell could not live (Latin, nux = a nut).

Obturator, from the Latin obturare = to seal, hence obturator foramen, the closed foramen.

Oedema, excess fluid in the tissue spaces (Greek, oidema = a swelling).

Olecranon, from the Greek, olekranon = the point of the elbow.

Olivo-, pertaining to the olive.

Omentum, peritoneum connecting the stomach with adjacent organs (Latin).

Opponens, opposing (Latin).

Orbicular, orbicularis, circular (Latin).

Osteoblasts, cells which are formed into bone (Greek, osteon = bone, and blastos = germ).

Osteoclasts, cells which destroy bone (Greek, osteon = bone, and klan = to break).

Osteology, from the Greek, osteon = bone, and logos = discourse.

Ovale, from the Latin, ovalis = egg-shaped.

Pancreas, from the Greek, pan = all, and kreas = flesh.

Papilla, a small elevation (Latin).

Para-, beside (Greek).

Parietal, pertaining to the walls of organs (Latin, parietalis).

Pasteur, Louis Pasteur, famous French chemist and bacteriologist, 1822–1895 (hence pasteurisation).

Patella, a plate (Latin).

Pecten, a comb (Latin).

Pectoralis, pertaining to the chest (Latin).

Pedicle, stalk-like (Latin, pes = foot).

Peduncles, a supporting part (Latin, pes = a foot).

Pelvis, basin (Latin).

Pepsin, an enzyme converting proteins into peptones (Greek, pepsis = digestion).

Peptone, formed from the breakdown of proteins (Greek, peptein = to digest).

Peri-, around (Greek).

Peristalsis, a wave of contraction passing along a tube (Greek, peristellein = to send round).

Peritoneum, from the Greek, peri = around and teinein = to stretch.

Pernicious, tending to be fatal (Latin, per = through, and neco = to kill).

Peroneus, pertaining to the fibula (Greek, perone = a brooch—the fibula is sometimes referred to as the brooch bone).

Phagocyte, a cell which destroys bacteria (Greek, phagein = to eat).

Phalanges, from the Greek, phalanx = in line of battle.

Pharyngeal, pertaining to the pharynx (Greek).

Phrenic, pertaining to the diaphragm (Greek).

Phytin, a phosphorus compound derived from plants (Greek, psuton = plant).

Pia, tender (Latin), pia mater = tender mother.

Piriformis, pear-shaped (Latin, pirum = a pear, forma = shape).

Pisiform, from the Latin, pisum = a pea, and forma = shape.

Placenta, the organ present in the pregnant uterus (womb) connecting mother with child, sometimes called the afterbirth (Latin, placenta = a flat cake).

Plantaris, from the Latin, planta = the sole of the foot.

Plasma, the fluid portion of the blood (Greek, plassein = to mould).

Platysma, from the Greek, platusma = a plate.

Pleura, a rib (Greek).

Poliomyelitis, an inflammation of the grey matter in the spinal cord (Greek, polios = grey, muelos = marrow).

Pollex, thumb (Latin)—hence pollicis.

Poly-, many (Greek).

Pons, a bridge (Latin).

Popliteal, from the Latin, poples = posterior part of knee.

Poupart, French anatomist, 1661–1709.

Profunda, deep (Latin, pro = for, and fundus = bottom).

Protein, a nitrogenous compound found in meat, vegetables, eggs, milk, etc.

Protoplasm, the first plasm (Greek, protos = first).

Psoas, from the Greek, psoa = loin.

Pterygoid, wing-shaped (Greek, pterugion = a wing).

Ptyalin, an enzyme found in the saliva (Greek, ptualon = spittle).

Purkinje, Hungarian physiologist, 1787–1850.

Pylorus, from the Greek, pule = a gate, and ouros = guard.

Radius, a spoke (Latin).

Ramus, a branch (Latin).

Ranvier, French pathologist, 1835–1922.

Receptaculum, receptacle (Latin).
Recessus, a cavity (Latin).
Rectus, straight (Latin).
Renal, from the Latin, ren = a kidney.
Restiform, rope-like, (Latin, restis = rope).
Recticulo-, from the Latin, rete = a net.
Retinaculum, a halter (Latin).
Rhomboideus, kite-shaped (Greek, rhombos = rhombus, and eidos = form).
Ringer, Sidney Ringer, English pharmacologist and physician, 1835–1910.
Risorius, from the Latin, risus = laughter.
Rolando, Italian anatomist, 1773–1831.
Rubro, pertaining to the red nucleus (Latin, ruber = red).

Sacciformis, sac-shaped (Latin, saccus = a sac, and forma = shape).
Sagittal, (Latin, sagitta = an arrow).
Saphenous, easily seen (Greek, saphenes = manifest).
Sarcolemma, a muscle sheath (Greek, sarx = flesh, and lemma = husk).
Sartorius, from the Latin, sartor = a tailor.
Scalene, from the Greek, skalenos = uneven.
Scaphoid, from the Latin scapha = a skiff (Greek, skaphe).
Scapula, the shoulder (Latin).
Scarpa, Italian anatomist, 1747–1832.
Schafer, British physiologist, 1850–1934.
Schwann, German anatomist, 1810–1882.
Scrotum, a pouch (Latin).
Sebaceous, from the Latin, sebum = suet.
Segmentation, division into small parts or segments (Latin, segmentum).
Semi-, from the Latin, semis = half.
Septum, a partition (Latin).
Sesamoid, named after the sesame seed (Greek).
Silvester, English physician, 1829–1908.
Soleus, pertaining to the sole (Latin).
Spermatozoa, the sperms in the semen which fertilise the ovum (Greek, sperma = semen).
Sphenoid, wedge-shaped (Greek, sphen = a wedge).
Spigelian, Spigelius, Flemish anatomist, 1578–1625.
Splenius, a bandage (Greek, splenion).
Squamous, scaly (Latin).
Stapes, a small stirrup-shaped bone (ossicle) in the middle ear (Latin).
Stapedius, a muscle attached to the stapes.
Sternum, from the Greek, sternon = the breast.
Styloid, pin-shaped (Latin, stylus = pin, and Greek, eidos = form).
Sub-, under (Latin).
Sustentaculum, a support (Latin).
Suture, a seam (Latin).
Sylvius, French anatomist, 1614–1672.
Symphysis, from the Greek, sun = together, and phuein = to grow.
Synapse, the junction between two nerve cells (from the Greek, sun = together, and aptein = to touch).

Synchondrosis, from the Greek, sun = together, and chondros = cartilage.

Syncytium, a multi-nucleated mass of protoplasm (from the Greek, sun = together, and kultos = cell).

Syndesmosis, from the Greek, sundesmos = a band.

Synovial, from the Greek, sun = with, and oon = egg (synovial fluid looks like white of egg).

Syringomyelia, abnormal cavitation in the spinal cord (Greek, surigx = a pipe, and muelos = marrow).

Systemic, affecting the body as a whole (Greek, sustema).

Systole, the stage of contraction of the heart muscle (Greek, sustole = contraction).

Taurocholate, a bile salt derived from the amino-acid taurine.

Tecto-, pertaining to the tectum (Latin, tectum = a roof).

Tentorium, resembling a tent (Latin).

Teres, round (Latin).

Terminale, placed at the end (Latin).

Testis, or testicle, the male sex gland (Latin, testis or testiculus).

Tetanus, sustained muscular contraction seen in lock-jaw (Greek, teinein = to stretch).

Tetany, muscle spasm (Greek, teinein = to stretch).

Thalamus, from the Greek, thalamos = a chamber.

Thenar, the palm of the hand (Greek).

Therapy, the treatment of disease (Greek).

Thrombin, a substance formed in the clotting of blood (Greek, thrombos = clot).

Thyroid, like a shield (Greek, thureos = a shield, and eidos = form).

Trachea, the windpipe (Greek, tracheia = rough).

Trachelo-, from the Greek, trachelos = neck.

Trapezius, table-shaped (Greek).

Tricuspid, having three cusps.

Triquetral, from the Latin, triquetrus = triangular.

Trochanter, from the Greek, troksis = a runner.

Trochlea, a pulley (Latin).

Trypsin, an enzyme converting proteins into peptones (Greek, tripsis = rubbing).

Tuberosity, from the Latin, tuberositas.

Urea, an end product of protein metabolism, excreted in the urine (Greek, ouron = urine).

Uric acid, an end product of nucleo-protein metabolism, excreted in the urine (Greek, ouron = urine).

Vagina, a sheath (Latin).

Valsalva, Italian anatomist, 1666–1723.

Varolii, Varolius—Italian anatomist, 1542–1575.

Vaso-dilator, something which dilates the blood vessels. The opposite of vaso-constrictor.

Vater, German anatomist, 1684–1751.

Vein, a vessel conveying blood towards the heart (Latin, vena).

Ventricle, from the Latin, ventriculus = a small cavity.

Vermiform, worm-like (Latin, vermis = worm, and forma = shape).

Vestibule, an antechamber (Latin, vestibulum).

Vestibulo-, pertaining to the vestibule.

Vincula, from the Latin, vinculum = a band.

Vitamin, a group of substances vital to life (from the Latin, vita = life) originally
   believed to be an amine.

Vitellin, derived from egg yolk (Latin, vitellus = yolk).

Volar, from the Latin, vola = the palm.

Xiphoid, from the Greek, xiphos = a sword, and eidos = shape.

INDEX

Abdominal zones, 298
Abscess, psoas, 168
Absorption, 413
Acetabulum, 51
Acetylcholine, 225, 367
Acid, lactic, 349
Acromegaly, 448
Actomyein, 343
Addison's disease, 447
Adenosine diphosphate, 340
  triphosphate, 340, 403
Adhesions, 376
Adrenaline, *see* Hormones.

Air
  alveolar, composition of, 380
  atmospheric, 380
  residual, 384
  tidal, 384
Alcohol, 408

Alimentary canal
  effect of exercise on, 391
  large intestine, 272, 418
    movements of, 416
  small intestine, 271, 417
    movements of, 417
  stomach, 270, 417
  swallowing, 417
Alveoli, 379
Amino-acids, essential, 414
Amylase, 411
Anal canal, 274
Anaphylaxis, 449

Angle
  carrying, 85
  of Louis, 33, 295
Ankle, surface markings at, 308
Anoxia, 385
Antibodies, 478
Antigens, 478
Antiprothrombin, 355
Antrum, mastoid, 292

Aponeurosis
  bicipital, 302
  definition, 117
  palmar, 151
  plantar, 176
Appendix, vermiform, 273, 300
Aqueduct cerebral, 190
Arc, reflex, 452

Arch
  aortic, 228, 298
  palmar, 237, 238, 304

Arches
  of foot, 112
  superciliary, 292

Arches—*continued*
  zygomatic, 292
Arrowroot, 406

Arteries
  aorta,
    abdominal, 239, 300
    arch of, 228
    ascending, 228
    thoracic, 238
  auricular, posterior, 231
  axillary, 235
  basilar, 234
  brachial, 236
  carotid, common, 228
  carotid, external, 230
  carotid, internal, 232
  carpal arch, anterior, 238
  carpal arch, posterior, 238
  cervical, transverse, 235
  coeliac, 239
  coronary, 228, 361
  dorsalis pedis, 242
  facial, 231
  femoral, 241, 309
  histology of, 15
  iliac, common, 240
  iliac, external, 240
  iliac, internal, 240
  innominate, 228
  intercostal, superior, 235
  lingual, 231
  lumbar, 240
  mammary, internal, 235
  maxillary, 231
  mesenteric, inferior, 240
  mesenteric, superior, 240
  occipital, 231
  ovarian, 240
  palmar-arch, deep, 238, 304
  palmar-arch, superficial, 237, 304
  pharyngeal, ascending, 231
  phrenic, inferior, 239
  plantar, lateral, 243
  plantar, medial, 243
  popliteal, 242, 310
  pulmonary, 227
  radial, 236
  renal, 240
  sacral, middle, 240
  subclavian, 233
  suprarenal, middle, 240
  suprascapular, 235
  temporal, superficial, 231
  testicular, 240
  thyroid, 231, 234
  thyrocervical, 234
  tibial, anterior, 242, 309, 311

33